MOUNT SINAI
EXPERT GUIDES
Psychiatry

T0258271

MOUNT SINAI EXPERT GUIDES

Psychiatry

EDITED BY

Asher B. Simon, MD
Assistant Professor of Psychiatry
Associate Director of Residency Training
Department of Psychiatry
Icahn School of Medicine at Mount Sinai
New York, NY, USA

Antonia S. New, MD
Professor of Psychiatry
Vice Chair for Education
Director of Residency Training
Department of Psychiatry
Icahn School of Medicine at Mount Sinai
New York, NY, USA

Wayne K. Goodman, MD
Esther and Joseph Klingenstein Professor
Chair, Department of Psychiatry and Behavioral Health System
Professor of Neuroscience
Icahn School of Medicine at Mount Sinai
New York, NY, USA

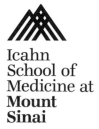

Icahn
School of
Medicine at
Mount
Sinai

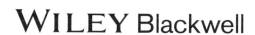

This edition first published 2017 © 2017 by John Wiley & Sons, Ltd.

Registered Office
John Wiley & Sons, Ltd, The Atrium, Southern Gate, Chichester, West Sussex, PO19 8SQ, UK

Editorial Offices
9600 Garsington Road, Oxford, OX4 2DQ, UK
The Atrium, Southern Gate, Chichester, West Sussex, PO19 8SQ, UK
111 River Street, Hoboken, NJ 07030-5774, USA

For details of our global editorial offices, for customer services and for information about how to apply for permission to reuse the copyright material in this book please see our website at www.wiley.com/wiley-blackwell

The right of the author to be identified as the author of this work has been asserted in accordance with the UK Copyright, Designs and Patents Act 1988.

All rights reserved. No part of this publication may be reproduced, stored in a retrieval system, or transmitted, in any form or by any means, electronic, mechanical, photocopying, recording or otherwise, except as permitted by the UK Copyright, Designs and Patents Act 1988, without the prior permission of the publisher.

Designations used by companies to distinguish their products are often claimed as trademarks. All brand names and product names used in this book are trade names, service marks, trademarks or registered trademarks of their respective owners. The publisher is not associated with any product or vendor mentioned in this book. It is sold on the understanding that the publisher is not engaged in rendering professional services. If professional advice or other expert assistance is required, the services of a competent professional should be sought.

The contents of this work are intended to further general scientific research, understanding, and discussion only and are not intended and should not be relied upon as recommending or promoting a specific method, diagnosis, or treatment by health science practitioners for any particular patient. The publisher and the author make no representations or warranties with respect to the accuracy or completeness of the contents of this work and specifically disclaim all warranties, including without limitation any implied warranties of fitness for a particular purpose. In view of ongoing research, equipment modifications, changes in governmental regulations, and the constant flow of information relating to the use of medicines, equipment, and devices, the reader is urged to review and evaluate the information provided in the package insert or instructions for each medicine, equipment, or device for, among other things, any changes in the instructions or indication of usage and for added warnings and precautions. Readers should consult with a specialist where appropriate. The fact that an organization or Website is referred to in this work as a citation and/or a potential source of further information does not mean that the author or the publisher endorses the information the organization or Website may provide or recommendations it may make. Further, readers should be aware that Internet Websites listed in this work may have changed or disappeared between when this work was written and when it is read. No warranty may be created or extended by any promotional statements for this work. Neither the publisher nor the author shall be liable for any damages arising herefrom.

Library of Congress Cataloging-in-Publication data are available

ISBN: 9781118654286

A catalogue record for this book is available from the British Library.

Wiley also publishes its books in a variety of electronic formats. Some content that appears in print may not be available in electronic books.

Cover image: iStock photo file #6124416 © David Marchal
Cover design by Ruth Bateson

Set in 8.5/12pt Frutiger by SPi Global, Pondicherry, India
Printed and bound in Malaysia by Vivar Printing Sdn Bhd

1 2017

Contents

Part 1: INTRODUCTION

Part 2: ADULT DISORDERS

Part 3: CHILD/ADOLESCENT DISORDERS

Part 4: GERIATRIC DISORDERS

Part 5: SPECIAL TOPICS

Contributors

Schahram Akbarian MD, PhD
Professor
Departments of Psychiatry and Neuroscience
Icahn School of Medicine at Mount Sinai
New York, NY, USA

Nelly Alia-Klein PhD
Associate Professor
Department of Psychiatry
Icahn School of Medicine at Mount Sinai
New York, NY, USA

Yadira Alonso MD
Fellow in Psychosomatic Medicine
Brigham and Women's Hospital
Harvard Medical School
Boston, MA, USA

Amy Aloysi MD MPH
Assistant Professor
Departments of Psychiatry and Neurology
Icahn School of Medicine at Mount Sinai
New York, NY, USA

Benjamin N. Angarita MD
Fellow in Child and Adolescent Psychiatry
Department of Psychiatry
Icahn School of Medicine at Mount Sinai
New York, NY, USA

Jacob M. Appel MD, JD, MPH
Assistant Professor
Department of Psychiatry
Icahn School of Medicine at Mount Sinai
New York, NY, USA

Hansel Arroyo MD
Assistant Professor
Department of Psychiatry
Director of Psychiatry and Behavioral
  Medicine, Institute for Advanced
  Medicine
Division of Consultation Psychiatry
Icahn School of Medicine at Mount Sinai
New York, NY, USA

Roy Bachar MD
Assistant Clinical Professor of Psychiatry and
  Staff Psychiatrist
Hackensack University Medical Center
At the Debra Simon Center for Integrative
  Behavioral Health and Wellness,
Maywood, NJ, USA
Adjunct Assistant Professor of Psychiatry
Department of Psychiatry
Mount Sinai Hospital
New York, NY, USA

Sharon M. Batista MD
Assistant Professor
Department of Psychiatry
Associate Director for Recruitment and
  Retention
Center for Multicultural and Community
  Affairs
Icahn School of Medicine at Mount Sinai,
New York, NY, USA

Anne F. Bird MD
Assistant Professor
Department of Psychiatry
Icahn School of Medicine at Mount Sinai
New York, NY, USA

Michael Brus MD
Assistant Professor
Department of Psychiatry
Icahn School of Medicine at Mount Sinai
New York, NY, USA

Katherine E. Burdick PhD
Chief of Neurocognitive Research
Department of Psychiatry
Professor of Psychiatry and Neuroscience
Icahn School of Medicine at Mount Sinai
New York, NY, USA

William Byne MD, PhD
Associate Professor
Department of Psychiatry
Icahn School of Medicine at Mount Sinai
New York, NY, USA

Joseph M. Cerimele MD, MPH
Acting Assistant Professor
Division of Population Health
Department of Psychiatry and Behavioral
    Sciences
University of Washington School
    of Medicine
Seattle, WA, USA

Dennis S. Charney MD
Anne and Joel Ehrenkranz Dean,
Icahn School of Medicine at Mount Sinai
President for Academic Affairs
Mount Sinai Health System
Professor
Departments of Psychiatry, Neuroscience
    and Pharmacology & Systems
    Therapeutics
Icahn School of Medicine at Mount Sinai
New York, NY, USA

Ivan Chavarria-Siles MD, PhD
Resident
Department of Psychiatry
Icahn School of Medicine at Mount Sinai
New York, NY, USA

Barbara J. Coffey MD, MS
Professor
Department of Psychiatry
Director of Child and Adolescent Psychiatry
    Fellowship Training
Icahn School of Medicine at Mount Sinai
New York, NY, USA

Jesse L. Costales MD
Fellow in Child and Adolescent Psychiatry
Department of Psychiatry
Icahn School of Medicine at Mount Sinai
New York, NY, USA

Thomas J. DePrima MD
Assistant Professor
Department of Psychiatry
Icahn School of Medicine at Mount Sinai
New York, NY, USA

Olanrewaju Dokun MD
Resident
Department of Psychiatry
Icahn School of Medicine at Mount Sinai
New York, NY, USA

Claudine Egol MD
Psychiatry Attending
Northport Veterans Affairs Medical Center
    Psychiatry Department
Northport, NY, USA

Amy L. Egolf MD
Chief Resident
Departments of Psychiatry and Medical
    EducationDirector, Psychosomatic Medicine
    Fellowship
Icahn School of Medicine at Mount Sinai
New York, NY, USA

Carrie L. Ernst MD
Associate Professor
Departments of Psychiatry and Medical
    EducationDirector, Psychosomatic
    Medicine Fellowship
Icahn School of Medicine at Mount Sinai
New York, NY, USA

Adriana Feder MD
Associate Professor
Department of Psychiatry
Associate Director for Research
World Trade Center Mental Health
    Program

Icahn School of Medicine at Mount Sinai
New York, NY, USA

Madeleine Fersh MD
Psychosomatic Medicine
Northwell Health
Glen Oaks, NY, USA

Zorica Filipovic-Jewell MD
Assistant Professor
Department of Psychiatry
Icahn School of Medicine at
    Mount Sinai
New York, NY, USA

Jennifer Finkel MD
Assistant Professor
Department of Psychiatry
Division of Consultation Psychiatry
Icahn School of Medicine at
    Mount Sinai
New York, NY, USA

Michael B. First MD
Professor of Clinical Psychiatry
Columbia University
New York State Psychiatric Institute
New York, New York, USA

Rachel Fischer MD
Resident
Department of Psychiatry
Icahn School of Medicine at Mount Sinai
New York, NY, USA

Amanda Focht MD
Acting Assistant Professor
Department of Psychiatry and Behavioral
    Sciences
University of Washington
Seattle, WA, USA

Sophia Frangou MD, PhD, FRCPsych
Professor
Department of Psychiatry
Icahn School of Medicine at Mount Sinai
New York, NY, USA

Joseph I. Friedman MD
Associate Professor
Department of Psychiatry
Icahn School of Medicine at Mount Sinai
New York, NY, USA

Brian Fuchs MD, MPH
Resident
Department of Psychiatry
Icahn School of Medicine at Mount Sinai
New York, NY, USA

Vilma Gabbay MD, MS
Associate Professor of Psychiatry and
    Neuroscience
Department of Psychiatry
Icahn School of Medicine at Mount Sinai
New York, NY, USA

Amir Garakani MD
Assistant Clinical Professor of Psychiatry
Icahn School of Medicine at Mount Sinai
    New York, NY, USA
Assistant Professor (Adjunct) of Psychiatry
Yale School of Medicine
New Haven, CT, USA

Suzanne Garfinkle MD, MSc
Assistant Professor
Departments of Psychiatry and Medical
    Education
Director, Academy for Medicine and the
    Humanities
Icahn School of Medicine at Mount Sinai
New York, NY, USA

Amy R. Glick MD
Fellow in Child and Adolescent Psychiatry
Department of Psychiatry
Icahn School of Medicine at Mount Sinai
New York, NY, USA

Joseph F. Goldberg MD
Clinical Professor of Psychiatry
Department of Psychiatry
Icahn School of Medicine at Mount Sinai
New York, NY, USA

Rita Z. Goldstein PhD
Professor
Departments of Psychiatry and Neuroscience
Director, Neuropsychoimaging of Addiction and
    Related Conditions (NARC) Research Program
Icahn School of Medicine at Mount Sinai
New York, NY, USA

Marianne Goodman MD
Clinical Professor
Department of Psychiatry
Icahn School of Medicine at Mount Sinai
New York, NY, USA

Wayne K. Goodman MD
Esther and Joseph Klingenstein Professor
Chair, Department of Psychiatry and
    Behavioral Health System
Professor of Neuroscience
Icahn School of Medicine at Mount Sinai
New York, NY, USA

Samuel P. Greenstein MD
Assistant Professor Department of Psychiatry
    and Behavioral Neuroscience
University of Cincinnati College of Medicine
Cincinnati, OH, USA

Dorothy E. Grice MD
Professor of Psychiatry
Chief, OCD and Related Disorders Program
Department of Psychiatry
Icahn School of Medicine at Mount Sinai
New York, NY, USA

Tobias B. Halene MD, PhD
Research Fellow
Department of Psychiatry
Icahn School of Medicine at Mount Sinai
New York, NY, USA

Thomas B. Hildebrandt PsyD
Associate Professor
Department of Psychiatry
Chief, Division of Eating and Weight Disorders
Icahn School of Medicine at Mount Sinai
New York, NY, USA

Yasmin L. Hurd PhD
Professor
Departments of Psychiatry and
    Neuroscience
Director, Center for Addictive Disorders
Icahn School of Medicine at Mount Sinai
New York, NY, USA

Dan V. Iosifescu MD, MSc
Director of Adult Psychopharmacology
Mount Sinai Behavioral Health System
Associate Professor of Psychiatry and
    Neuroscience
Icahn School of Medicine at Mount Sinai
New York, NY, USA

Iliyan Ivanov MD
Assistant Professor
Division of Child and Adolescent Psychiatry
Department of Psychiatry
Icahn School of Medicine at Mount Sinai
New York, NY, USA

Robert J. Jaffe MD
Assistant Professor of Psychiatry
Associate Training Director
Child and Adolescent Psychiatry
Icahn School of Medicine at Mount Sinai
New York, NY, USA

Amy L. Johnson MD
Assistant Professor of Psychiatry
New York-Presbyterian Hospital
Weill Cornell Medical College
New York, NY, USA

Brandon D. Johnson MD
Assistant Professor
Department of Psychiatry
Icahn School of Medicine at
    Mount Sinai
New York, NY, USA

Adam Karz MD
Consult Liaison Psychiatrist
Swedish Medical Group
Seattle, WA, USA

Craig L. Katz MD
Associate Professor
Departments of Psychiatry and Medical
    Education
Director
Program in Global Mental Health
Icahn School of Medicine at Mount Sinai
New York, NY, USA

Charles H. Kellner MD
Professor
Department of Psychiatry
Chief of Geriatric Psychiatry for the Mount
    Sinai Behavioral Health System
Director, ECT Service
Icahn School of Medicine at Mount Sinai
New York, NY, USA

Nigel I. Kennedy MD, PhD
Resident Physician-Scientist
Department of Psychiatry
Icahn School of Medicine at Mount Sinai
New York, NY, USA

Kim Klipstein MD
Associate Director
Department of Psychiatry
Director, Behavioral Medicine and Consultation
    Psychiatry, Mount Sinai Health System
Icahn School of Medicine at Mount Sinai
New York, NY, USA

Alexander Kolevzon MD
Professor of Psychiatry and Pediatrics
Clinical Director, Seaver Autism Center
Director, Child Behavioral Health and
    Science Center, Mount Sinai Health
    System
Department of Psychiatry
Icahn School of Medicine at Mount Sinai
New York, NY, USA

Anna B. Konova PhD
Clinical Assistant Professor
NYU Langone School of Medicine;
Staff Psychiatrist
VA NY Harbor Healthcare System
New York, NY, USA

Michal Kunz MD
Director of Clinical Services
Kirby Forensic Psychiatric Center
New York, NY, USA

Mary M. LaLonde MD, PhD
Child and Adolescent Psychiatrist
Private Practice
Scarsdale, NY, USA

Kyle A.B. Lapidus MD, PhD
Assistant Professor
Department of Psychiatry
Stony Brook University
Stony Brook, NY, USA

Amy Lehrner PhD
Assistant Professor
Department of Psychiatry
Icahn School of Medicine at Mount Sinai
New York, NY, USA
Clinical Psychologist, Trauma & Readjustment
    Services (PTSD)
James J. Peters VA Medical Center
Bronx, NY, USA

Evan Leibu MD
Assistant Professor
Department of Psychiatry
Icahn School of Medicine at Mount Sinai
New York, NY, USA

John Leikauf MD
Clinical and Research Fellow
Child and Adolescent Psychiatry
Department of Psychiatry and Behavioral
    Sciences
Stanford University School of Medicine
Palo Alto, CA, USA

Marc S. Lener MD
Clinical Research Fellow
National Institute of Mental Health
Bethesda, MD, USA

Sabina Lim MD, MPH
Vice-President and Chief of Strategy, Behavioral
    Health, Mount Sinai Health System

Associate Professor
Department of Psychiatry
Icahn School of Medicine at Mount Sinai
New York, NY, USA

Maria Linden MD
Assistant Professor
Department of Psychiatry
Icahn School of Medicine at Mount Sinai
New York, NY, USA

Daniella Loh MD
Assistant Professor
Department of Psychiatry
Icahn School of Medicine at Mount Sinai
New York, NY, USA

Sara Lozyniak MD
Child Psychiatry Fellow
Cambridge Health Alliance
Harvard Medical School
Cambridge, MA, USA

Matthew F. Majeske MD
Assistant Professor
Department of Psychiatry
Icahn School of Medicine at Mount Sinai
New York, NY, USA

Jane Martin PhD
Assistant Professor of Psychiatry
Director, Neuropsychology Service
Director, Psychology Training
Department of Psychiatry
Icahn School of Medicine at Mount Sinai
New York, NY, USA

Stacy McAllister MD
Resident in Child and Adolescent
    Psychiatry
Children's Hospital of Philadelphia
Philadelphia, PA, USA

Daniel McGonigle MD
Assistant Proffessor
Department of Psychiatry
Icahn School of Medicine at Mount Sinai
New York, NY, USA

Nathaniel Mendelsohn MD
Fellow in Forensic Psychiatry
New York University School of Medicine
New York, NY, USA

Paul A. Mitrani MD, PhD
Assistant Professor of Psychiatry
Director, Child and Adolescent Outpatient
    Psychiatry
Director, Child and Adolescent Consultation
    and Liaison
Stony Brook University School of Medicine
Stony Brook, NY, USA

Rachel Moster MD
Assistant Professor of Psychiatry
Columbia University Medical Center
New York, NY, USA

James W. Murrough MD
Assistant Professor
Director
Mood and Anxiety Disorders Program
Assistant Professor of Psychiatry and
    Neuroscience
Icahn School of Medicine at Mount Sinai
New York, NY, USA

Thomas P. Naidich MD
Professor
Departments of Radiology, Neurosurgery,
    and Pediatrics
Icahn School of Medicine at Mount Sinai
New York, NY, USA

Eric J. Nestler MD, PhD
Director for Academic and Scientific Affairs
Director, Friedman Brain Institute
Nash Family Professor of Neuroscience
Departments of Neuroscience, Psychiatry, and
    Pharmacological Sciences
Icahn School of Medicine at Mount Sinai
New York, NY, USA

Judith Neugroschl MD
Assistant Professor
Icahn School of Medicine at Mount Sinai
New York, NY, USA

Antonia S. New MD
Professor of Psychiatry
Vice Chair for Education
Director of Residency Training
Department of Psychiatry
Icahn School of Medicine at Mount Sinai
New York, NY, USA

Jeffrey H. Newcorn MD
Associate Professor of Psychiatry and
  Pediatrics
Director, Division of ADHD and Learning
  Disorders
Icahn School of Medicine at
  Mount Sinai
New York, NY, USA

Violeta Nistor MD
Geriatric Psychiatrist
Western Carolina Psychiatric Associates
Greenwood, SC, USA

Betsy O'Brien MD
Assistant Professor
Department of Psychiatry
Icahn School of Medicine at Mount Sinai
New York, NY, USA

John O'Brien MD
Professor
Department of Psychiatry
Icahn School of Medicine at Mount Sinai
New York, NY, USA

Alkesh Patel MD, FASAM
Assistant Clinical Professor
Department of Psychiatry
Icahn School of Medicine at Mount Sinai
New York, NY, USA

M. Mercedes Perez-Rodriguez MD, PhD
Assistant Professor
Department of Psychiatry
Medical Director, Psychosis Research
  Integrating Science and Medicine
  (PRISM)
Icahn School of Medicine at Mount Sinai
New York, NY, USA

Laura Powers MD
Fellow in Child and Adolescent Psychiatry
Icahn School of Medicine at Mount Sinai
New York, NY, USA

Laura C. Pratchett PsyD
Assistant Clinical Professor
Department of Psychiatry
Icahn School of Medicine at Mount Sinai
New York, NY, USA
Clinical Psychologist, Trauma &
  Readjustment Services (PTSD)
James J. Peters VA Medical Center
Bronx, NY, USA

Erica Rapp MD
Instructor
Department of Psychiatry
University of Colorado
Aurora, CO, USA

Timothy Rice MD
Assistant Professor
Department of Psychiatry
Icahn School of Medicine at Mount Sinai
New York, NY, USA

Silvana Riggio MD
Professor
Departments of Psychiatry and Neurology
Icahn School of Medicine at Mount Sinai
New York, NY, USA

Gloria J. Rodriguez MD
Assistant Professor
Department of Psychiatry
Icahn School of Medicine at Mount Sinai
New York, NY, USA

Jake Rosenberg MD
Fellow in Addiction Psychiatry
Department of Psychiatry
University of Pennsylvania School of
  Medicine
Philadelphia, PA, USA

Manuela Russo MD
Postdoctoral Fellow
Department of Psychiatry

Icahn School of Medicine at
   Mount Sinai
New York, NY, USA

Diana Samuel MD
Assistant Clinical Professor
Department of Psychiatry
Associate Director of CPEP
Columbia University Medical Center/
   New York-Presbyterian Hospital
New York, NY, USA

Mary Sano PhD
Director
Alzheimer's Disease Research Center
Professor
Department of Psychiatry
Associate Dean of Clinical Research
Icahn School of Medicine at
   Mount Sinai
New York, NY, USA
James J. Peters VAMC
Bronx, NY, USA

Mariana Schmajuk MD
Fellow in Psychosomatic Medicine
Columbia University Medical Center/
   New York-Presbyterian Hospital
New York, NY, USA

Naomi Schmelzer MD
Assistant Professor of Psychiatry
Brigham and Women's Hospital
Boston, MA, USA

Jan Schuetz-Mueller MD
Assistant Professor
Director of Inpatient Services
Department of Psychiatry
Icahn School of Medicine at Mount Sinai
New York, NY, USA

Matthew Shear PhD
Instructor in Psychiatry
Eating and Weight Disorders Division
Weil Cornell Medical College
White Plains, NY, USA

Akhil Shenoy MD, MPH
Assistant Professor
Department of Psychiatry
Icahn School of Medicine at Mount Sinai
New York, NY, USA

Larry J. Siever MD
Director, Mental Illness Research, Education
   and Clinical Center
James J. Peters VA Medical Center
Bronx, NY, USA

Michael E. Silverman PhD
Assistant Professor
Department of Psychiatry
Icahn School of Medicine at Mount Sinai
New York, NY, USA

Asher B. Simon MD
Assistant Professor of Psychiatry
Associate Director of Residency Training
Department of Psychiatry
Icahn School of Medicine at Mount Sinai
New York, NY, USA

Pamela Sklar MD, PhD
Professor of Psychiatry, Neuroscience,
   Genetics and Genomic Sciences
Chief, Division of Psychiatric Genomics
Departments of Psychiatry and
   Neuroscience
Icahn School of Medicine at Mount Sinai
New York, NY, USA

Stephen Snyder MD
Associate Clinical Professor of Psychiatry
Department of Psychiatry
Icahn School of Medicine at Mount Sinai
New York, NY, USA

Steven M. Southwick MD
Glenn H. Greenberg Professor of Psychiatry,
   PTSD and Resilience
Yale University School of Medicine and Yale
   Child Study Center
National Center for PTSD
New Haven, CT, USA

Icahn School of Medicine at Mount Sinai
New York, NY, USA

Emily Stern PhD
Assistant Professor of Psychiatry and
    Neuroscience
Departments of Psychiatry and Neuroscience
Icahn School of Medicine at Mount Sinai
New York, NY, USA

Nicholas S. Stevens MD
Chief Resident
Department of Psychiatry
Icahn School of Medicine at Mount Sinai
New York, NY, USA

Katharine A. Stratigos MD
Assistant Clinical Professor of Psychiatry
Whitaker Developmental Neuropsychiatry
    Scholar
Columbia University Department of Psychiatry
New York State Psychiatric Institute
New York, NY, USA

Devendra S. Thakur MD
Assistant Professor of Psychiatry
Geisel School of Medicine at Dartmouth College
Hanover, NH, USA

Allison K. Ungar MD
Resident
Department of Psychiatry
Icahn School of Medicine at Mount Sinai
New York, NY, USA

Ellen Vora MD
Psychiatrist
Eleven Eleven Wellness Center and One
    Medical Group
New York, NY, USA

Le-Ben Wan MD, PhD
Clinical Instructor
Department of Psychiatry
New York University School of Medicine
New York, NY, USA

Alison Welch MD
Assistant Professor of Psychiatry
Department of Psychiatry
Icahn School of Medicine at Mount Sinai
New York, NY, USA

Hiwot Woldu MD
Clinical Assistant Professor of Psychiatry
New York University School of Medicine
Adjunct Clinical Assistant Professor of
    Psychiatry
Icahn School of Medicine at Mount Sinai
New York, NY, USA

Rachel Yehuda PhD
Director, Mental Health Patient
    Care Center
James J. Peters VA Medical Center
Bronx, NY
Professor of Psychiatry and Neuroscience
Director, Traumatic Stress Studies
    Division
Icahn School of Medicine at Mount Sinai
New York, NY, USA

Rachel Zhuk MD
Resident
Department of Psychiatry
Icahn School of Medicine at Mount Sinai
New York, NY, USA

Series Foreword

Now more than ever, immediacy in obtaining accurate and practical information is the coin of the realm in providing high quality patient care. The Mount Sinai Expert Guides series addresses this vital need by providing accurate, up-to-date guidance, written by experts in formats that are accessible in the patient care setting: websites, smartphone apps, and portable books. The Icahn School of Medicine, which was chartered in 1963, embodies a deep tradition of pre-eminence in clinical care and scholarship that was first shaped by the founding of the Mount Sinai Hospital in 1855. Today, the Mount Sinai Health System, comprised of seven hospitals anchored by the Icahn School of Medicine, is one of the largest healthcare systems in the United States, and is revolutionizing medicine through its embracing of transformative technologies for clinical diagnosis and treatment. The Mount Sinai Expert Guides series builds upon both this historical renown and contemporary excellence. Leading experts across a range of disciplines provide practical yet sage advice in a digestible format that is ideal for trainees, mid-level providers, and practicing physicians. Few medical centers in the USA could offer this type of breadth while relying exclusively on its own physicians, yet here no compromises were required in offering a truly unique series that is sure to become embedded within the key resources of busy providers. In producing this series, the editors and authors are fortunate to have an equally dynamic and forward-viewing partner in Wiley Blackwell, which together ensures that healthcare professionals will benefit from a unique, first-class effort that will advance the care of their patients.

Scott L. Friedman, MD
Series Editor
Fishberg Professor of Medicine
Dean for Therapeutic Discovery
Chief, Division of Liver Diseases
Icahn School of Medicine at Mount Sinai
New York, NY, USA

Preface

As the editors of this volume, we have made our careers in psychiatric clinical care, education, and research. We bring a broad perspective to the several dozen chapters that follow.

The knowledge base that informs the clinical practice of psychiatry continues to expand, not only in quantity of data but also in the fields from which it draws. We sought to consolidate this growth into a handbook that is approachable, and we have prioritized clinically immediate and useful content rather than in-depth coverage. As editors of this Expert Guide, we have chosen to include information that is clearly evidence-based as well as that which has been backed by the clinical experience of our experts. We have selected our faculty at Mount Sinai to present their respective fields in a manner that should be easily-digestible by the busy hospitalist, the psychiatrist in practice, the non-psychiatric practitioner, the new graduate, and the psychiatric trainee. While the text is not meant to be exhaustive, it should provide a useful starting point – a pocket guide – for directing practitioners on their approaches to patients with common conditions.

We have departed slightly from the format of the Mount Sinai Expert Guides Series, in that we have included a substantial amount of conceptual material. We felt this necessary as the field of psychiatry (1) lacks much of the clearly-defined evidence and algorithms of other medical disciplines, (2) mandates an inherently creative, adaptive, and flexible approach to patient care, and (3) requires that a conceptual knowledge of psychopharmacology, neuroscience, psychotherapy, and documentation informs daily clinical practice. Thus, in the layout of this volume, there is some necessary squeezing of a square peg into a round hole. We hope that as psychiatric research and practice further develop and as non-psychiatric medicine begins to realize and internalize a greater focus on mental health care, such procrustean manipulation will be seen as a thing of the past.

The introductory chapters that follow include an overview of diagnostic systems, neuroscience, psychological and lab testing, neuromodulation, psychotherapy, and clinical documentation. The 26 chapters covering clinical disorders provide high-yield and salient aspects of the major syndromes one encounters in clinical practice. The concluding Special Topics section reflects the practice of psychiatry in distinctive settings and with special populations.

We would like to express our gracious appreciation to the individuals who contributed to this volume as well as to Dr. Scott Friedman, Dr. Dennis Charney, and our colleagues at Mount Sinai.

We are also deeply thankful to our families who facilitated and tolerated (as any author knows) the production process: Katy, Evie, Phoebe, Benjamin, Emma, Becca, Gillian, and Aida.

Asher B. Simon MD
Antonia S. New MD
Wayne K. Goodman MD
Icahn School of Medicine at Mount Sinai
New York, NY, USA

List of Abbreviations

ABA   applied behavior analysis
ACC   anterior cingulate cortex
ACO   accountable care organization
ACT   acceptance and commitment therapy
ACTH   adrenocorticotropic hormone
AD   Alzheimer's disease
ADHD   attention deficit hyperactivity disorder
ADI   Autism Diagnostic Interview-Revised
ADLs   activities of daily living
ADOS   Autism Diagnostic Observation Schedule
AED   anti-epileptic drug
ALB   albumin
Alk Phos   alkaline phosphatase
ALT   alanine aminotransferase
AMPA   α-amino-3-hydroxy-5-methyl-4-isoxazolepropionic acid
AN   anorexia nervosa
ANC   absolute neutrophil count
AOT   assisted outpatient treatment
ARRA   American Recovery and Reinvestment Act
ASD   autism spectrum disorder
ASPD   antisocial personality disorder
ASQ   Ages and Stages Questionnaire
ASSIST   Alcohol, Smoking, and Substance Involvement Screening Test
AST   aspartate aminotransferase
AUDIT   Alcohol Use Disorder Identification Test
AvPD   avoidant personality disorder
BA   Brodmann Area
BD   bipolar disorders
BDD   body dysmorphic disorder
BDI   Beck Depression Inventory
BDNF   brain-derived neurotrophic factor
BDSS   Brief Bipolar Disorder Symptom Scale
BED   binge-eating disorder
bid   twice a day
BISS   Bipolar Inventory of Symptoms Scale
BMI   body mass index
BN   bulimia nervosa
BP   blood pressure
BPD   borderline personality disorder
BPRS   Brief Psychiatric Rating Scale
BUN   blood urea nitrogen
CAARMS   Comprehensive Assessment of At-Risk Mental States
CAGE-AID   CAGE-Adapted to Include Drugs
CAMS   Collaborative Assessment and Management of Suicidality
CAT   cognitive analytic therapy
CBC   complete blood count

CBCL	Child Behavior Checklist
CBIT	comprehensive behavioral intervention for tics
CBT	cognitive behavioral therapy
CD	conduct disorder
CDI	Child Depression Inventory
CDR	Clinical Dementia Rating scale
CDRS-R	Children's Depression Rating Scale-Revised
CES	cranial electrotherapy stimulation
CES-DC	Center for Epidemiological Studies Depression Scale Modified for Children
CGI	Clinical Global Impressions Scale
CGI-S	Clinical Global Impressions Scale-Severity
CHF	congestive heart failure
CIWA-Ar	Clinical Institute Withdrawal Assessment for Alcohol, Revised
CJD	Creutzfeldt–Jacob disease
CMV	cytomegalovirus
CNS	central nervous system
COPD	chronic obstructive pulmonary disease
COWS	Clinical Opiate Withdrawal Scale
CPK	creatinine phosphokinase
CPT	cognitive processing therapy
Cr	creatine
CREB	cAMP response element-binding protein
CRH	corticotropin-releasing hormone
CSDD	Cornell Scale for Depression in Dementia
CSF	cerebrospinal fluid
CST	cortico-striatal-thalamic
CT	computed tomography
CVA	cerebrovascular accident
CVLT	California Verbal Learning Test
CXR	chest x-ray
DA	dopamine
DAI	diffuse axonal injury
DALYs	disability-adjusted life years
DBS	deep brain stimulation
DBT	dialectical behavior therapy
DBT-CM	dialectical behavior therapy, corrections modified
DE	delayed ejaculation
DEXA	dual energy x-ray absorptiometry
DHEA	dehydroepiandrosterone
DIB-R	Diagnostic Interview for Borderline Personality Disorder
DLBD	diffuse Lewy body dementia
DLPFC	dorsolateral prefrontal cortex
DMDD	disruptive mood dysregulation disorder
DNMT	DNA methyltransferases
DSM	*Diagnostic and Statistical Manual of Mental Disorders*
DST	dexamethasone suppression test
DTI	diffusion tensor imaging
dTMS	deep transcranial magnetic stimulation
DTS	Davidson Trauma Scale
DUP	duration of untreated psychosis
DUST	Drug Use Screening Tool
EBV	Epstein–Barr virus
eCB	endocannabinoid
ECT	electroconvulsive therapy

ED	erectile dysfunction
EDE	Eating Disorder Examination
EDI	Eating Disorders Inventory
EEG	electroencephalogram
EKG	electrocardiogram
E/M	evaluation and management
EMDR	eye movement desensitization and reprocessing
EMRs	electronic medical records
EMTALA	Emergency Medical Treatment and Labor Act
EpCS	epidural cortical stimulation
EPS	extrapyramidal symptoms
ER	emergency room/extended-release
ERP	exposure and response-prevention
ESR	erythrocyte sedimentation rate
ETOH	ethanol
FDA	Food and Drug Administration
FFT	family focused therapy
FGA	first-generation antipsychotic
fMRI	functional magnetic resonance imaging
FOD	female orgasmic disorder
FSIAD	female sexual interest/arousal disorder
FTLD	frontotemporal lobar degeneration
GABA	γ-aminobutyric acid
GAD	generalized anxiety disorder
GBI	General Behavioral Inventory
GC/MS	gas chromatography/mass spectrometry
GDS	Geriatric Depression Scale/Global Deterioration Scale
GGTP	gamma-glutamyl transpeptidase
GHQ	General Health Questionnaire
GI	gastrointestinal
GnRH	gonadotropin releasing hormone
GPPPD	genito-pelvic pain-penetration disorder
GWAS	genome-wide association studies
H&P	history and physical
HAM-A	Hamilton Anxiety Rating Scale
HAM-D	Hamilton Depression Rating Scale
HbA1c	hemoglobin A1c
HCG	human chorionic gonadotropin
HCR-20	Historical Clinical Risk
HD	hoarding disorder
HDAC	histone deacetylase
HDE	humanitarian device exemption
HDL	high density lipoprotein
HDRS	Hamilton Depression Rating Scale
HHS	(Department of) Health and Human Services
HIPAA	Health Insurance Portability and Accountability Act of 1996
HIV	human immunodeficiency virus
HPA	hypothalamic-pituitary-adrenal
HR	heart rate
HRT	habit reversal training/therapy
HSV	herpes simplex virus
5-HT	5-hydroxytryptamine (serotonin)
IADLs	instrumental activities of daily living
ICU	intensive care unit

ID	intellectual disability
IDS	Inventory for Depressive Symptoms
IED	intermittent explosive disorder
IES-R	Impact of Events Scale-Revised
IL	interleukin
INR	international normalized ratio
iPS	induced pluripotent stem (cells)
IPSRT	interpersonal/social rhythm therapy
IPT	interpersonal psychotherapy
IQ	intelligence quotient
IR	immediate-release
IRB	institutional review board
KSADS-MRS	Kiddie Schedule for Affective Disorders and Schizophrenia, Mania Rating Scale
LC	locus coeruleus
LC-NE	locus coeruleus–norepinephrine
LDL	low density lipoprotein
LFT	liver function tests
LH	luteinizing hormone
LOC	loss of consciousness
LSD	lysergic acid diethylamide
MADRS	Montgomery Asberg Depression Rating Scale
MAOI	monoamine oxidase inhibitor
MASC	Multidimensional Anxiety Scale for Children
MAST	Michigan Alcohol Screening Test
MBSR	mindfulness-based stress reduction
MBT	mentalization based therapy
M-CHAT-R	modified checklist for autism in toddlers, revised
MCI	mild cognitive impairment
MCV	mean corpuscular volume
MDAC	Mental Disability Advocacy Center
MDD	major depressive disorder
MDE	major depressive episode
MDMA	3,4-methylenedioxy-methamphetamine
MDQ	Mood Disorders Questionnaire
MHSDD	male hypoactive sexual desire disorder
MI	myocardial infarction/motivational interviewing
MMPI	Minnesota Multiphasic Personality Inventory
MMSE	mini mental status examination
MoCA	Montreal Cognitive Assessment
mPFC	medial prefrontal cortex
MR	mental retardation
MRI	magnetic resonance imaging
MSE	mental status exam
MST	magnetic seizure therapy/multisystemic treatment
MT	motor threshold
MTFC	multidimensional treatment foster care
NASSA	noradrenergic and specific serotonergic antidepressant
NCD	neurocognitive disorder
NCSE	non-convulsive status epilepticus
NE	norepinephrine
NGO	non-governmental organization
NIMH	National Institute of Mental Health
NMDA	N-methyl-D-aspartate
NMS	neuroleptic malignant syndrome

NPH	normal pressure hydrocephalus
NPI	Neuropsychiatric Inventory
NPY	neuropeptide Y
NRT	nicotine replacement therapy
NSAIDs	non-steroidal anti-inflammatory drugs
OCD	obsessive-compulsive disorder
ODD	oppositional defiant disorder
OFC	orbitofrontal cortex
PAD	psychiatric advance directive
PAG	periaqueductal gray matter
PANDAS	pediatric autoimmune neuropsychiatric disorders associated with streptococcal infections
PANS	pediatric acute-onset neuropsychiatric syndrome
PCL	PTSD Checklist
PCL-R	Psychopathy Checklist, Revised
PCOS	polycystic ovarian syndrome
PCP	phencyclidine
PCS	post-concussive syndrome
PD	panic disorder/Parkinson's disease
PDE5	phosphodiesterase type 5
PDEQ	Peritraumatic Dissociative Experiences Questionnaire
PE	prolonged exposure/premature ejaculation
PET	positron emission tomography
PFA	psychological first aid
PHI	protected health information
PHQ	patient health questionnaire
PMS	Phelan–McDermid syndrome
PNS	paraneoplastic syndrome
prn	*pro re nata*, as needed
PT	prothrombin time
PTA	posttraumatic amnesia
PTSD	posttraumatic stress disorder
PTT	partial thromboplastin time
PVD	provoked vestibulodynia
qd	once a day (daily)
qhs	every night at bedtime
qid	four times a day
QIDS-SR	Quick Inventory of Depressive Symptomatology
RPR	rapid plasma reagin
rTMS	repetitive transcranial magnetic stimulation
SAD	social anxiety disorder
SAMe	*S*-adenosylmethionine
SCARED	Screen for Child Anxiety Related Emotional Disorders
SGA	second-generation antipsychotic
SHIM	Sexual Health Inventory for Men
SIADH	syndrome of inappropriate antidiuretic hormone secretion
SIPS	Structured Interview for Prodromal Syndromes
SIQ	Suicidal Ideation Questionnaire
SJW	St. John's Wort
SLE	systemic lupus erythematosus
SN	substantia nigra
SNRI	serotonin–norepinephrine reuptake inhibitor
SP	specific phobia
SSD	sub-syndromal delirium/Social Security Disability benefits

SSRI	serotonin-selective reuptake inhibitor
ST	seizure threshold
SUD	substance use disorder
TBI	traumatic brain injury
TCA	tricyclic antidepressant
tDCS	transcranial direct current stimulation
TFP	transference focused psychotherapy
TIBC	total iron-binding capacity
tid	three times a day
TMS	transcranial magnetic stimulation
TNF	tumor necrosis factor
TP	total protein
TSH	thyroid stimulating hormone
TSQ	Trauma Screening Questionnaire
TTM	trichotillomania
UTI	urinary tract infection
vlPFC	ventrolateral prefrontal cortex
VNS	vagus nerve stimulation
VTA	ventral tegmental area
WAIS	Wechsler Adult Intelligence Scale
WCST	Wisconsin Card Sorting Test
Y-BOCS	Yale–Brown Obsessive Compulsive Scale
YGTS	Yale Global Tic Severity Scale
YLDs	years lived with disabilities
YMRS	Young Mania Rating Scale

About the Companion Website

This book is accompanied by a companion website:

www.mountsinaiexpertguides.com/psychiatry

The website includes:
- Advice for patients
- Case studies
- ICD codes
- Interactive MCQs
- Links to video clips

To check out the Mount Sinai series homepage, go to:

www.mountsinaiexpertguides.com

PART 1

Introduction

CHAPTER 1

DSM-5

Evan Leibu[1] and Michael B. First[2]
[1] Icahn School of Medicine at Mount Sinai, New York, NY, USA
[2] Columbia University, New York, NY, USA

OVERALL BOTTOM LINE

- DSM-5 involves multiple changes to the DSM-IV.
- DSM remains a categorical and descriptive method of categorizing symptoms into specified syndromes.
- Diagnostic groupings were reorganized to reflect common putative mechanisms and risk factors.
- The order of the diagnostic groupings attempts to reflect the developmental lifespan.

Discussion of topic and guidelines

The *Diagnostic and Statistical Manual of Mental Disorders* (DSM), first published in 1952, has undergone multiple revisions, the most recent being DSM-5, released in May of 2013. Multiple changes have been made, including changes to diagnostic classes, the addition and removal of diagnoses, and modification of previous diagnoses.

Despite these changes, DSM-5 remains a mainly categorical and descriptive method of classifying symptoms. Clinical diagnosis continues to be based on sets of symptoms that are clustered into heterogeneous syndromes, which often overlap among disorders. With the exception of those disorders for which the etiology is at least partially known (e.g., trauma and stress-related disorders, substance-induced disorders, disorders due to another medical condition), DSM disorders continue to be classified without regard to etiology.

Some of the major changes of DSM-5 from DSM-IV include the removal of the multiaxial system and the inclusion of ICD-10-CM diagnostic codes to ensure compliance with the Health Insurance Portability and Accountability Act of 1996 (HIPAA). Even though it was not possible to modify disorder definitions to reflect the burgeoning understanding of underlying pathophysiological mechanisms, diagnostic groupings were reorganized to reflect common putative mechanisms and risk factors. Moreover, the order of the diagnostic groupings attempts to reflect the developmental lifespan with diagnoses that occur early in the developmental process coming earlier in the classification.

Brief overviews of significant changes made to the diagnostic categories are outlined here in the same order in which they appear in DSM-5.

Neurodevelopmental disorders

- Intellectual Disability
  - Formerly called mental retardation, severity is no longer determined by IQ range but by impairment in adaptive functioning.

Mount Sinai Expert Guides: Psychiatry, First Edition. Edited by Asher B. Simon, Antonia S. New, and Wayne K. Goodman.
© 2017 John Wiley & Sons, Ltd. Published 2017 by John Wiley & Sons, Ltd.
Companion website: www.mountsinaiexpertguides.com/psychiatry

- Global Developmental Delay
  - A new diagnosis for individuals under age 5 with intellectual impairment who are unable to undergo systematic assessment due to age.
- Social (Pragmatic) Communication Disorder
  - A new diagnosis for individuals with deficits in social communication in the absence of other symptoms of autism spectrum disorder or Intellectual Disability.
- Autism Spectrum Disorder
  - This new category reflects the dimensional view that autistic symptoms occur across a spectrum and replaces the DSM-IV diagnoses of Autistic Disorder, Asperger's Disorder, Childhood Disintegrative Disorder, Rett's Disorder, and Pervasive Developmental Disorder Not Otherwise Specified.
- Attention-Deficit/Hyperactivity Disorder
  - The onset requirement has been changed from before age 7 years to prior to age 12. A comorbid diagnosis with autism spectrum disorder is now allowed. The symptom threshold has been lowered for adults from six to five symptoms.
- Specific Learning Disorder
  - The DSM-IV diagnoses of reading disorder, mathematics disorder, and disorder of written expression have been combined. Impairments in specific academic domains are indicated with specifiers.

Schizophrenia spectrum and other psychotic disorders
- Delusional Disorder
  - Delusions no longer have to be non-bizarre.
- Schizophrenia
  - Individuals with Schizophrenia now must evidence at least one of the first three items from Criterion A (i.e., delusions, hallucinations, and disorganized speech). In addition, the designation of certain symptoms (e.g., bizarre delusions) as being of special diagnostic significance has been dropped. Subtypes of Schizophrenia (i.e., paranoid, disorganized, catatonic, undifferentiated, and residual) have been removed and replaced with symptom-based severity dimensions.
- Schizoaffective Disorder
  - Schizoaffective disorder now requires that symptoms meeting criteria for a major mood episode be present for the majority of the disorder's total lifetime duration.
- Catatonia
  - Diagnostic criteria for a catatonia syndrome, which can apply to psychotic and mood disorders and etiological medical conditions, are now provided.

Bipolar and related disorders
- Bipolar Disorders
  - Increased activity or energy with elevated or irritable mood is now required for a manic or hypomanic episode. The mixed type of manic episode has been removed in favor of a more broadly defined mixed features specifier that can also apply to depressive episodes.

Depressive disorders
- Disruptive Mood Dysregulation Disorder
  - A new diagnosis, characterized by severe and recurrent temper outbursts that are superimposed on a baseline of chronic irritability, has been added to address the misuse of the bipolar disorder diagnosis for chronically irritable children. This diagnosis should only be used

in children between ages 6 and 18. It is considered more severe than oppositional defiant disorder and should not be comorbidly diagnosed.

- Major Depressive Disorder
  - To cover the common presentation of comorbid anxiety symptoms, an "anxious distress" specifier (which also can be applied to manic or hypomanic episodes) is provided if anxiety symptoms are present for most days. The bereavement exclusion has been removed and replaced by a note suggesting the exercise of clinical judgment.
- Persistent Depressive Disorder
  - This new diagnosis highlights the prognostic significance of chronicity (i.e., duration of at least 2 years) and incorporates the DSM-IV diagnosis of dysthymia along with chronic forms of major depressive disorder.
- Premenstrual Dysphoric Disorder
  - Premenstrual Dysphoric Disorder, for women with disabling mood symptoms that start in the week prior to the onset of menses and remit within a week post-menses, has been promoted from the DSM-IV research appendix.

Anxiety disorders

- Separation Anxiety Disorder
  - Separation Anxiety Disorder has moved from the DSM-IV section of Disorders usually first diagnosed in Infancy, Childhood, or Adolescence and now aims to also encompass adults with anxiety resulting from separation from important attachment figures.
- Agoraphobia, Specific Phobia, and Social Anxiety Disorder (Social Phobia)
  - The requirement that patients recognize their fears as excessive has been replaced by a clinical judgment that the fears are out of proportion to the actual danger. To reflect the transient nature of normal fears, symptoms must be present for a minimum of six months.
- Social Anxiety Disorder (Social Phobia)
  - The "performance only" specifier replaces the DSM-IV "generalized" specifier.
- Panic Attack
  - A "with panic attacks" specifier can be applied to any disorder to indicate the comorbid presence of panic attacks.
- Panic Disorder and Agoraphobia
  - These are now completely separate diagnoses, in contrast to the DSM-IV approach which offered three diagnoses for the various combinations.

Obsessive-compulsive and related disorders

- Obsessive-Compulsive Disorder
  - Obsessive-Compulsive Disorder has been removed from Anxiety Disorders and now is part of a group of disorders that are related on a range of diagnostic validators. A tic related specifier identifies a predominantly familial form with early onset and characteristic obsessions and compulsions (symmetry and ordering).
- Body Dysmorphic Disorder
  - Delusional forms are no longer considered to be a type of Delusional Disorder but are characterized as BDD with absent insight.
- Hoarding Disorder
  - This new disorder describes a persistent difficulty with discarding possessions that results in cluttered active living areas, compromising their intended use.
- Excoriation (Skin-Picking) Disorder
  - This new disorder comprises compulsive skin picking that results in lesions.

Trauma- and stressor-related disorders
- Reactive Attachment Disorder/Disinhibited Social Engagement Disorder
  - These two disorders, originally subtypes of DSM-IV reactive attachment disorder, occur as a result of extremely pathogenic care during early life.
- Posttraumatic Stress Disorder
  - The exposure to trauma requirement has been broadened to include occupational exposure to aversive details of the trauma and no longer requires that the person's response involve intense fear, helplessness, or horror. Avoiding reminders of the trauma is now required for a diagnosis. Additional items include irritable, aggressive, or self-destructive behavior and persistent negative alterations in cognitions and moods. An alternative criteria set is available for children age 6 or younger.
- Acute Stress Disorder
  - The criteria de-emphasize the previous need for dissociative symptoms as a hallmark of the disorder.
- Adjustment Disorders
  - Adjustment Disorders are now included in the Trauma and Stressor-Related Disorders and no longer constitute a major diagnostic class.

Dissociative disorders
- Dissociative Identity Disorder
  - Symptoms can now be observed by others or self-reported. In addition, gaps in recall include everyday events and are not restricted to traumatic events.
- Dissociative Amnesia
  - This now includes the subtype Dissociative Fugue, which has been eliminated as a discrete diagnosis.
- Depersonalization/Derealization Disorder
  - Derealization symptoms have been added to both the name and definition of this disorder.

Somatic symptom and related disorders
- Somatic Symptom Disorder
  - The concept of "somatoform" (i.e., psychological symptoms taking the form of somatic symptoms) has been eliminated, as has the DSM-IV requirement that the symptoms be medically unexplained. It is now defined in terms of distressing somatic symptoms accompanied by excessive thoughts, feelings, or behaviors related to the symptoms.
- Illness Anxiety Disorder
  - This new disorder is for those cases of DSM-IV hypochondriasis that occur in the absence of somatic symptoms. Those with somatic symptoms are to be diagnosed as Somatic Symptom Disorder.

Feeding and eating disorders
- Avoidant/Restrictive Food Intake Disorder
  - This is a reformulated version of the DSM-IV Feeding Disorder of Infancy or Early Childhood that can now be applied to adults as well. It is defined by an eating or feeding disturbance leading to significant low weight or nutritional deficiency.
- Anorexia Nervosa
  - The amenorrhea requirement has been eliminated.
- Bulimia Nervosa
  - The number of binge eating episodes has been reduced to once weekly.

- Binge-Eating Disorder
  - This new disorder is characterized by recurrent binge eating without abnormal compensatory behavior. It has been promoted from the DSM-IV research appendix.

Sleep-wake disorders

- Insomnia and Hypersomnolence Disorder
  - These disorders combine the DSM-IV diagnoses of primary insomnia/hypersomnia, insomnia/hypersomnia related to another mental disorder, and sleep disorder due to medical condition. Etiological factors are now indicated using specifiers.
- Breathing-Related Sleep Disorders
  - Breathing-Related Sleep Disorders are now divided in to three disorders: obstructive sleep apnea hypopnea, central sleep apnea, and sleep-related hypoventilation.
- Rapid Eye Movement Sleep Behavior Disorder
  - This new disorder occurs when individuals have REM sleep without muscle atonia resulting in the acting out of parts of the dream (e.g., kicking, flailing).
- Restless Legs Syndrome
  - A new disorder involving an urge to move the legs which is usually accompanied by uncomfortable and unpleasant sensations in the legs.

Sexual dysfunctions

- Female Sexual Interest/Arousal Disorder
  - A new diagnosis in the DSM-5 which combines the previous diagnoses of female hypoactive sexual desire disorder and female hypoactive arousal disorders due to frequent concurrence of these phases in women.
- Genito-Pelvic Pain/Penetration Disorder
  - A new DSM-5 disorder which merges the previous DSM-IV diagnoses of vaginismus and dyspareunia.
- Sexual Aversion Disorder
  - This diagnosis has been removed from DSM-5.

Gender dysphoria

- Gender Dysphoria
  - A new diagnostic class and disorder in the DSM that highlights dysphoria regarding gender incongruence and separates issues of gender identity from the paraphilias and sexual dysfunctions where they were classified in the DSM-IV.

Disruptive, impulse-control, and conduct disorders

- Oppositional Defiant Disorder
  - This disorder can now be diagnosed comorbidly with conduct disorder because of evidence that these disorders can occur independently and have different life trajectories.
- Conduct Disorder
  - The disorder has a new specifier, "with limited prosocial emotions," that identifies a subgroup with a more severe form of the disorder and a worse treatment response.
- Intermittent Explosive Disorder
  - Verbal aggression is now included within the construct of aggressive outbursts.

Substance-related and addictive disorders

- Gambling Disorder
  - The substance-related disorders chapter has been expanded to include gambling disorder, reflecting research which shows that similar brain reward pathways are activated.
- Substance Use Disorders
  - The DSM-IV substance abuse and substance dependence categories have been combined to form a single Substance Use disorder category, reflecting the dimensional nature of substance use.

Neurocognitive disorders

- Major and Mild Neurocognitive Disorder
  - The DSM-IV diagnoses of dementia and amnestic disorders are subsumed under the newly named entity called major neurocognitive disorder. Mild neurocognitive disorder is a new category for neurocognitive problems that reflect an only "modest" decline in functioning.

Personality disorders

- The criteria for personality disorders have not changed from those in DSM-IV. An alternative hybrid dimensional/categorical approach to the diagnosis of personality disorders was developed for DSM-5 but was rejected because of concerns about its reliability, validity, and clinical utility. It is included in a section called "Emerging Measures and Models".

Paraphilic disorders

- There are minor changes in criteria from DSM-IV. Paraphilias can now be specified as "in remission."

Reading list

American Psychiatric Association. Diagnostic and Statistical Manual of Mental Disorders, 5th edn. Arlington, VA: American Psychiatric Publishing, 2013.

Barnhill JW. DSM-5 Clinical Cases. Arlington, VA: American Psychiatric Publishing, 2013.

First MB. DSM-5 Handbook of Differential Diagnosis. Arlington, VA: American Psychiatric Publishing, 2013.

Kupfer DJ, Kuhl EA, Wulsin L. Psychiatry's integration with medicine: the role of DSM-5. Ann Rev Med 2013;64:385–392.

Wakefield JC, First MB. Placing symptoms in context: the role of contextual criteria in reducing false positives in Diagnostic and Statistical Manual of Mental Disorders diagnoses. Compr Psychiatry 2012;53(2):130–9.

CHAPTER 2

Research Domain Criteria (RDoC)

Tobias B. Halene and Vilma Gabbay

Icahn School of Medicine at Mount Sinai, New York, NY, USA

OVERALL BOTTOM LINE
- The heterogeneity of psychiatric conditions has contributed to the failure to identify biomarkers and develop personalized treatments.
- The challenge is that psychiatric conditions defined by the *Diagnostic and Statistical Manual of Mental Disorders* (DSM) are based on a cluster of symptoms which most likely derive from different etiologies.
- A strategy developed by the National Institute of Mental Health (NIMH) called "Research Domain Criteria' or "RDoC" addresses this limitation by redefining "mental disorders into dimensions or components of observable behaviors that are more closely aligned with the biology of the brain."
- Until better alternatives are available, the DSM remains the widely accepted standard for the clinical diagnosis and treatment of psychiatric disorders.

Discussion of topic and guidelines

Despite extensive research into the biology of psychiatric conditions over the past 50 years, almost nothing is known about their pathogenesis and no biological markers have proven to be diagnostic tools.
- This creates a barrier for the development of new and personalized treatments.
- The major challenge may be the current categorical classification of psychiatric disorders, based exclusively on symptom clusters which often overlap across disorders but likely represent distinct etiologies.

It has been argued that psychiatric symptoms exist on a continuum ranging from lesser to greater severity rather than as binary categories of "present" or "absent" as currently defined by the DSM diagnostic system. Consequently, DSM-defined syndromes are highly heterogeneous and show excessive comorbidity with one another. The NIMH strategic plan introduced Research Domain Criteria (RDoC) to address the limitations of the categorical DSM diagnostic system. It posits that mental disorders are based on dimensions of observable behavior and their related neurobiological systems. RDoC is currently used only as a research framework, but it is envisioned that it will become a diagnostic system once specific behaviors are linked to specific alterations in biological markers, genes, and neural circuitry.

Mount Sinai Expert Guides: Psychiatry, First Edition. Edited by Asher B. Simon, Antonia S. New, and Wayne K. Goodman.
© 2017 John Wiley & Sons, Ltd. Published 2017 by John Wiley & Sons, Ltd.
Companion website: www.mountsinaiexpertguides.com/psychiatry

RDoC "Guiding principles"

1. Mental disorders involve brain circuits and these circuits underlie specific domains of cognition, emotion, or behavior. Each domain is not just dichotomous (as in "ill" versus "healthy") but spans a continuum of function ranging from normal to abnormal.
2. Instead of starting with a categorical definition, the classification system envisioned by RDoC will be generated from the neurobiology of symptoms.
3. The domains will be better understood and defined by studying them on different levels ("units of analysis") such as molecular, genetic, cellular, neural circuits, physiological, behavioral, and self-reports.

RDoC has proposed five research domains

1. Negative Valence Systems (fear, anxiety, threat, loss, frustration);
2. Positive Valence Systems (reward learning, reward valuation, habit);
3. Cognitive Systems (attention, perception, working memory, cognitive control);
4. Systems for Social Processes (attachment formation, social communication, perception of self, perception of others);
5. Arousal/Modulatory Systems (arousal, circadian rhythms, sleep and wakefulness).

Major depressive disorder (MDD) is a good example of how RDoC could change research

- Per DSM, MDD diagnosis requires the presence of 5 of 9 symptoms, (one of which must be sadness or anhedonia).
- This results in significant heterogeneity and symptomatic overlap with other psychopathologies.
- Patients with milder symptoms often do not meet full diagnostic criteria and often are excluded from research studies.
- There are high rates of mixed mood, anxiety, and somatic symptom clusters and current diagnostic criteria do not capture that most symptoms lie on a continuum ranging from lesser to greater severity.
- An RDoC approach would target a specific symptom or specific brain function regardless of the categorical diagnosis.
  - For example, for MDD or mood disorder, anhedonia severity or its underlying reward circuitry would be the target of investigation. A studied sample might then include patients with a wide range of anhedonia severity with a wide range of psychiatric conditions.
  - Studies might then include patients that have different diagnoses under DSM but share a specific symptom or trait of interest.

If successful, RDoC could become the foundation of a classification system

- Clinicians could base diagnosis and treatment for patients not only on clinical evaluations but also on data from imaging, genetic testing, and laboratory observation to determine prognosis and most importantly appropriate treatment.
- A challenge for an alternative classification is clinical practicality: while dimensional models appear to represent biology better than categorical models, the latter are better adjusted to clinical practice as they allow information to be conveyed in a concise manner.

- RDoC has yet to fulfill the NIMH's vision and prove that it can produce results that apply to clinical practice. Clinical diagnoses continue to be made through the categorical DSM system for the present.

Reading list

NIMH Research Domain Criteria (RDoC), Draft 3.1, June 2011. Available at http://www.nimh.nih.gov/research-priorities/rdoc/nimh-research-domain-criteria-rdoc.shtml

The National Institute of Mental Health Strategic Plan, August 2008. Available at http://www.nimh.nih.gov/about/strategic-planning-reports/index.shtml

Additional material for this chapter can be found online at:
www.mountsinaiexpertguides.com/psychiatry

This includes advice for patients.

CHAPTER 3

Functional Neuroanatomy

James W. Murrough, Amy R. Glick, Nicholas S. Stevens, and Thomas P. Naidich
Icahn School of Medicine at Mount Sinai, New York, NY, USA

OVERALL BOTTOM LINE
- Mental states and complex behavior arise from tightly regulated electrochemical activity within discrete neural circuits in the brain.
- Psychiatric disorders reflect a particular set of disturbances within specific neural circuits.
- The concept of the limbic system refers to an interconnected set of brain regions responsible for the generation and expression of emotion.
- Cortico-striatal-thalamic (CST) circuits represent a series of parallel closed loops interconnecting specific areas of cortex and subcortex and are a major organizing principle of behavioral neuroanatomy.
- The projecting monoamine systems – noradrenergic, serotonergic, and dopaminergic systems – are critical components of behavioral neuroanatomy and are the primary sites of action of most pharmacological treatments in psychiatry.

Discussion of topic and guidelines
Introduction

Mental states and complex behavior arise from tightly regulated electrochemical activity within discrete neural circuits in the brain. Psychiatric disorders, in turn, can be understood as arising from dysfunction within specific neural circuits. Psychiatric disorders, as currently defined in the *Diagnostic and Statistical Manual of Mental Disorders*, appear to reflect a unique constellation of abnormal functioning within a subset of brain circuits. Specific circuits map to functional domains (of behavior, emotion, cognition) rather than to the psychiatric syndromes themselves. For example, in patients with major depressive disorder (MDD), dysfunction within distinct circuits appears to underlie the observed alterations in mood, motivation, psychomotor function, anxiety, attention, or neuroendocrine functioning, respectively. The specific character of an individual patient's illness can be understood as the unique involvement of a particular circuit interacting with the nature of the disordered circuitry specific to that patient. Further, the dysfunctional circuitry characteristic of a specific behavioral abnormality (e.g., motivation or fear response) is expected to be present across diagnostic categories (e.g., MDD, anxiety disorders, schizophrenia).

Our knowledge of functional neuroanatomy rests largely on neuronal tracing studies conducted in non-human primates and other animals. The development of noninvasive *in vivo* functional neuroimaging – including functional magnetic resonance imaging (fMRI) – provides new opportunities to test specific functional anatomical hypotheses in patients with psychiatric disorders. In this chapter, we provide a brief overview of selected aspects of functional

---

Mount Sinai Expert Guides: Psychiatry, First Edition. Edited by Asher B. Simon, Antonia S. New, and Wayne K. Goodman.
© 2017 John Wiley & Sons, Ltd. Published 2017 by John Wiley & Sons, Ltd.
Companion website: www.mountsinaiexpertguides.com/psychiatry

neuroanatomy relevant to psychiatric disorders. A firm grasp of basic functional neuroanatomy will provide the student of psychiatry and behavioral science with a solid footing on which to develop additional knowledge regarding psychiatric nosology, cognitive science, and neuropsychopharmacology.

The limbic system and related structures

- In Latin, "limbus" means border. Anatomically, the limbic system refers to a ring of structures organized about the medial aspect of the cerebral hemispheres.
- It refers to an interconnected set of brain regions responsible for the generation and expression of emotion.
- Structures originally described as part of the limbic system included:
  - bilateral cingulate and parahippocampal gyri;
  - amygdalae;
  - hippocampi;
  - anterior and medial thalami;
  - hypothalami.
- Subsequent research demonstrated important connections between these core limbic structures and additional cortical and subcortical regions (Figures 3.1 and 3.2), including:
  - medial and orbital prefrontal cortices (mPFC and OFC, respectively);
  - insulae;
  - striata;
  - periaqueductal gray matter (PAG).

The amygdala

- Animal and human imaging studies have consistently implicated the amygdala in:
  - fear;
  - novelty-related processes.
- Abnormal functioning of the amygdala features prominently in models of mood and anxiety disorders.
  - The amygdala – a collection of nuclei deep within antermedial temporal lobe – has emerged as a key structure in neurocircuitry models of psychiatric disease. Sensory information is

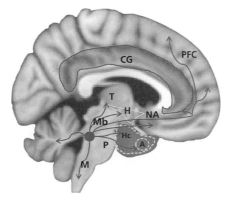

KEY:

PFC, prefrontal cortex
CG, cingulate gyrus
T, thalamus
H, hypothalamus
Hc, hippocampus
A, amygdala
Mb, midbrain
P, pons
M, medulla
NA, nucleus accumbens

Figure 3.1 The limbic system and related structures. Midline sagittal view depicting core limbic structures. The hippocampi and amygdalae lie deep to temporal cortex, illustrated here by dotted lines. Also shown is a schematic depiction of the ascending noradrenergic system with fibers originating in the locus coeruleus. Two additional monoamine systems – the serotonergic and dopaminergic systems – have been omitted for clarity.

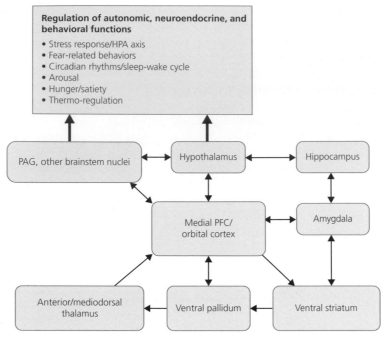

Figure 3.2 Cortico-striatal-thalamic circuitry involving the medial prefrontal cortex. Cortico-striatal-thalamic (CST) circuitry centering on medial prefrontal cortex (PFC) and medial aspects of orbital cortex important for emotional behavior and psychiatric disorders. Also shown are select anatomical connections between components of the CST circuitry and core limbic structures. Projection from hypothalamus to ventral striatum is not shown.

received by the basolateral nucleus, processed, and then forwarded to the central nucleus (the primary output region of the amygdala).
- Amygdala activation in response to threat stimuli has been demonstrated to be elevated in patients with posttraumatic stress disorder (PTSD).
- The amygdala has extensive reciprocal projections to the mPFC, medial aspects of the OFC, hippocampus, hypothalamus, and ventral striatum (including the nucleus accumbens).
- Interactions between the mPFC and the amygdala appear to be critical for adaptive fear conditioning and extinction.

The hippocampus
- The hippocampus plays a key role in memory formation and is a primary site of pathology in Alzheimer's disease.
  - The hippocampus also exerts a regulatory influence over the amygdala and the hypotha-lamic-pituitary-adrenal (HPA) axis via a negative feedback system (see further on).
  - Hippocampal volumes are reduced in some studies of MDD and PTSD.
- The hippocampus is a complex structure composed of functionally and molecularly distinct subregions enfolded within the medial temporal lobe.
  - Information enters the hippocampus through the entorhinal cortex, is passed to the dentate gyrus through the perforant pathway, continues to the CA3 region through the mossy fibers and eventually terminates in the subiculum, which is the major output region of the hippocampus.

The hypothalamus

- The hypothalamus is a complex set of nuclei lying ventral to the thalamus. It exerts critical control over many neurovegetative, neuroendocrine, and autonomic functions, including the sleep-wake cycle, hunger/satiety, thermo-regulation, and the stress response.
  - The hypothalamus sits as the control center of the HPA axis and has dense reciprocal connections with the amygdala, hippocampus, mPFC/OFC, ventral striatum, and brainstem visceromotor nuclei.
  - In response to stress, the paraventricular nucleus of the hypothalamus releases corticotropin-releasing factor to stimulate the anterior pituitary to release adrenocorticotropic hormone (ACTH).
  - ACTH stimulates the adrenal gland to secrete cortisol into the systemic circulation, regulating diverse behavioral and physiological responses to stress.
  - Cortisol negatively regulates HPA axis activity via glucocorticoid receptors in the hypothalamus and mineralocorticoid receptors in the hippocampus.
  - Dysregulation of the HPA axis has been consistently implicated in MDD, PTSD, and other psychiatric disorders.

Cortico-striatal-thalamic circuits

- The concept of a series of parallel closed circuits or loops interconnecting specific areas of cortex and subcortex has emerged as a major organizing principle of behavioral neuroanatomy.
- These circuits can be described generally as cortico-striatal-thalamic (CST) circuits and are defined by specific cortical-subcortical connections.
  - Fibers originate in a discrete region of the PFC and project to a specific region of striatum, which in turn projects through the pallidum to specific relay nuclei in the thalamus, from which thalamic fibers project back to the originating region of cortex.
  - The fibers are divided in characteristic patterns, with preservation of the relative topography at each level of the circuits (i.e., medial fibers remain medial in each structure).
  - An important early observation supporting the functional importance of this organization was that a lesion anywhere along a given circuit produced similar behavioral deficits, whereas a lesion in a parallel circuit would produce a distinct deficit.
- Three well-described CST circuits relevant to psychiatry are presented further on.

The dorsolateral prefrontal cortex circuit

- The dorsolateral PFC (DLPFC) circuit is critical to executive function (e.g., organizing, planning, attention).
  - Lesions to the DLPFC classically result in deficits in the Wisconsin Card Sorting task, in strategy generation, and in learning tasks.
  - Dysfunction within the DLPFC and related circuitry has been consistently implicated in schizophrenia and other disorders with prominent cognitive deficits.
  - More recently, cognitive neuroimaging studies have highlighted the DLPFC as an important region for certain types of cognitive control of emotion.
  - In this circuit, projections originate in the DLPFC, pass through the dorsal striatum, dorsomedial pallidum and anterior and mediodorsal thalamus, and project back to the DLPFC. The DLPFC also has important reciprocal cortico-cortical connections with the mPFC and OFC which are in turn tightly linked to the limbic system (see previously).

The orbitofrontal cortex circuit

- The orbitofrontal circuit plays a key role in social behavior, impulse control, and stimulus-reward associations.
  - Lesions to the OFC circuit result in marked personality changes, including irritability, mood lability, and tactlessness, for example in the famous case of Phineas Gage.
  - The OFC and related circuitry has been implicated in numerous psychiatric disorders, including obsessive-compulsive disorder, mood disorders, substance use disorders, and pathological gambling.
  - Projections originate in the OFC and connect specific regions of ventromedial striatum, ventral pallidum, and inferomedial sectors of mediodorsal thalamus (Figure 3.2). Medial aspects of the OFC are highly interconnected with the limbic system (see previously). More central and caudal aspects have cortico-cortical connections with unique regions including primary olfactory and gustatory cortex.

The anterior cingulate cortex circuit

- The anterior cingulate cortex (ACC) is critically involved in a variety of cognitive and emotional processes, including motivation, error detection, attention, and autonomic functions.
- Neurons in Brodmann Area (BA) 24 of the ACC project to ventral striatum and ventral pallidum, which in turn project to mediodorsal and midline thalamus.
- Classically, bilateral ACC lesions produce akinetic mutism, apathy, and immobility.
- The ACC is a complex structure that manifests a cognitive-emotional division along its dorsal-ventral axis. The dorsal ACC, located superior to the genu of the corpus callosum, is associated with cognitive processes including attention and is anatomically related to lateral PFC. Dysfunction within this region has been implicated in attention deficit-hyperactivity disorder (ADHD), among other disorders. In contrast, the ventral ACC (including rostral BA 24 and subgenual ACC) is more related to the mPFC, medial OFC, and limbic system. The term mPFC can be used to describe the ventral ACC, ventromedial PFC and more rostral related areas including the medial part of BA 10. The ventral ACC – and related mPFC/OFC networks – is strongly implicated in MDD and other mood and anxiety disorders. Hypermetabolism or overactivity in response to emotional stimuli is observed within the ventral ACC in MDD, which is then normalized with successful treatment.

Projecting monoamine systems

In addition to the limbic system and CST circuitry reviewed above, the projecting monoamine systems – the noradrenergic, serotonergic, and dopaminergic systems – are critical components of behavioral neuroanatomy and are the primary site of action of most pharmacological treatments in psychiatry. Monoaminergic transmission arises primarily from small groups of widely projecting neurons located in the brainstem. These include the norepinephrine (NE)-producing neurons in the locus coeruleus (LC); the serotonin (5-HT)-producing neurons in the raphe nuclei; and the dopamine (DA)-producing neurons in the ventral tegmental area (VTA) and substantia nigra (SN). These systems innervate diffuse cortical and subcortical regions and generally serve a modulatory function. They are critical to such global functions as arousal, attention, and mood.

The noradrenergic system

Stimulation of NE receptors in the amygdala enhances the encoding of novelty or threat-related information and sensitization of this system has been implicated in models of PTSD and other anxiety disorders. Norepinephrine-producing neurons in the LC project widely to neocortex, striatum, and regions of the limbic system, including the amygdala (Figure 3.1). The LC receives inputs from mPFC and OFC and the firing rate of LC neurons varies with level of arousal and in response to stress, threat, and novelty.

The serotonergic system

Serotonin is critical to regulaitry mood, sleep and arousal, and the serotonin transporter is a primary site of action of the serotonin-selective reuptake inhibitor (SSRI) antidepressant drugs. Serotonin-producing neurons in the brainstem raphe project to an impressive array of brain regions including the cortex, thalamus, striatum, hippocampus, and dopaminergic midbrain nuclei.

The dopaminergic system

Dopamine (DA)-producing neurons play a key role in reward and motivation. These neurons in the VTA project to the forebrain via two primary pathways: the mesolimbic and mesocortical pathway. The mesolimbic pathway carries dopaminergic fibers from the VTA to the ventral striatum/nucleus accumbens, to the amygdala, and to other limbic targets. The mesolimbic pathway is also believed to be the main site of action of antipsychotic drugs on positive symptoms of schizophrenia. The mesocortical pathway carries fibers to the neocortex where DA modulates attention, working memory, and other cognitive processes. Schizophrenia may be characterized by a relative deficit of cortical DA, accounting for the cognitive and negative symptoms of the disorder. The mesocortical pathway is also believed to be the primary site of action of stimulant medication for the treatment of ADHD. Discussion of another important DA pathway – the nigrostriatal pathway – is beyond the scope of this chapter.

Conclusion

We have provided a brief overview of selected aspects of functional neuroanatomy relevant to psychiatric disorders. We have discussed in some detail the concept of the limbic system, of parallel cortico-striatal-thalamic circuits and of the monoamine systems critical to neuropsychopharmacology. The reader is directed to the suggested reading list for further details.

Reading list

Alexander GE, DeLong MR, Strick PL. Parallel organization of functionally segregated circuits linking basal ganglia and cortex. Annu Rev Neurosci 1986;9:357–81.

Cummings JL, Mega MS. Neuropsychiatry and Behavioral Neuroscience. Oxford: Oxford University Press, 2003.

Murrough JW, Schiller D, Charney DS. Neurocircuitry of anxiety disorders: focus on panic disorder and post-traumatic stress disorder. In: Rankovic Z, Bingham M, Nestler EJ, Hargreaves R (eds). Drug Discovery for Psychiatric Disorders. Cambridge: RSC Publishing, 2012.

Naidich TP, Castillo M, Cha S, Smirniotopoulos JG (eds). Imaging of the Brain. Philadelphia: Elsevier Saunders, 2013.

Nestler EJ, Hyman SE, Malenka RC (eds). Molecular Neuropharmacology: A Foundation for Clinical Neuroscience, 2nd edn. New York: McGraw Hill, 2009.

Price JL, Drevets WC. Neurocircuitry of mood disorders. Neuropsychopharmacology 2010;35(1):192–216.

Additional material for this chapter can be found online at:
www.mountsinaiexpertguides.com/psychiatry

This includes multiple choice questions.

CHAPTER 4

Translational Neuroscience in Clinical Psychiatry

Ivan Chavarria-Siles, Emily Stern, Schahram Akbarian, Pamela Sklar, and Eric J. Nestler

Icahn School of Medicine at Mount Sinai, New York, NY, USA

OVERALL BOTTOM LINE
- Most psychiatric disorders are highly polygenic; the number of genes contributing to these disorders is in the thousands, and many of the genes are shared among different disorders.
- Epigenetic modifications may contribute to many psychiatric disorders; certain environmental factors may hijack the brain's epigenetic machinery and, in combination with genetic predispositions, produce the behavioral manifestations of these disorders. (Epigenetics is explained further on.)
- Animal models of complex heterogeneous psychiatric disorders are valuable preclinical tools with which to investigate the neurobiological basis of the disorder. However, a perplexing problem is how to assess some of the core symptoms of psychiatric disorders, which are uniquely human traits.
- The goal of psychiatric neuroimaging is to integrate neuroimaging data in humans with information obtained from genetics and the study of animal models, including non-human primates, with the expectation that such multidisciplinary work will increasingly reveal the neural circuits that underlie the behavioral abnormalities that define psychiatric disorders.

Genetics of psychiatric disorders

Most psychiatric disorders have a strong genetic component; heritability estimates are as high as 80% for schizophrenia and bipolar disorder, 60% for alcohol dependence, and 40% for major depression and panic disorder (Owen et al., 2000). As of today, little is known about the specific genes that comprise the genetic risk for any psychiatric illness. Early strategies to identify such factors focused on associating changes in one or a small number of particular genes with a psychiatric illness, but those studies were limited in retrospect by an insufficient appreciation of the genetic complexity underlying psychiatric illness. Genome-wide association studies (GWAS) have made clear that these disorders are influenced by many genetic variants (each with a very small effect size). Few if any of these genetic factors, almost all of which have required large, well-powered studies for their discovery and replication, are deterministic (Sullivan et al., 2012).

The clinical phenotype definitions remain rooted in observational diagnostic concepts from the late 19th century without firm genetic or biological foundation. The definitions in use describe highly heritable clinical entities, as measured in family and twin studies, which have allowed researchers to apply successfully genetic methods. However, we can expect substantial overlap of

---

Mount Sinai Expert Guides: Psychiatry, First Edition. Edited by Asher B. Simon, Antonia S. New, and Wayne K. Goodman.
© 2017 John Wiley & Sons, Ltd. Published 2017 by John Wiley & Sons, Ltd.
Companion website: www.mountsinaiexpertguides.com/psychiatry

genetic susceptibility across, and substantial heterogeneity within, diagnostic categories (Craddock and Sklar, 2013). DSM-5, like the two preceding editions, places disorders in discrete categories that are based largely on symptoms. Over the past decade, many psychiatrists have proposed dimensional approaches informed by genetics and biology, but they are not in practice yet (Adam, 2013). A strength of the DSM classification system has been to establish "reliability" (each edition has ensured that clinicians use the same terms in the same ways); this reliability has standardized the way diagnoses are made and has facilitated the development of evidence-based treatments. To improve on this, the National Institute of Mental Health (NIMH) has launched the Research Domain Criteria (RDoC) project to transform diagnosis by incorporating genetics, imaging, cognitive science, and other levels of information to lay the foundation for a new classification system.

Since 2010, there have been a series of major findings in the genetics of autism, schizophrenia, and bipolar disorder. These include identifying an important role for copy number variants (missing or added sections of DNA). These variants often have a large effect on disease risk, contain many genes, and are shared across many diseases (e.g., autism spectrum disorder, intellectual disability, epilepsy, and schizophrenia). In addition, multiple genome-wide significant findings in schizophrenia and bipolar disorder now exist and are beginning to highlight underlying molecular pathways as well as overlapping risk genes. Surprisingly, the number of genes contributing to the risk for a psychiatric illness is likely in the many thousands, thus defining these as "highly polygenic" disorders. These studies have also clarified that the risk for particular illnesses may not be independent; for example, it is clear that there is shared genetic risk between schizophrenia and bipolar disorder. While both disorders share the heightened risk for psychotic symptoms, it is as yet unknown why one individual presents with the severe mood symptoms of bipolar disorder while another presents with the flattening of mood of schizophrenia. Interestingly, some of the genes implicated in schizophrenia and bipolar disorder also confer risk for autism, which is even more surprising. These results represent an important step towards the goal of moving beyond descriptive syndromes in psychiatry, and towards a nosology informed by disease cause (Sullivan et al., 2012).

The overlap of genetic factors in major psychiatric disorders (i.e., copy number variant, polygenes, and calcium-channel genes) confirms previously reported evidence of abundant overlap of symptoms in human complex disorders. Thus, the same gene variant might contribute to the risk of different diseases, possibly based on other genetic factors, on environmental exposures, or on epigenetic mechanisms, the topic of the following paragraphs.

Epigenetics in psychiatric disorders

Epigenetics refers to the potentially heritable, but environmentally modifiable regulation of gene function and expression that is mediated through non-DNA-encoded mechanisms. Thus, the structure of chromatin, the mixture of DNA and proteins in a cell nucleus, is critical for gene transcription, DNA replication, DNA recombination, and DNA repair. The availability of DNA to be transcribed into RNA and then proteins is modulated by a host of epigenetic mechanisms that alter the structure of chromatin and provide binding sites for a wide variety of regulatory proteins. The orchestrated organization of epigenetic factors, including DNA methylation, histone acetylation and methylation, non-coding RNAs (ncRNAs), and their associated chromatin proteins, is essential for cellular differentiation during development (Berdasco and Esteller, 2013).

Evidence derived mostly from animal research suggests that the alterations in the availability of DNA to be transcribed into proteins may underlie many psychiatric disorders. Accordingly, a recent hypothesis is that certain environmental factors hijack the brain's epigenetic machinery and, in combination with genetic predispositions, produce the behavioral manifestations of these disorders.

In fact, it has been demonstrated that, during the lifetime of monozygotic twins, there is a profound accumulation of epigenetic differences, likely because of different life experiences as well as random events during development.

Epigenetic dysregulation has been associated with depression; for example, systemic or intra-cerebral administration of histone deacetylase (HDAC) inhibitors, which increase histone acetylation and promote gene expression, either alone or in combination with standard antidepressants, improved antidepressant responses in several animal models. Several studies have reported increased histone acetylation or phosphoacetylation in several brain regions after exposure to acute or chronic stress in both mice and rats, suggesting that this represents an adaptive change that helps an animal cope with the stress (Sun et al., 2013). This represents a model by which life events (e.g., stress) can change the expression of genes and thereby change the risk or presentation of illness.

Schizophrenia and bipolar disorder have also been examined for disease-associated epigenetic changes; several dozen sites with DNA methylation alterations have been found across the genome in psychotic disorders, some of which were sex specific. Loci with significant epigenetic differences between affected individuals and controls contained genes involved in brain development and neurotransmitter pathways, which had previously been associated with psychotic illness. Perturbations of DNA methylation in psychosis may also result from the abnormal activity of DNA methyltransferases (DNMT) or changes in the levels of methyl-group donors and cofactors affecting DNA methylation. DNMT genes have been reported to be upregulated in the prefrontal cortex of patients with schizophrenia and bipolar disorder. Differences in patterns of histone modifications have also been found in major psychosis. As well, antipsychotic medications have been shown to produce epigenetic changes in the brain, although it is still unclear whether their therapeutic effects are a direct consequence of these epigenetic alterations (Labrie et al., 2012).

Animal and cell based models in psychiatric disorders

Animal models of complex heterogeneous psychiatric disorders are valuable preclinical tools with which to investigate the neurobiological basis of the disorder. They offer a unique means of studying causation among molecular, cellular, circuit, and behavioral phenomena. However, a perplexing problem is how to assess some of the core symptoms of psychiatric disorders (like thoughts, feelings, hallucinations), which are uniquely human traits. In general, most behaviors studied in animal models represent performance in tasks designed to have translational relevance to core symptoms. A further problem with animal models of psychiatric disorders is that there is no current "gold standard" medication available to treat all symptoms of a disorder that can be used as a definitive positive control in preclinical studies. Useful animal models should have the appropriate triad of face (symptom homology), construct (replicate the etiology), and predictive (show the expected pharmacological response, or lack of it) validity to the clinical disorder being modeled (Nestler and Hyman, 2010; Jones et al., 2011).

Given the subjective nature of most psychiatric symptoms and the lack of valid biomarkers, establishing links between clinical variables and animal end points cannot currently be done without a large degree of interpretation. The majority of mutant mouse models have been so far developed in the context of the "common variant" hypothesis, whereby the genetic risk for a psychiatric disorder is hypothesized to reflect the additive or multiplicative influence of several alleles (i.e., genetic variations) with small effect plus perhaps an environmental exposure such as stress. However, the lack of a highly penetrant mutation of strong effect associated with psychiatric disorders is one of the primary causes for the lack of valid psychiatric animal models (Nestler and Hyman, 2010; Berton et al., 2012).

Optogenetics

Cognitive and social deficits lie at the core of many neuropsychiatric diseases and are among the behavioral symptoms not adequately treated with today's pharmacological interventions. Despite significant advances in identifying genes and epigenetic factors that affect cognition and social behavior, understanding how molecular and cellular events lead to behavioral abnormalities has been technically difficult. Optogenetic and related techniques have in recent years provided unprecedented means to establish such causal connections (Tye and Deisseroth, 2012). In optogenetics, ion channels, pumps, or receptors that can be activated by light are expressed in a specific brain region or even a specific type of nerve cell within that region (those genes are transgenically transferred in animals). The activity of these proteins is then controlled with a fiberoptic cable into the targeted brain area. In this manner, it is possible to experimentally increase or decrease the activity of nerve cells with subsecond temporal resolution.

Use of light-controlled neurons and brain circuits has made possible the elucidation of the cellular and circuit mechanisms underlying normal cognitive and social behavior as well as abnormalities produced in animal models (Yizhar, 2012). Applying such tools to non-human primates with parallel studies of numerous other behavioral domains (mood, reward, motivation, motor function, etc.) will be especially important in defining brain circuits involved in particularly complex behaviors such as those that characterize most mental illnesses.

Induced pluripotent stem (iPS) cells

Studies of postmortem brain tissue from individuals with a psychiatric disorder have contributed importantly to our current knowledge of mental illness (Deep-Soboslay et al., 2011). Nevertheless, such studies are limited by the lack of access to sufficient numbers of brains obtained at the time of disease onset and the long postmortem intervals between death and brain tissue fixation. Recently the generation of so-called induced pluripotent stem (iPS) cells and related technology has made it possible to induce neuron-like cells (perhaps even a type of neuron, such as one producing dopamine versus glutamate) *in vitro* from fibroblasts or other peripheral cells obtained from a patient with a mental disorder. This permits the creation in a laboratory of neuronal networks that can be used to test the effect of experimental manipulations on the networks. In theory, induced neuron-like cells from patients, compared to those from healthy control subjects, should show genetically and perhaps some epigenetically determined cellular and molecular abnormalities related to the pathogenesis of the illness. If so, these neuron-like cells could provide powerful new platforms for drug screening. While studies of iPS cells and induced neurons remain at early stages of development, there is considerable excitement for their potential in psychiatric research (Brennand et al., 2012).

Brain imaging and cognitive neuroscience in psychiatry

Magnetic resonance imaging (MRI) technology is a noninvasive procedure that allows the *in vivo* study of the human brain. MRI is a powerful tool used for characterizing individual differences in brain anatomy, function, and connectivity. The use of structural and functional MRI technology has become a standard procedure in evaluating most neurological conditions. While MRI and other neuroimaging modalities cannot yet be utilized to diagnose a psychiatric condition, they are being employed widely in research to investigate the biological basis of mental illness and its treatment. A particularly exciting line of research in psychiatric neuroimaging investigates the way functional MRI measures can be used to predict treatment response. A growing number of studies have identified patterns of brain activity that distinguish patients who respond to treatments (both medication and therapy) from those who do not. Down the line, this approach may help identify those patients most likely to receive benefit from a given type of treatment, in line with the growing field of personalized medicine. Another way in which neuroimaging can directly inform clinical care is by associating differential patterns of neural functioning with various symptom dimensions within a psychiatric disorder. Psychiatric disease heterogeneity is a common problem in designing treatments and understanding biological mechanisms. Neuroimaging endophenotypes related to specific symptoms may eventually be targeted by neuromodulation and cognitive training treatments tailored to a specific neural signature to enhance the validity of psychiatric diagnosis.

Cognitive neuroscientists and geneticists have recently come together to investigate the relationship between brain-relevant genetic variants and neural functioning. The development of novel statistical methods has allowed this new field of imaging genetics to map genes that have been associated with cognitive processes with specific brain structures and functional networks. Most brain structural measurements have been found to be highly heritable, suggesting a strong genetic component. Unfortunately, there is a lack of consistency in neuroimaging genetics studies of psychiatric disorders to date. This may be due to small samples and effect sizes, and future work will require greater capability to acquire high-quality scans in combination with novel imaging-genetics approaches.

Finally, a goal of many investigations of psychiatric neuroimaging is to integrate neuroimaging data in humans with information obtained from the study of animal models, including importantly the use of non-human primates, through optogenetics, electrophysiological recordings from several brain areas of behaving animals, and related approaches. The expectation is that such multidisciplinary work will increasingly reveal the neural circuits that underlie the behavioral abnormalities that define psychiatric disorders.

Future directions

There has never been a more exciting time for neuroscience and genetics. We have learned an enormous amount over the past decade about how the brain functions and how an individual's genetic and epigenetic constitution influences neural function and complex behavior. The experimental approaches described very briefly outline the ways in which we can now increasingly translate this impressive knowledge into better diagnostic tests and treatments for mental illness.

Reading list/references

Adam D. Mental health: On the spectrum. Nature 2013;496:416–8.

Berdasco M, Esteller M. Genetic syndromes caused by mutations in epigenetic genes. Hum Genet 2013;132:359–83.

Berton O, Hahn CG, Thase ME. Are we getting closer to valid translational models for major depression? Science 2012;338:75–9.

Brennand KJ, Simone A, Tran N, Gage FH. Modeling psychiatric disorders at the cellular and network levels. Mol Psychiatry 2012;17:1239–53.

Craddock N, Sklar P. Genetics of bipolar disorder. Lancet 2013; 381:1654–62.

Deep-Soboslay A, Benes FM, Haroutunian V, Ellis JK, Kleinman JE, Hyde TM. Psychiatric brain banking: three perspectives on current trends and future directions. Biol Psychiatry 2011;69:104–12.

Jones CA, Watson DJ, Fone KC. Animal models of schizophrenia. Br J Pharmacol 2011;164:1162–94.

Labrie V, Pai S, Petronis A. Epigenetics of major psychosis: progress, problems and perspectives. Trends Genet 2012;28:427–35.

Nestler EJ, Hyman SE. Animal models of neuropsychiatric disorders. Nat Neurosci 2010;13:1161–9.

Owen MJ, Cardno AG, O'Donovan MC. Psychiatric genetics: back to the future. Mol Psychiatry 2000;5:22–31.

Sullivan PF, Daly MJ, O'Donovan M. Genetic architectures of psychiatric disorders: the emerging picture and its implications. Nat Rev Genet 2012;13:537–51.

Sun H, Kennedy PJ, Nestler EJ. Epigenetics of the depressed brain: role of histone acetylation and methylation. Neuropsychopharmacology 2013;38:124–37.

Tye KM, Deisseroth K. Optogenetic investigation of neural circuits underlying brain disease in animal models. Nat Rev Neurosci 2012;13:251–66.

Yizhar O. Optogenetic insights into social behavior function. Biol Psychiatry 2012;71:1075–80.

Additional material for this chapter can be found online at:
www.mountsinaiexpertguides.com/psychiatry

This includes multiple choice questions.

CHAPTER 5

Neuropsychological Assessment and Psychological Tests

Katherine E. Burdick, Manuela Russo, and Jane Martin
Icahn School of Medicine at Mount Sinai, New York, NY, USA

OVERALL BOTTOM LINE
- Neuropsychological assessment and psychological tests can be fundamental components of the complete psychiatric evaluation and provide the clinician with critical information about a patient's cognitive functioning, severity of psychopathology, and underlying personality traits.
- A neuropsychological assessment consists of a series of standardized psychometric measures designed to examine both general cognitive capacity as well as more specific cognitive domains, including processing speed, attention, working memory, verbal and visual learning, and executive functioning.
- Psychological tests are administered to gather information about potential psychopathological symptoms and personality characteristics, and may include symptom scales, personality tests, and projective tests.

Introduction

As a discipline, neuropsychology focuses on psychological and behavioral processes in relationship to brain structure and function. Originally, neuropsychological data were derived primarily from patients with structural lesions in specific areas of the brain, resulting in difficulties or performance deficits on tasks associated with cognitive skills such as attention, learning, and memory. As advancing technology in neuroimaging is allowing for functional assays of brain activation patterns and studies of how one neural region interacts with other regions (e.g., connectivity), the neuropsychological field has since expanded considerably to incorporate a multitude of neurological and psychiatric illnesses that are brain-based but not linked to specific lesions.

In clinical settings, the current purpose of neuropsychological assessments is to determine which brain functions (or aspects of them) are impaired or, in some cases, enhanced. A comprehensive neuropsychological assessment is warranted in psychiatric practice in several situations:

1. to identify and quantify cognitive impairments or functional incapacity, so as to determine a baseline level of functioning and set realistic treatment goals;
2. to rule out structural compromise or "organicity," as a complement to a neurological examination and/or brain imaging and electroencephalogram (EEG);
3. to evaluate an unexpected change in cognitive performance, personality, or functional capacity, including when reported by the patient or by caregivers/clinicians.

Mount Sinai Expert Guides: Psychiatry, First Edition. Edited by Asher B. Simon, Antonia S. New, and Wayne K. Goodman.
© 2017 John Wiley & Sons, Ltd. Published 2017 by John Wiley & Sons, Ltd.
Companion website: www.mountsinaiexpertguides.com/psychiatry

In a neuropsychological assessment, a patient's performance on a series of standardized psychometric measures (pencil and paper tests and computerized tasks) is compared with normative data collected from demographically-matched individuals, and the results are interpreted by a trained clinician. Critical to interpretation is the inclusion of a thorough clinical interview, including psychiatric diagnoses, family history, medical history, and a detailed account of childhood milestones and educational history. In patients with psychiatric illnesses, current symptom severity must be assessed, as this can significantly influence performance on cognitive measures.

Neuropsychological assessment

A comprehensive neuropsychological assessment typically includes measures of general cognitive capacity as well as more specific cognitive domains.

General cognitive ability/intelligence

The intelligence quotient (IQ) is a widely used measure that indicates one's level of general intellectual capacity and is most commonly tested by the Wechsler Adult Intelligence Scale (WAIS; several revisions have been made, the current version is WAIS-IV). Age-appropriate versions have also been developed to allow for estimates of IQ in infants, children, and adolescents. IQ is represented on a standardized scale relative to age-matched normative samples. Standard scores have a mean value of 100 and a standard deviation (SD) of ±15, with "average performance" ranging between 85 and 115. IQ scores are often used as a reference point for how an individual is expected to perform on other cognitive tasks; however, average IQ does not necessarily imply integrity or normality in other neurocognitive domains (e.g., attention). For this reason, a neuropsychological battery generally includes additional tests to assess specific cognitive functions.

Specific cognitive domains

Processing speed, attention, working memory, verbal and visual learning, and executive functions are common areas of investigation.

- *Processing speed* refers to how quickly cognitive activities can be executed. The WAIS Digit Symbol subtest is among the most widely used to assess processing speed and requires the subject to fill in as many empty squares as quickly as possible by using a key that matches numbers to symbols.
- *Attention* reflects the conscious processing of information and includes several component parts: vigilance (sustained attention), orienting (attentional shifting), and detection (selective attention; cognitive control). Sustained attention can be measured by the Continuous Performance Test-Identical Pairs Version, during which the subject is asked to press a button on a computer pad each time a series of letters (flashing on the screen) is immediately followed by the exact same series of letters. Selective attention/cognitive control assessments often require that the subject resolve conflicting information among different stimuli; this can be measured using the Stroop test, where incongruent information (e.g., a color word "red" printed in green ink) requires active inhibition of an automated response.
- *Working memory* incorporates cognitive activities involved in the temporary storage and active manipulation of information during the process of learning and comprehension. In the WAIS Digit Span Backward, the examiner reads aloud a string of numbers after which the subject must respond by providing the same string of numbers in the reverse order.
- *Learning* is commonly subdivided into three processes: encoding, storage, and retrieval. *Encoding* requires a person to register and combine information. *Storage* is the active transfer of information from short-term banks to longer-term memories and is processed by a variety of

strategies (e.g., rehearsal of newly learned information). *Retrieval* represents the active recall of previously stored data. The California Verbal Learning Test (CVLT) requires a person to attend to and remember a list of 16 words presented repeatedly. Initial performance indicates encoding, and performance after a 20-minute delay indicates retrieval.

- *Executive functions* incorporate a number of higher-order cognitive functions, such as set-shifting, abstract thinking, concept formation, and planning and decision-making. The Wisconsin Card Sorting Test (WCST) requires that the subject deduce, without *a priori* instruction, the rules for sorting cards into stacks based upon some unknown construct (e.g., color or shape). During the test, the subject is provided feedback as to whether each sorting response is correct or incorrect, after which s/he can either continue with or change the current strategy, thus measuring cognitive flexibility.

Psychological assessment

It is essential that a neuropsychological assessment be complemented by an evaluation of the person's mental status. Psychological tests (e.g., symptom scales, personality tests, and projective tests) are often administered to gather information about potential psychopathological symptoms and personality characteristics.

Psychopathological ratings

An evaluation of psychopathology provides the clinician with information about the presence of relevant clinical signs and symptoms, such as anxiety, depression, mania, and psychosis. The Hamilton Depression Rating Scale (HDRS) is an example of a widely-used clinically-relevant scoring instrument which estimates the severity of current depressive symptoms: no depression (scores of 0–7); mild depression (8–16); moderate depression (17–23); and severe depression (≥24). Several similar scales have been devised to assess for mania, anxiety, OCD, and positive and negative symptoms in psychosis. In clinical practice it is often practical to utilize self-report ratings such as the Beck Depression Inventory (BDI) to track a patient's progress in treatment.

Assessment of personality

Considered a gold standard measure of personality, the Minnesota Multiphasic Personality Inventory (MMPI) comprises 567 true/false statements of how a person would "generally describe himself." A trained psychologist is able to derive a personality profile by evaluating a subject's scores on 10 subscales derived from the data: Hypochondriasis (various and vague concerns about bodily functioning), Depression (low mood and hopelessness), Hysteria (poor physical health and neuroticism), Psychopathic Deviance (social deviation, lack of acceptance of law and authority), Masculinity/Femininity (rejection/adherence to stereotypical gender roles), Paranoia (suspiciousness and delusional thinking), Psychasthenia (excessive doubts, compulsions, obsessions), Schizophrenia (bizarreness, emotional and social withdrawal, abnormal perception), Hypomania (mild degree of elated mood, psychomotor activity, flight of ideas), and Social Introversion (tendency to withdraw). This measure is widely used in forensic settings.

Projective tests

Developed based upon psychoanalytic theories, these tests are based on the assumption that unconscious and partially-unconscious components of personality (i.e., dissonant and/or unacceptable emotions, thoughts, fears, needs, and internal conflicts) can be revealed through a subject's response to ambiguous stimuli. In short, a person fills in the gaps and projects his/her own feelings/thoughts when trigged by an ambiguous stimulus. The Rorschach Inkblot Test is among the most popular and consists of 10 symmetrical vague inkblot figures/cards (five in gray-scale, two in black and red, and three in multicolor). The subject is shown one figure at a time and asked what s/he sees. The figure can be rotated as the person chooses, and multiple answers can be given for each figure. Different criteria are used for scoring and include popularity (how frequently the answer is given by other people), location (does the respondent incorporate all or only part of the figure), attention to color, form quality, and content of response. The most popular objective method for scoring is the Exner Comprehensive System, which must be interpreted by a trained psychologist.

Conclusion

Neuropsychological assessment and psychological testing can be fundamental components of a comprehensive psychiatric evaluation. They provide the clinician with critical information about a patient's cognitive functioning, severity of psychopathology, and underlying personality traits. Comprehensive evaluations allow the clinician to identify not only weaknesses or impairments but also strengths and can help in detailing concrete recommendations for treatment planning.

Reading list

Anastasi A, Urbina S. Psychological Testing, 7th edn. Upper Saddle River, NJ: Prentice Hall, 1997.

Lezak MD. Neuropsychological Assessment, 2nd edn. New York: Oxford University Press, 1983.

Snyder PJ, Nussbaum PD. Clinical Neuropsychology. Washington, DC: American Psychological Association, 1998.

Spreen O, Strauss EA. Compendium of Neuropsychological Tests, 2nd edn. New York: Oxford University Press, 1998.

Wechsler D. The Wechsler Adult Intelligence Scale – Revised Manual. New York: The Psychological Corporation, 1981.

Additional material for this chapter can be found online at:
www.mountsinaiexpertguides.com/psychiatry

This includes a case study and multiple choice questions.

CHAPTER 6

Clinical Use of Laboratory Tests, Brain Imaging, and Biomarkers

Carrie L. Ernst and James W. Murrough
Icahn School of Medicine at Mount Sinai, New York, NY, USA

OVERALL BOTTOM LINE
- Although the interview and mental status examination are the primary tools used to make diagnoses in psychiatry, laboratory testing and neuroimaging are essential for working up patients presenting with neuropsychiatric sign/symptoms, ruling out non-psychiatric etiologies, and monitoring psychotropic medications and side effects.
- Currently, the availability of laboratory and imaging studies that can meaningfully help clinical psychiatrists with early identification, management, and prevention of psychiatric disorders is limited. However, ongoing research into genetic and biological markers may ultimately result in an increased arsenal of valuable tools for the clinical psychiatrist.

Discussion of topic and guidelines
General approach to utilizing laboratory and other assessment tools
- A thorough history and physical (H&P) – including medical and psychiatric histories, mental status exam, and neurological exam – remains the first and most important step in evaluating a patient presenting with neuropsychiatric signs/symptoms.
- Use the H&P to guide decisions about laboratory testing.
- Before ordering a test, consider how it will change clinical management.
- Avoid ordering unnecessary tests.
- Consult colleagues in other specialties for advice about appropriate use and interpretation of tests.

Screening and health maintenance
Presently, there are no consensus guidelines regarding the use of laboratory tests to screen *otherwise medically healthy* patients presenting with *only* psychiatric complaints. Several studies have suggested that the following tests may be useful in such patients:
- serum glucose;
- blood urea nitrogen (BUN);
- creatinine (Cr) clearance;
- urinalysis;
- thyroid function (in females >50 or with symptoms of thyroid disease);

Mount Sinai Expert Guides: Psychiatry, First Edition. Edited by Asher B. Simon, Antonia S. New, and Wayne K. Goodman.
© 2017 John Wiley & Sons, Ltd. Published 2017 by John Wiley & Sons, Ltd.
Companion website: www.mountsinaiexpertguides.com/psychiatry

- EKG (if H&P suggests cardiovascular disease, or before prescribing medications known to affect cardiac function);
- pregnancy test (before prescribing medications that carry risk of congenital anomalies);
- urine toxicology screen (if presentation suggests active substance use).

As many psychiatric patients do not receive regular health maintenance examinations, psychiatrists may be faced with the task of delivering preventive care, which may include screening for diabetes, dyslipidemia, hypertension, obesity, and sexually transmitted diseases, as well as providing counseling about healthier lifestyle choices. Associated laboratory tests that psychiatrists might order should be dictated by a patient's specific presentation, and abnormalities may prompt referral to a primary care physician for further management.

Patients in several high-risk categories may require more extensive laboratory testing:
- elderly;
- cognitive impairment;
- immunocompromised;
- substance use;
- significant medical comorbidity;
- institutionalized (nursing home, prison, shelter);
- homeless;
- acute change in mental status;
- late-onset new neuropsychiatric symptoms;
- suspicion of overdose.

Diagnosis

Table 6.1 reviews commonly used laboratory tests and indications for use in patients presenting with neuropsychiatric symptoms. This list is not intended to be comprehensive. Since there are no clinically reliable biomarkers for diagnosing psychiatric illnesses, laboratory tests are generally used to rule out the many non-psychiatric illnesses that may be producing the patient's symptoms. (Non-psychiatric illnesses that can present with prominent neuropsychiatric symptoms are reviewed in subsequent chapters.)

Additional diagnostic studies

- *Cerebrospinal fluid (CSF)*
  - Lumbar puncture to evaluate patients presenting with new or atypical neuropsychiatric symptoms, *particularly* if there is evidence of cognitive impairment, seizures, or other neurological signs/symptoms. It can detect infectious, inflammatory, and neoplastic etiologies.
  - Lumbar puncture should *not* be performed until after head CT has ruled out conditions that can cause increased intracranial pressure.
- *Neuroimaging*
  - CT and MRI can show structural brain abnormalities, and should be considered in patients with neuropsychiatric symptoms that are atypical for any known psychiatric disorders.
  - CT with or without contrast is useful for rapid screening for stroke, hemorrhage, tumor, or mass, though there is disagreement in the literature regarding its indications in psychiatric patients.
  - CT should be done for patients presenting with focal neurological symptoms, recent head injury, and EEG abnormalities, and probably also for initial dementia work-ups and those with known history of abnormal CT findings who present with acute mental status change.

Table 6.1 Commonly used laboratory tests and indications for use in patients presenting with neuropsychiatric symptoms.

Test	Indication	Comments
Hematological		
Hemoglobin, hematocrit	• Fatigue • Impaired cognition	
White blood cells	• Psychotropic medications • Rule out infection (e.g., in intravenous drug use)	• Leukocytosis: lithium, neuroleptic malignant syndrome (NMS), infection • Leukopenia/agranulocytosis: clozapine, carbamazepine, phenothiazines
Platelets	• Psychotropic medications	• Thrombocytopenia: valproate, carbamazepine, antipsychotics • Impaired platelet aggregation and bleeding risk with SSRIs
Iron studies (ferritin, TIBC, iron)	• Fatigue • Impaired cognition	
Mean corpuscular volume	• Fatigue • Impaired cognition • Especially if alcoholic and/or poor nutritional status	• Elevated: alcohol use, vitamin B_{12} and folate deficiency, HIV
Coagulation factors (PT, PTT, INR)	• Assessment of hepatic synthetic function • Concomitant anticoagulant therapy and highly protein-bound psychotropics	Elevated PT in cirrhosis
Serum chemistries		
Liver function tests (LFT): ALT, AST, Alk Phos, GGTP, bilirubin	• General neuropsychiatric work-up • *Evaluation of liver disease severity, impairing metabolism of many psychotropics* • Alcohol • Delirium • Hepatotoxic psychotropic medications (e.g., valproate, carbamazepine, olanzapine)	• Elevated AST: hepatic disease (in alcoholic liver disease AST:ALT ratio is ≥2:1), heart failure, eclampsia • Elevated ALT: hepatic disease • Decreased AST and ALT in pyridoxine (vitamin B_6) deficiency • Elevated Alk Phos: many diseases including hepatic, bone, and hyperparathyroidism; phenothiazine use • Elevated bilirubin: hepatic disease • Elevated GGTP: alcohol use, hepatobiliary disease
Albumin (ALB); total protein (TP)	• General neuropsychiatric work-up • Prior to use of highly protein-bound psychotropics in patients with liver disease	• *Low levels result in high fraction of unbound (active) drug which may result in more active and side effects* • Elevated ALB: dehydration • Elevated TP: dehydration, inflammation, chronic infection, multiple myeloma • Decreased ALB, TP: cirrhosis/hepatic disease, malnutrition, renal disease

Table 6.1 (*Continued*)

Test	Indication	Comments
Renal function (BUN, Cr, Cr clearance)	• General neuropsychiatric work-up • *Evaluation of renal disease severity impairing excretion of many psychotropics* • Prior to use of renally-excreted psychotropics (e.g., lithium, gabapentin, topiramate)	• Elevated Cr: renal disease • Elevated BUN: renal disease, dehydration; often results in delirium • Follow 24-hour Cr clearance in patients taking lithium
Sodium	• General neuropsychiatric work-up • Psychotropic medications • Delirium	• Decreased: SIADH, polydipsia, carbamazepine, oxcarbazepine, SSRIs • Hyponatremia associated with delirium
Potassium	• General neuropsychiatric work-up • Eating disorders • Psychogenic vomiting	• Decreased: purging, laxative or diuretic abuse, psychogenic vomiting, associated with weakness, fatigue, cardiac arrhythmias
Chloride	• General neuropsychiatric work-up • Eating disorders • Psychogenic vomiting	• Decreased: purging, psychogenic vomiting
Bicarbonate	• General neuropsychiatric work-up • Eating disorders • Panic disorder	• Decreased: hyperventilation • Increased: purging, laxative abuse
Phosphorus	• General neuropsychiatric work-up • Eating disorders	• Decreased: purging, hyperparathyroidism • Increased: hypoparathyroidism, acute porphyria
Magnesium	• General neuropsychiatric work-up • Delirium • Alcohol	• Decreased: associated with alcohol, agitation, delirium, seizures, coma
Calcium	• General neuropsychiatric work-up • Mood disorders • Psychosis • Eating disorders • Delirium	• Decreased: laxative abuse, hypoparathyroidism, renal failure; associated with depression, delirium, irritability • Increased: hyperparathyroidism, bone metastases; associated with depression, delirium, psychosis
Glucose	• General neuropsychiatric work-up • Delirium • Fatigue • Psychotropic medications	• Elevated or low levels associated with delirium, agitation, anxiety

(*Continued*)

Table 6.1 (*Continued*)

Test	Indication	Comments
Ammonia	• General neuropsychiatric work-up • Delirium • Liver disease	• Elevated: hepatic encephalopathy, liver failure, GI bleed
Pancreatic function (amylase, lipase)	• Alcohol use disorder • Eating disorder • Psychotropic medication (e.g., valproate)	• Elevated: pancreatitis, purging (amylase only)
Creatinine phosphokinase (CPK)	• Delirium • Antipsychotics	• Elevated: NMS, intramuscular injection, restraints, rhabdomyolysis, long period of immobility
Endocrine/metabolic		
HbA1c	• Second generation antipsychotics • Symptoms of diabetes or poorly adherent diabetic	• If on second generation antipsychotics, monitor at baseline, 12 weeks, and annually
Lipids (fasting cholesterol, triglycerides, HDL, LDL)	• Second generation antipsychotics • Health maintenance	• If on second generation antipsychotics, monitor at baseline, 12 weeks, and annually
Cortisol	• Neuropsychiatric work-up • Symptoms of Cushing's or Addison's • Mood disorders • Psychosis	
Pregnancy test (beta-HCG)	• Prior to prescribing medications associated with congenital anomalies	
Catecholamines (urinary homovanillic acid, plasma vanillylmandelic acid)	• Panic attacks, anxiety	• Elevated: pheochromocytoma
Testosterone profile	• Poor libido • Impaired sexual function • Depression • Fatigue • Aggression	• Elevated: anabolic steroid abuse • Decreased: many medical causes
Prolactin	• Antipsychotics • Poor libido, menstrual irregularities, galactorrhea	• Elevated: antipsychotics; post-seizure; prolactinoma
Thyroid function (TSH, free T_4)	• General neuropsychiatric work-up • Weight change, fatigue, heat/cold intolerance • Depression, anxiety • Dementia • History of thyroid disease • Lithium	

Table 6.1 (*Continued*)

Test	Indication	Comments
Parathyroid hormone	• Thyroidectomy • Anxiety • Psychosis • Delirium • Cognitive impairment	
Vitamins (serum)		
Folate	• Dementia • Delirium • Fatigue • Alcohol	
B_{12}	• Dementia • Delirium • Mood disorder • Psychosis • Alcohol • Malnutrition • Elevated MCV	
Thiamine (B_1)	• Delirium • Dementia • Alcohol • Malnutrition • Abnormal gait, eye movements	
Metal assays and environmental toxins		
Copper studies (serum and urine copper; serum ceruloplasmin)	• Neuropsychiatric symptoms with liver disease • Delirium	
Lead	• Unexplained depression, neuropsychiatric symptoms, and somatic complaints in conjunction with possible lead exposure	
Mercury	• Unexplained mood, cognitive symptoms, and somatic complaints in conjunction with possible mercury exposure	
Autoimmune studies		
Erythrocyte sedimentation rate (ESR)	• Neuropsychiatric work-up	• When elevated, is nonspecific sign of infectious, inflammatory, autoimmune, or neoplastic disease

(Continued)

Table 6.1 (*Continued*)

Test	Indication	Comments
Antinuclear antibody	• New cognitive or psychiatric symptoms and physical symptoms suspicious for lupus (e.g., fatigue, joint pain, malar rash, fever, anemia in women of childbearing age)	• Found in most patients with lupus; can also be positive in patients with a variety of autoimmune diseases and drug-induced lupus (phenothiazines, anticonvulsants)
Infectious disease testing		
HIV (ELISA to screen and Western blot to confirm)	• Neuropsychiatric symptoms in high-risk patient	
Rapid plasma reagin (RPR)	• Neuropsychiatric symptoms in high-risk patient	• False positive in patients with various autoimmune conditions
Epstein–Barr virus (EBV)	• Chronic fatigue • Refractory depression	
Hepatitis C core antibody	• Intravenous drug use • High-risk sexual practices • Unexplained hepatic disease	
Urine studies		
Urinalysis	• Neuropsychiatric screening • Delirium • Cognitive change in elderly	
Myoglobin	• Substance use disorder • Antipsychotics	• Elevated: NMS, restraints, PCP, cocaine or LSD intoxication
Catecholamines, metanephrines, vanillylmandelic acid	• Anxiety/panic • Tachycardia, hypertension, flushing	• Elevated: pheochromocytoma
Toxicology		
Urine toxicology screen	• Known or suspected substance use • Intoxication with unknown substance • Altered mental status	• Standard screen typically includes amphetamines, barbiturates, benzodiazepines, cannabis, cocaine, phencyclidine, and opiates; can get false negatives or positives; substances detectable in urine for different periods of time
Blood alcohol level	• Altered mental status • Agitation • Psychosis • Lethargy • Dysarthria	
Salicylate level (serum)	• Suspected salicylate overdose (includes psychosis, delirium, acid-base abnormalities, tachypnea, tinnitus, vomiting) • Overdose of unknown substance	
Acetaminophen level (serum)	• Suspected acetaminophen overdose • Overdose of unknown substance	• Need to follow at intervals for at least 96 hours post-ingestion if plasma acetaminophen concentration indicates potential hepatotoxicity; may produce fatal hepatic necrosis

- Other indications for CT, debated in the literature, include prolonged catatonia, first episode psychosis, unexplained delirium, and late-onset (age >50) presentation of new psychiatric symptoms.
- Brain MRI is more sensitive than CT and does not involve radiation exposure but is more expensive and time-consuming. MRI is especially useful for detecting vascular brain disease, demyelinating disease, neurodegenerative disorders, small seizure foci, and periventricular white matter hyperintensities.
- *Electroencephalogram (EEG)*
  - There are no clear guidelines for the use of EEG in routine evaluations of psychiatric patients.
  - EEG is generally used in patients with altered mental status to rule out a non-psychiatric etiology (e.g., complex partial seizure, status epilepticus, delirium). It may also be helpful in evaluating a patient with new-onset psychosis and episodic behavioral disturbance, and it can help rule out specific non-psychiatric etiologies in cases of malingering, somatic symptom disorders, and suspected catatonia.

Treatment monitoring

Laboratory testing is advised *before* prescribing medications to ensure that there are no abnormalities that might render such treatment unsafe. *During* treatment, serum levels of some medications (e.g., valproate, carbamazepine, lithium, tricyclic antidepressants, clozapine) are used to monitor compliance, efficacy, variations in metabolism, and safety/toxicity. Laboratory testing can also screen for medication-induced end-organ damage and other adverse effects (e.g., metabolic syndrome, renal disease, cardiac arrhythmias). See Table 6.2 for recommendations.

Investigational biological markers
General characteristics of a biomarker

Although definitions can vary, a biomarker is commonly regarded as a quantifiable biological measure that provides information regarding a disease state or treatment response in a given individual. Examples of *diagnostic biomarkers* can be found in the characteristic distribution of lesions on MRI in multiple sclerosis, or the presence of rheumatoid factors (auto-antibodies directed against a portion of immunoglobulin G) in rheumatoid arthritis. *Treatment biomarkers* provide the clinician with information regarding the likelihood of a particular treatment outcome, such as the manner in which the treatment regimen for a given oncology patient is guided by specific markers expressed by the tumor. Despite intensive research, a reliable and clinically useful biomarker in psychiatry has not yet been developed.

For a biomarker to be useful, it must: (1) provide meaningful information about a disease state or treatment response, (2) possess good sensitivity and specificity, and (3) be relatively easy to measure and be cost effective. An early example of a candidate biomarker in psychiatry is the dexamethasone suppression test (DST) for major depressive disorder. Despite considerable research implicating hypothalamic-pituitary-adrenal axis dysregulation in depression, and the fact that the DST is relatively easy to implement and analyze, poor sensitivity and specificity in psychiatric populations with depression has limited widespread adoption of this test into clinical practice.

However, advances in pathophysiological models of psychiatric illness, as well as advances in our ability to measure specific biological functions, provide hope for the identification of clinically useful psychiatric biomarkers in the near future. Further on we briefly review examples of future candidate biomarkers.

Table 6.2 Treatment monitoring.

Medication	Serum drug levels	Pretreatment screening	Monitoring during maintenance treatment
Antidepressants			
Tricyclics	• If unexpected clinical response to a standard dose, check level to confirm rapid or slow metabolizers • Use level to document adequacy of exposure before terminating a trial • Imipramine/desipramine: established therapeutic window 175–300 ng/mL • Nortriptyline: established therapeutic window 50–150 ng/mL; toxic at >500 ng/mL	• EKG for patients >40, with cardiac disease, or on other medications that prolong QT interval	• EKG if start other medications that prolong QT interval, or as clinically appropriate
SSRIs	• Not routinely used	• Before starting citalopram or escitalopram: EKG for patients >40, with cardiac disease, or on other medications that prolong QT interval • Check platelets if history of blood dyscrasias	• In patients taking citalopram or escitalopram, EKG if start other medications that prolong QT interval, or as clinically appropriate • Check sodium level if fatigue, cognitive impairment, delirium, seizure • Check platelets if signs of increased bleeding
Anticonvulsants and lithium			
Lithium	• Acute mania: 0.6–1.2 mEq/L • Maintenance: 0.8–1.0 mEq/L • Likely toxic: >1.5 mEq/L	• Electrolytes, BUN, Cr, TSH, T_4, CBC, urinalysis, beta-HCG • 24-hour Cr clearance if known renal disease • EKG for patients >40 or with cardiac disease	• At start of therapy, lithium level every 5 days to adjust dose • Once on stable dose, check level every 3–6 months or if signs of toxicity • Cr after achieving therapeutic blood level, then TSH, BUN, Cr, every 6–12 months or if signs of renal or thyroid toxicity emerge • 24-hour Cr clearance if increased serum Cr or unexplained increased lithium level • EKG as needed for patients >40 or with cardiac disease

Drug	Levels/Comments	Baseline labs	Monitoring
Valproate	• Acute mania: 50–150 µg/mL • Maintenance: optimal levels not established	• CBC with platelets, LFT, beta-HCG	• Drug level, CBC with platelets, and LFT every 3–6 months or sooner if side effects • Amylase and lipase if symptoms of pancreatitis • Ammonia if altered mental status, lethargy
Carbamazepine	• Epilepsy range: 4–12 µg/mL • No established correlation between anti-epileptic levels and psychotropic effects • Guide dosage by clinical response and toxicity; carbamazepine auto-induces own metabolism, so may need to check levels and raise dose	• CBC with platelets, LFT, BUN, Cr, beta-HCG • Consider EKG for patients >40, with cardiac disease, or on other medications that prolong QT interval	• CBC with platelets every 2 weeks for the first 2 months, then every 3 months • LFT, BUN, sodium, Cr
Gabapentin	• None	• BUN, Cr	• Dose adjustment needed if renal impairment
Antipsychotics			
Clozapine	• Sources suggest that at least 350 ng/mL is considered necessary to achieve therapeutic response in refractory schizophrenia	• EKG • CBC, including ANC • Some sources suggest chest X-ray to rule out pretreatment myocarditis and heart failure	• CBC with ANC: Weekly for first 6 months, bi-weekly for second 6 months, then monthly thereafter
All other antipsychotics	• Not clinically meaningful although preliminary reference range of 20–50 ng/mL has been suggested for olanzapine	• EKG • Fasting blood glucose and lipids for second generation antipsychotics	• EKG if start other medications that prolong the QT interval or as clinically appropriate • Fasting blood glucose and lipids at 12 weeks, then annually to monitor patients taking second generation antipsychotics; more frequently if significant weight gain or symptoms suggestive of diabetes • CPK, electrolytes, BUN, Cr, and CBC if signs of NMS • Prolactin if menstrual irregularities, decreased libido, sexual dysfunction, galactorrhea

Example candidate biomarkers in psychiatry

Some markers of disease may be present *before* the onset of clinically significant illness, thereby representing a risk or vulnerability factor. Identifying such disease markers is a major focus of current research efforts and has the potential to make a large impact on clinical care by allowing the clinician to initiate treatment at an earlier stage in the illness, thereby preventing further disease progression.

An example candidate diagnostic marker is the *in vivo* imaging of the amyloid beta peptide using positron emission tomography (PET) at an early stage of Alzheimer's disease (AD). The beta-amyloid imaging agent, florbetapir, a fluorine-18 radiolabeled small-molecular tracer, was approved in 2012 by the US FDA for use in brain PET scans to evaluate cases of suspected AD. This test is not, however, able to establish or predict a diagnosis of AD, and it is most useful in ruling out AD. Additionally, the clinical use of this test is limited by restrictive labeling imposed by the FDA and uncertainty regarding payer reimbursement. CSF levels of tau and other proteins in AD are also being explored as candidate biomarkers. The ultimate clinical utility of these assays awaits further study.

There is growing evidence implicating dysregulated inflammatory signaling in the pathogenesis of major depressive disorder and bipolar disorder. Studies demonstrate elevations in peripheral inflammatory markers in the depressed state and improvement in these markers with treatment. Specific pro-inflammatory cytokines most strongly implicated include interleukin (IL)-6 and tumor necrosis factor (TNF)-alpha. While there is meta-analytic support for these alterations, abnormal levels of inflammatory markers are not universally observed in patients and the potential sensitivity, specificity, and clinical utility of these markers are not yet clear. Other biomarkers being investigated in mood disorders include neuroendocrine (cortisol, cortisol releasing factor) and growth factor markers [brain-derived neurotrophic factor (BDNF), insulin-like growth factor (IGF-1), vascular endothelial growth factor (VEGF)]. Some authors have suggested that a biomarker panel made up of many tests – yielding a "biosignature" – may provide improved test characteristics.

An example of a potential treatment biomarker in psychiatry is activity within the anterior cingulate cortex (ACC) predicting antidepressant response in patients with major depressive disorder. Higher baseline activity within rostral and ventral aspects of the ACC is associated with a higher likelihood of response to treatment across multiple studies and treatment modalities, including medications, neurostimulation, and psychotherapy. Most neuroimaging studies have not provided information regarding differential response to different treatments, however. Further research is required to determine the sensitivity, specificity, and clinical utility of these approaches.

Additional promising avenues for biomarker development in psychiatry not discussed here include genetic polymorphisms associated with diagnosis or treatment, epigenetic markers including DNA methylation and histone modification, and advanced neuroimaging analytic approaches including pattern classification based on machine learning algorithms.

Reading list

Hales RE, Yudofsky SC, Roberts LW, Kupofer DJ. American Psychiatric Publishing Textbook of Psychiatry, 6th edn. Arlington, VA: American Psychiatric Publishing, 2014.

Labbate LA, Fava M, Rosenbaum JF, Arana GW. Handbook of Psychiatric Drug Therapy, 6th edn. Philadelphia, PA: Lippincott Williams & Wilkins, 2009.

Pizzagalli DA. Frontocingulate dysfunction in depression: toward biomarkers of treatment response. Neuropsychopharmacology 2011;36:183–206.

Sadock BJ, Sadock VA, Ruiz P. Kaplan & Sadock's Comprehensive Textbook of Psychiatry, 9th edn. Philadelphia, PA: Lippincott Williams & Wilkins, 2009.

Schmidt HD, Shelton RC, Duman RS. Functional biomarkers of depression: diagnosis, treatment, and pathophysiology. Neuropsychopharmacology 2011;36:2375–94.

Additional material for this chapter can be found online at:
www.mountsinaiexpertguides.com/psychiatry

This includes a case study and multiple choice questions.

CHAPTER 7

Neuromodulation Treatments

Kyle A.B. Lapidus[1], Nigel I. Kennedy[2], Wayne K. Goodman[2], and Charles H. Kellner[2]
[1] Stony Brook University, Stony Brook, NY, USA
[2] Icahn School of Medicine at Mount Sinai, New York, NY, USA

OVERALL BOTTOM LINE

- Electroconvulsive therapy (ECT) is a highly effective treatment for severe and medication-resistant major depression; this treatment has been established as the standard of care based on decades of research and successful treatment outcomes in depression as well as in acute mania, psychosis, catatonia, and neuroleptic malignant syndrome.
- Surgical treatment options in psychiatry include deep brain stimulation (DBS), which has a humanitarian device exemption (HDE) from the Food and Drug Administration (FDA) in treatment-refractory patients with obsessive-compulsive disorder (OCD), and vagus nerve stimulation (VNS), accepted by the FDA since 2005 as an adjunctive treatment in patients with major depression who have failed to respond to at least four medication trials.
- Multiple non-surgical neuromodulation treatment options exist. Transcranial magnetic stimulation (TMS) and deep TMS are both recognized by the FDA for patients with major depressive disorder (MDD) who have failed to respond to one or more antidepressant medications. Transcranial direct current stimulation (tDCS) has limited supporting evidence but a growing research base in the treatment of MDD, tinnitus, and auditory hallucinations, and as an adjunct to stroke rehabilitation. Magnetic seizure therapy (MST), epidural cortical stimulation (EpCS), and cranial electrotherapy stimulation (CES) are less well researched and have not been shown to be effective in the treatment of neuropsychiatric illnesses.

Discussion of topic and guidelines
Overview and need

Psychiatric disorders remain clinically challenging, and despite several decades of treatment advances there have been few significant innovations or paradigm-shifting developments in psychopharmacological treatments. Even with adequate dosing and perfect patient adherence, pharmacological treatments, which are not without considerable side effects, may still fail to provide sufficient resolution of symptoms for many patients. Further, when current treatments are effective, there is often a significant delay in onset of efficacy for weeks to months, during which time patients continue to suffer and are at risk for adverse illness outcomes, including suicide. In addition, a variety of psychiatric illnesses lack any approved, evidence-based somatic treatments (e.g., personality disorders, hoarding). There is a great public health need for new therapies that address persistent symptoms, reduce functional impairment, and improve quality of life. Ideally, novel therapies will prove to have efficacy across diagnoses by treating particular symptom domains.

Mount Sinai Expert Guides: Psychiatry, First Edition. Edited by Asher B. Simon, Antonia S. New, and Wayne K. Goodman.
© 2017 John Wiley & Sons, Ltd. Published 2017 by John Wiley & Sons, Ltd.
Companion website: www.mountsinaiexpertguides.com/psychiatry

Electroconvulsive therapy (ECT)

ECT has been widely used for decades to provide highly effective acute and maintenance treatment for patients with severe and/or refractory depression. ECT is also effective for mania, catatonia, psychosis, and NMS. Performed under full general anesthesia, with oxygen supplementation and muscle relaxation, ECT is usually given 2–3 times per week until remission of symptoms occurs. Studies of refinements in techniques to further reduce side effects, particularly memory loss, are currently underway. A variety of electrode placement options (e.g., right unilateral, bifrontal, bifrontotemporal) and stimulus dosing regimens are available. Stimulus parameters that can be modified to enhance seizure efficacy include frequency, pulse width, and duration. Specific anesthetics can also affect seizure production. In many cases initial treatment is performed using right unilateral electrode placement, although in particularly acute or severe cases, bilateral electrode placement may be advised from the outset (bilateral should also be considered if there has been no response to unilateral). "Dose titration" is used to minimize cognitive impact of the treatment, and involves identifying an individual's seizure threshold (ST) and subsequently treating at a multiple of ST (usually 6× ST for unilateral and 1.5–2.5× ST for bilateral). An acute course of ECT usually involves 6–12 treatments and is individualized based on the patient's response. For many patients, continuation and maintenance outpatient ECT may be recommended to help prevent relapse.

Circuit-based treatments

As our understanding of molecular neuroscience has grown, so has our knowledge of the circuitry that may be altered in psychiatric illnesses, and when patients have shown limited responses to other available therapies, circuit-based and neuromodulatory treatments may have an expanding role. Initial circuit-based treatments used ablative techniques (e.g., surgical lysis, thermolytic, radiation) to destroy brain tissue, producing an irreversible lesion in the selected pathway. Since then, therapeutic neuromodulation, which is the application of electricity and electromagnetic fields to reversibly affect neuronal function, has become an area of increasing interest.

Surgical neuromodulation

Surgical neuromodulation involves the delivery of electrical signals via implanted devices to influence brain activity.

Deep brain stimulation (DBS) has been a widely used neurosurgical approach for intractable movement disorders such as Parkinson's disease and is now being actively studied for various psychiatric illnesses. DBS usually involves bihemispheric intracranial implantation of electrodes, with the neurostimulator placed in the chest or abdomen. Following implantation, the psychiatrist can noninvasively program the neurostimulator (parameters include pulse width, frequency, amplitude, and polarity at individual contacts) to optimize response and minimize side effects. The rationale for studying DBS in OCD is based on numerous factors, including the limited number of effective pharmacotherapies, the apparent effectiveness of ablative treatments, and the understanding of this disorder in terms of circuit dysfunction. DBS has yielded clearer results in the treatment of OCD than in other psychiatric disorders, leading the FDA to grant an HDE for its use for this condition. For OCD, the FDA provided an indication for bilateral stimulation of the anterior limb of the internal capsule as an adjunct to medication or alternative to capsulotomy for chronic, severe, treatment-resistant OCD that had failed to respond to at least three SSRIs. Despite ongoing trials for other psychiatric disorders (e.g., MDD), DBS lacks FDA status beyond its use in OCD. Because DBS involves craniotomy, neurosurgical risks are an important consideration and include infection, hemorrhage, and edema, with risk of severe neurological sequelae or death. In addition, programming parameter-related risks include induction of hypomania and impulsivity.

These programming-related risks are generally rapidly reversible with adjustment of programming parameters.

Vagus nerve stimulation (VNS) is a surgical neuromodulatory treatment that targets the left ascending branch of the vagus nerve. Despite limited efficacy in controlled trials, this treatment has been sanctioned by the FDA since 2005 as an adjunctive treatment for patients with MDD who have failed four or more standard treatments. However, this treatment's invasiveness coupled with limited efficacy has led to reduced clinical interest.

Transcranial magnetic stimulation (TMS)

Repetitive transcranial magnetic stimulation (rTMS), as delivered by Neuronetics' NeuroStar® and the more recently sanctioned Magstim® Rapid[2] systems, received initial FDA clearance in 2008 and is indicated for patients with MDD who have failed to respond to at least one antidepressant medication in the current episode. To use rTMS in MDD, a coil is positioned over the left dorsolateral prefrontal cortex (DLPFC). Before treatment, the motor threshold (MT) is determined at the point of maximal sensitivity. Then the coil is moved 5.5 cm anterior to the position of maximal MT and treatment is provided at 120% MT. A treatment session lasts for 37.5 minutes and consists of the following repeated cycle: 4 seconds of 10 Hz pulses are followed by a 26-second quiet period; a total of 3000 pulses are delivered. In a full course of acute treatment for MDD, rTMS is applied 5 days per week for 4–6 weeks. Although no other psychiatric indications are currently approved, a TMS device manufactured by Cerena™ has received clearance for use in patients with migraines.

Deep transcranial magnetic stimulation (dTMS) uses a different coil design to produce fields at greater depth from the skull surface. As delivered by a Brainsway™ device for patients with MDD, dTMS received FDA clearance in 2013 under a 510(k) (see http://www.fda.gov/MedicalDevices/ProductsandMedicalProcedures/DeviceApprovalsandClearances/510kClearances/) showing "substantial equivalence" with the NeuroStar® TMS system, although the efficacy in clinical trials appears to be higher using dTMS. Treatment with dTMS is also similar to rTMS with MT determination followed by treatment at 120% MT 5 days per week for at least 4 weeks in an acute course. Additional studies of dTMS for other indications, including bipolar disorder, OCD, posttraumatic stress disorder (PTSD), and smoking cessation, are underway.

Transcranial direct current stimulation (tDCS)

tDCS, an alternative noninvasive neuromodulation technique, involves targeted placement of anode and cathode electrodes on the scalp to provide current across brain regions. The passage of low electrical currents (0.5–2 mA) through the target tissue does not directly induce neuronal stimulation but rather affects the threshold required to generate an action potential in the stimulated neurons. The overall efficacy of tDCS is unclear given the heterogeneity and small sample sizes of many published studies. However, tDCS is a relatively novel therapy and remains an area of active research. There have been promising studies using tDCS as a treatment for MDD, tinnitus, craving in addiction, stroke rehabilitation, chronic pain, and auditory hallucinations in schizophrenia.

Summary

With a large evidence base and a long history of clinical utility, ECT remains the most effective somatic treatment for severe depression. A growing evidence base supports the clinical benefit of ECT in treating other psychiatric diagnoses. Emerging device-based electrical manipulation of neuronal and circuit function provides an important and urgently needed option for many patients with psychiatric illnesses. Evidence for the efficacy of DBS as a treatment for OCD is continually growing, and DBS is evolving from a research protocol to a surgical standard of care.

Additionally, DBS is being studied as an effective treatment for other neuropsychiatric conditions including Tourette's syndrome, with promising results. These treatments show not only great promise for the development of targeted treatments, but also utility in increasing understanding of psychiatric illnesses by highlighting key circuits that may be dysfunctional. At the time of writing a range of devices are sanctioned by the FDA, providing additional therapeutic options for patients with variations in disease severity and levels of treatment resistance.

Reading list

Abrams R. Electroconvulsive Therapy, 4th edn. Oxford: Oxford University Press, 2002.

American Psychiatric Association Task Force. The Practice of Electroconvulsive Therapy: Recommendations for Treatment, Training, and Privileging. Arlington, VA: American Psychiatric Association Publishing, 2001.

Fink M. Convulsive Therapy: Theory and Practice. Philadelphia, PA: Lippincott Williams & Wilkins, 1979.

Goodman WK, Alterman RL. Deep brain stimulation for intractable psychiatric disorders. Ann Rev Med 2012;63:511–24.

Kellner CH. Brain Stimulation in Psychiatry: ECT, DBS, TMS, and Other Modalities. Cambridge: Cambridge University Press, 2012.

Schwartz CM. Electroconvulsive and Neuromodulation Therapies. Cambridge: Cambridge University Press, 2009.

Suggested websites

International Neuromodulation Society. http://www.neuromodulation.com/

International Society for ECT and Neurostimulation. http://www.isen-ect.org/

Additional material for this chapter can be found online at:
www.mountsinaiexpertguides.com/psychiatry

This includes advice for patients, a case study, and multiple choice questions.

CHAPTER 8

General Principles of Psychotherapy

Asher B. Simon and Michael Brus

Icahn School of Medicine at Mount Sinai, New York, NY, USA

OVERALL BOTTOM LINE
- Psychotherapy is an effective treatment for a variety of conditions.
- Targeted symptom/syndrome-specific approaches are common.
- Most psychotherapies utilize the principle that symptoms reflect enduring maladaptive patterns in cognitions, emotions, behaviors, and relationships, and that each of these areas is intimately connected with the others.
- The therapeutic alliance is a feature common to all effective psychotherapies and is correlated with clinical outcome.

Discussion of topic and guidelines

At this point in my existence, I cannot imagine leading a normal life without both taking lithium and having had the benefits of psychotherapy. Lithium prevents my seductive but disastrous highs, diminishes my depressions, clears out the wool and webbing from my disordered thinking, slows me down, gentles me out, keeps me from ruining my career and relationships, keeps me out of a hospital, alive, and makes psychotherapy possible. But, ineffably, psychotherapy heals. It makes some sense of the confusion, reins in the terrifying thoughts and feelings, returns some control and hope and possibility of learning from it all…that I might someday be able to contend with all of this. No pill can help me deal with the problem of not wanting to take pills; likewise, no amount of psychotherapy alone can prevent my manias and depressions. I need both. It is an odd thing, owing life to pills, one's own quirks and tenacities, and this unique, strange, and ultimately profound relationship called psychotherapy.

Jamison K. An Unquiet Mind. New York, Vintage Books, 1996

Psychotherapy is a talking and relationship-based treatment that opens up the brain and mind to new experiences and potential meanings. In restricting feelings, thoughts, and actions, psychopathology usually limits an individual's flexibility, resulting in a painful repetition of maladaptive functioning and a failure to see or exercise choice. A goal of all psychotherapies is to increase the range of behaviors available to the patient for the purpose of modifying maladaptive patterns. Psychotherapy, and the doctor–patient relationship therein, exists as an actual new life experience that takes advantage of the brain's flexibility and plasticity. As an example, consider any illusion: at first, you perceive one image or "reality," but if you allow yourself openness to alternatives, different possibilities emerge. While nothing changes in the scene, how you organize the incoming stimuli allows you to experience a fuller range of possibilities.

Mount Sinai Expert Guides: Psychiatry, First Edition. Edited by Asher B. Simon, Antonia S. New, and Wayne K. Goodman.
© 2017 John Wiley & Sons, Ltd. Published 2017 by John Wiley & Sons, Ltd.
Companion website: www.mountsinaiexpertguides.com/psychiatry

While multiple forms of psychotherapy have been developed to treat the wide spectrum of psychopathology, the two largest families are cognitive behavioral therapy (CBT) and psychodynamic psychotherapy. They remain relatively divergent, despite increasing efforts toward integration. Rather than highlighting specific techniques and enumerating similarities and differences, this chapter will describe some concepts and assumptions underlying each modality. In fact, many features are similar across psychotherapies, and therapists from divergent schools tend to resemble each other in their practices as they mature; in other words, the more experienced the therapist, the less clear may be the distinctions in terms of the nature of their interventions. This speaks to possible underlying mechanisms of action which may not be accounted for by specific technique.

Uses of psychotherapy
- Stand-alone treatment of some psychiatric symptoms and syndromes (see Table 8.1).
- Improving level of functioning.
- Addressing specific life problems (e.g., support, relationships, stresses, phase of life).
- Addressing general problematic patterns (e.g., self-esteem, inhibitions, feeling stuck, behaviors).
- Strengthening adherence to other treatments.
- Augmenting treatment in non-psychiatric conditions.
  - Has been found to improve nausea, pain, depression, anxiety, and survival in different cancers; improves medical stability and disease indices in children with diabetes.
- Augmenting psychopharmacologic treatments.
  - Psychotherapy can facilitate readjustment, recovery, and integration into family and community, increasing resilience and decreasing risks of morbidity and mortality.

Efficacy
- Psychotherapy is as effective as many other medical interventions, with effect sizes often larger than in other medical treatment trials.
  - CBT has the most evidence from randomized controlled trials.
  - Although historically a long-term treatment measured in years, briefer forms of psychodynamic psychotherapy have been developed and show efficacy.

Table 8.1 Applications of common types of psychotherapy.

Type of therapy	Condition(s) treated
Cognitive behavioral therapies	Depression, generalized anxiety, panic, psychosis, personality disorders, chronic fatigue, PTSD, eating disorders, ADHD, bipolar, insomnia
• Systematic desensitization; flooding	• Phobias
• Exposure and response-prevention (ERP)	• OCD
• Dialectical behavior therapy (DBT)	• Borderline personality, persistent emotional dysregulation, suicidality and self-harm
• Acceptance and commitment therapy (ACT)	• Coping with chronic illness/pain, stress, depression
• Schema therapy (includes elements of CBT and psychodynamic)	• Personality disorders, depression, relationship issues
Psychodynamic psychotherapies	Panic, personality disorders, "complex mental disorders," relationship issues, depression, anxiety, improve self-understanding
• Interpersonal psychotherapy (IPT)	• Depression
• Transference-focused psychotherapy	• Borderline and narcissistic personality
• Mentalization-based therapy	• Borderline personality

Core features common to both CBT and psychodynamic psychotherapy

- Therapeutic alliance.
  - Rapport; safety/trust; genuineness; validation; confidentiality; empathy.
  - The strength of the therapeutic relationship is correlated with outcome across schools of psychotherapy.
- Consistent boundaries; treatment frame; focus on adherence.
- Educating the patient as to the process of therapy.
- Finding patterns to explain and address problems; activating self-awareness and self-reflection.
- Developing formulations.

Therapeutic alliance

Providing a supportive and collaborative relationship underlies efficacy across all psychotherapies. The therapist's attitude of validation includes genuine interest, acceptance, caring, and compassion and avoids anger, contempt, and disgust. The therapeutic alliance, also based on empathy, allows the patient the safety to engage in necessary emotional processing; it can also serve as an affect-regulating mechanism in and of itself, enabling patients to effectively put themselves at risk and reveal their inner thoughts and feelings. Validation – accepting a patient's experience as valid – does not mean agreement; rather, it is an acknowledgment of what the patient is experiencing in the moment, that the experience is what it is. In this way, the therapist can help patients notice, label, and reflect on their emotional experiences.

Psychodynamic principles

Psychodynamic psychotherapy has existed for over 100 years, and the lexicon has become part of everyday language. A rigid psychosexual focus has given way to a more modifiable focus on relationships and self-esteem that is more reflective of contemporary society and individual symptoms; the applied therapy has been transformed, with various refinements developed for different conditions. Further on we present some core contemporary psychodynamic concepts (many of which have been validated by cognitive, affective, and social neuroscience), including unconscious processing, repeated relationship patterns, internal conflict, and self-esteem regulation. However, the field has been restricted by too little research about optimal techniques, an incomplete scientific backing for other underlying assumptions, and few controlled studies of outcomes.

Of note, these theoretical concepts are presented first because they may often underlie many other forms of psychotherapy as well (despite other forms employing different clinical techniques).

The goals of psychodynamic psychotherapy include greater insight into one's motivations/responses, ability to tolerate conflicting emotional states, flexibility in work, love, and play, feeling of meaning in one's life, capacity to seek and maintain relationships, and reduced vulnerability for relapse.

Unconscious (automatic) processing

Many mental processes operate outside of conscious awareness and reflect experiences from one's past and unconscious perceptions in the present; individual rewards and fears influence the activation thresholds for these processes which are felt by the individual to be automatic. For example, subliminal stimuli can trigger cortical processes, resulting in both rapid and long-lasting effects on the neural networks underlying emotional responses, conscious feelings, autonomic responses, memory formation, memory access, thoughts, value judgments and choices, motivational states, motor actions, goal-directed behaviors, and conscious awareness. Additionally, these resulting effects are often related to the personal meaning of the subliminal stimulus to a specific patient; associative networks are unique to the individual. In effect, Ms. A may (1) respond to a subliminal stimulus that has no effect on Ms. B, (2) act without knowing why, and (3) give retrospective/intuitive reasons for her behavior. Actions can be initiated without conscious awareness of both the goal and/or how one's behavior has been motivated. In short, what feels like an action may, in fact, be a reaction. Psychodynamic psychotherapists help patients recognize these processes to enable more conscious choice over potential responses.

Repeated relationship patterns

During development the external world is transcribed into enduring neuronal associational networks that can persist independently of the original context and act as a guide during similar emotional contexts later in life. In short, early experiences create a template. Helping an individual adapt to a particular environment with the greatest economy, these networks also allow the brain to make rapid predictions in response to early sensory stimuli; in this way they not only reflect prior experiences, they actively construct one's experience of the present, as a form of self-fulfilling prophecy and reinforcing the pattern (e.g., feeling, thinking, behaving, interpersonal relating). These biased responses can be powerful enough to override true interpretation of the incoming sensory information, and this misrepresentation of what is real often goes unnoticed. While these templates allow for economy and rapidity of functioning, rigidity may lead to trouble, as we use the past to understand and construct present experience. This is the basis of the concept of transference: the unconscious activation of (past-derived) templates/patterns when encountering someone or something in the present. A form of transference may also be called implicit relational knowing. Emotionally-charged past experiences are especially powerful, and present-day stimuli (conscious and unconscious) activate these implicit memory traces and shape current perceptions, thoughts, and feelings. Transference feelings "feel real." (In fact, the neural signature of an activated memory can be very similar to that of true external stimuli.) Patients have transferences to providers, medications, procedures, etc. (e.g., "I'm experiencing something that is hurting me..."), and these may affect adherence and response (e.g., placebo, nocebo).

The therapist's in-session and *in vivo* focus on the transference as a way to help the patient understand and change relationship patterns is perhaps what most separates psychodynamic psychotherapy from other forms of psychotherapy. The therapy becomes a laboratory in which the patient can examine feelings and thoughts s/he experiences toward another person within the safety of the therapeutic alliance; it is an opportunity to address problematic relationship patterns.

Countertransference is a reflection of how the patient's affective, cognitive, and behavioral cues activate associational networks in the doctor. General categories include empathy (i.e., emotional contagion; doctor experiences the patient's feelings) and role responsiveness (i.e., doctor feels similar to what other people in the patient's life have felt in response to the patient). Countertransference is used to assist in understanding the emotional reality of the patient.

Psychological conflict

People can have multiple feelings, thoughts, or behaviors about a given stimulus or event; these responses are both conscious and unconscious and are often not in harmony. In the simplest sense, conscious conflict is found when one desires something but also fears it, or desires two contradictory things. Going a level deeper, one can consider the interactions of the reward-based "approach/motivation" and the fear-based "avoidance/withdrawal" network. It is noteworthy that the activation of many desires and fears is unconscious in origin, and some of them may not be in keeping with one's specific concept of oneself. When this occurs, a psychodynamic tenet holds that such internal conflict is managed by the mind's altering its focus to allow only the non-dissonant aspects to reach conscious awareness. In effect, some internal conflicts (conscious and unconscious) are tolerable by an individual, while others are so dissonant with one's view of oneself that they result in a narrowed scope of attention to avoid recognizing the conflict.

A major part of psychodynamic psychotherapy is helping patients explore and persevere through their full emotional ranges, whether the emotions are troubling, contradictory, illogical, or difficult to express.

Self (emotional) homeostasis

As above, one's mind unconsciously avoids or distorts certain perceptions/thoughts/feelings to preserve one's sense of constancy, one's emotional equilibrium, and one's self-esteem. These unconscious processes have been called "defense mechanisms," but they can also be considered implicit self-homeostasis as they help maintain a coherent view of oneself. These mechanisms are woven throughout all experiences, and help keep dissonance at bay. They become pathological when activated rigidly or at inappropriate times. For example, patients might inadvertently (read: unconsciously) omit crucial information from a history; others might keep forgetting to make an appointment to address a concerning lump. Defense mechanisms can be as simple as unknowingly reinterpreting an event, selectively attending to only part of a situation, forgetting something important, refusing to acknowledge something, etc., all for the unconscious goals of regulating negative emotions, justifying inappropriate behavior, maintaining certain beliefs, preserving self-image, being able to forgive others, and maintaining a relationship. It is not the automatic and habitual activation of defenses which is a problem; rather it is the rigid use of a limited repertoire that causes distress and may reflect pathology.

Patients often misrepresent their own experiences, even to themselves. These constructed representations of experience reflect not only what is actually happening but also how they need to see themselves or certain life events. The psychodynamic therapist focuses on the specific thoughts/feelings/perceptions/memories that the patient obscures, the ways they are obscured, and why the patient seemed to need to employ the given defense. These techniques provide the therapist a window on behaviors that may be inexplicable from other vantage points. In some ways, the psychodynamic psychotherapist's focus on the patient's use of defense mechanisms is not unlike the CBT therapist's focus on automatic thoughts.

Cognitive behavioral therapy (CBT)

Based on the principle that thoughts, behaviors, and emotions influence each other and that pathological learning and information processing underlie psychiatric symptoms, CBT primarily targets maladaptive thinking and behavioral dysfunctions. An overall tenet is that distorted cognitive appraisals of stimuli provoke emotional distress that guides problematic behaviors which then increase the likelihood of another potentially negative event; cognitive processing is itself also affected by emotional and behavioral experiences. For example, a negative appraisal of an event may precipitate sadness, which may lead to social withdrawal, furthering negativity and leading to associated behavioral inclinations which create further loneliness. This basic CBT model has been graphically represented as a vicious circle (Figure 8.1; see Wright et al., 2006 in the reading list).

Although this way of thinking about mental suffering goes back to the Stoic philosophers, it was formally developed by Aaron Beck in the 1960s and has since been elaborated into numerous subtypes. The original model focused primarily on cognitive distortions, but as other clinicians began to incorporate behavioral theories from academic psychology into their psychotherapies (e.g., phobic

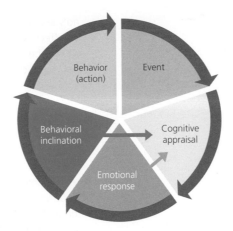

Figure 8.1 The CBT circle.

desensitization, relaxation training), a more unified model of CBT resulted. The therapist helps patients appraise, question, and modify their maladaptive thoughts and behavioral patterns in order to reduce symptoms and meet clearly defined clinical or functional goals. The CBT therapist takes an active, directive teaching mode, and leads skill rehearsal within sessions and assigns homework to be done between sessions. CBT strongly emphasizes the therapeutic relationship as a collaborative enterprise designed to help patients solve problems and reduce symptoms.

CBT has been modified to effectively treat many different conditions, such that there is no longer a one-size-fits-all model. However, in this limited space, we address the general principles of CBT as a therapeutic modality.

There are two major levels of dysfunctional information processing: (1) automatic thoughts and (2) core beliefs incorporated into schemas. Automatic thoughts arise rapidly in response to a given stimulus (e.g., "She hates me" is the thought if one's wife is angry). They may be irrational or based on illogical premises. Although they lead to emotional responses and behavioral actions, automatic thoughts are often out of a patient's awareness at the start of therapy, and patients are therefore taught how to recognize these thoughts.

Schemas are more foundational and include an individual's basic beliefs (e.g., "I am unlovable"), often influencing how one understands and acts in the world. Developed through early childhood experiences and refined throughout life, schemas allow for conservation of attentional resources, rapid decision-making, and adaptation to expected situations. The brain captures experience and physically inscribes it as memory, a primary function of which is to help the person make sense of the present and predict the future. Nothing is truly experienced *de novo*; rather, all perceptual inputs, stimuli, and experiences are organized according to the underlying templates, schemas, and internal working models which comprise a given individual's previous life experiences (which are themselves formed in concert with a person's neurobiological make-up). Although they frequently facilitate ease of functioning, maladaptive schemas may underlie and maintain pathology. Well-known maladaptive schemas in depression include attributing negative events to oneself, globalizing negative things that are limited in scope, and not attending to positive stimuli. Patients with certain anxiety disorders disproportionately direct their attention to threatening stimuli, leading to a narrowed scope of attention, an over-interpretation of danger, and a subjectively diminished ability to deal with things. Common to both anxiety and depression are an increased use of automatic information processing when under stress (i.e., vicious circle), leading to a reduced cognitive capacity for real-time problem-solving, and resultant demoralization.

Beck and colleagues identified six main types of cognitive errors that routinely appear in maladaptive thoughts:

1. mental filter: screening out evidence that does not fit a predetermined conclusion;
2. arbitrary inference: reaching a conclusion in the absence of evidence, or despite evidence to the contrary;
3. overgeneralization: reaching a broad conclusion based on a few isolated incidents;
4. magnification and minimization: exaggerating or reducing the importance of an event or situation;
5. personalization: relating random external events to oneself, often taking on excessive blame or responsibility as a result;
6. all-or-nothing thinking: forming judgments about the self, people, or experiences that are "all good" or "all bad."

Of course, helping patients correct cognitive errors is more complicated and subtle than simply pointing them out in a didactic fashion, and therapists use a variety of techniques to help patients assess the validity and utility of their thoughts. Chief among these is Socratic questioning (also called "guided discovery"), in which the therapist asks the patient a series of open-ended questions designed to foster the patient's curiosity and/or dissonance (e.g., "What is the evidence for and against the truth of your thought? What is an alternative perspective on the situation? What is the worst that could happen, and how would you cope with this outcome? What is the effect of believing your thought? If a friend had this thought, what advice would you give her?"). With a focus on specific here-and-now problems in the patient's life, CBT is highly agenda-driven, and with the high degree of collaboration between patient and therapist, there is a significantly empirical tone to the work. The therapist listens for *in vivo* distorted cognitions and automatic thoughts, which the therapist–patient team then focuses on as data to unpack and address. Moments of high emotion are particularly salient, as an in-session mood shift frequently reveals a preceding automatic thought. Role-play and imagery are used to elicit automatic thoughts as well as practice new skills. Patients are taught to use "thought records" between sessions to identify, document, and address distorted cognitions and their emotional and behavioral sequelae. Symptom rating scales are commonly employed for both patient and therapist to complete. Action plans may be developed to target behavioral dysfunctions. Behavioral techniques often used include graded task assignments to break patterns of avoidance, breathing techniques and relaxation, hierarchical exposure, behavioral activation, scheduling pleasant events, and others.

CBT may be used in both a short- and long-term manner, depending on the conditions being treated (e.g., 12 weekly sessions for panic disorder vs 1–2 years for personality disorders). While CBT emphasizes present problems instead of childhood patterns, the latter often emerge as underlying schemas are addressed. Additionally, a focus on specific, well-defined goals, and active problem-solving does not preclude addressing chronic diffuse dysfunctions.

Reading list

Beck JS. Cognitive Behavior Therapy: Basics and Beyond, 2nd edn. New York: Guilford Press, 2011.

Lynch TR, Trost WT, Salsman N, Linehan MM. Dialectical behavior therapy for borderline personality disorder. Annu Rev Clin Psychol 2007;3:181–205.

Shedler J. That Was Then, This is Now: An Introduction to Contemporary Psychodynamic Therapy. Accessed from http://www.jonathanshedler.com/PDFs/Shedler%20(2006)%20That%20was%20then,%20this%20is%20now%20R9.pdf on March 20, 2011.

Shedler J. The efficacy of psychodynamic psychotherapy. Am Psychol 2010;65(2):98–109.

Wachtel PL. Psychotherapy at ground level. In: Inside the Session: What Really Happens in Psychotherapy. Washington, DC: American Psychological Association, 2011, pp. 3–31.

Wachtel PL. Therapeutic Communication: Knowing What to Say When, 2nd edn. New York: Guilford Press, 2011.

Wright JH, Basco MR, Thase ME. Learning Cognitive-Behavior Therapy: An Illustrated Guide. Arlington, VA: American Psychiatric Publishing, 2006.

Wright JH, Turkington D, Sudak D, Thase ME. High-Yield Cognitive-Behavior Therapy for Brief Sessions: An Illustrated Guide. Arlington, VA: American Psychiatric Publishing, 2010.

Suggested websites

Academy of Cognitive Therapy. www.academyofct.org

American Psychological Association, Understanding psychotherapy and how it works. http://www.apa.org/helpcenter/understanding-psychotherapy.aspx

Psychiatry Online, Textbook of Psychotherapeutic Treatments. http://psychiatryonline.org/doi/book/10.1176/appi.books.9781585623648

Additional material for this chapter can be found online at:
www.mountsinaiexpertguides.com/psychiatry

This includes advice for patients and multiple choice questions.

CHAPTER 9

Clinical Documentation: What to Include in the Psychiatric Record

Amanda Focht[1], Gloria J. Rodriguez[2], and Brian Fuchs[2]
[1]University of Washington, Seattle, WA, USA
[2]Icahn School of Medicine at Mount Sinai, New York, NY, USA

OVERALL BOTTOM LINE
- Documentation is an integral and required part of patient care.
- Documenting risk assessment requires careful consideration.
- While electronic medical records (EMRs) facilitate documentation and collaboration, copying and pasting of records does not meet documentation standards.
- Information in the medical record must be carefully safeguarded to ensure patient confidentiality.
- Psychotherapy notes are not part of the medical record, but there is a unique set of standards governing their use and release.

Discussion of topic and guidelines
Introduction

The medical record plays an essential role in clinical practice (and institutional operations) and serves multiple overlapping purposes. Although some specific record-keeping is unique to the practice of psychiatry, most is shared among every medical specialty, including the stated objective to memorialize patient encounters and provide a record of all aspects of relevant patient information (e.g., history, exam, diagnosis, laboratory and other diagnostic tests, considerations of risk, clinical consultations, treatment plan, response to treatment, and case formulation). The medical record also serves to:

1. document clinical reasoning;
2. document risk and benefit discussions related to therapeutic interventions;
3. communicate clinical information among providers;
4. provide a record of clinical case discussions with members of the care team, and former and future providers;
5. document discussions with family and involved others;
6. record significant events in the course of patient care;
7. document patient consent to or refusal of treatment;
8. document consent for release of information to others;
9. enable research in performance improvement and quality assurance;
10. justify payment from third-party payers;
11. provide evidence of best practice and compliance with care, regulatory, and accrediting standards;
12. function as the treatment record in legal action.

Mount Sinai Expert Guides: Psychiatry, First Edition. Edited by Asher B. Simon, Antonia S. New, and Wayne K. Goodman.
© 2017 John Wiley & Sons, Ltd. Published 2017 by John Wiley & Sons, Ltd.
Companion website: www.mountsinaiexpertguides.com/psychiatry

Electronic medical records (EMRs)

The implementation of EMRs by institutions and individual providers occurred rapidly following the passage of the American Recovery and Reinvestment Act (ARRA) of 2009, which includes substantial financial incentives and penalties related to using EMRs. Widespread electronic documentation has meant a greater reliance on templates and standardized notes – frequently including checklists and drop-down menus – meant to ensure a thorough assessment and complete documentation to enhance patient care and ensure compliance with regulatory agencies and third-party payers. With goals being to improve safety, efficiency, and the quality of care, advantages of EMRs include improved convenience in accessing, sharing, and reviewing patient information and more efficient clinical encounters with faster documentation.

While the accessibility of records to all relevant providers can enhance the delivery of care through improved sharing of information and clinical coordination, making the psychiatric record transparent across care domains is complex, given the stigma surrounding psychiatric illnesses and patients' potential privacy concerns. While it limits collaboration and opposes some stated goals of the EMR, some institutions may offer the opportunity for patients to opt out of having their psychiatric records be so transparent. Providers are advised to communicate with patients about the extent of visibility of this information.

A common argument against EMRs is that template-based and standardized formats discourage complete and independent documentation by each contributing clinician. We urge practitioners to include all relevant patient information, even if not prompted in templated sections, and use free text narrative as may be necessary to best document certain aspects of care.

Additionally, the ability to copy and paste material is a potentially dangerous pitfall and is *not* an acceptable standard. Such duplication creates a poor record of patient care and is potentially dangerous in cases when erroneous information is carried forward and amplified. Duplication is not accepted by regulatory and accreditation agencies and may lead to citation and financial penalty, as well as liability in cases of legal action.

Confidentiality

The Health Insurance Portability and Accountability Act (HIPAA) and the ARRA set forth federal regulations concerning information designated as protected health information (PHI). The following list outlines general considerations in the safeguarding of PHI:

1. PHI is defined as demographic, financial, clinical, or psychosocial information that is linked to something identifying a particular individual (e.g., name, medical record number, social security number, etc.).
2. A provider may not use information s/he has legitimate access to for any purpose other than performing her/his job or taking care of patients.
3. Disclosure of information from the medical record should adhere to the minimum necessary standard: the minimum information needed to achieve the task at hand.
4. Written authorization must be obtained from the patient or personal representative to disclose PHI for purposes other than treatment, payment, institutional operations, institutional review board (IRB)-approved research, or as required by law.
5. Information about anyone other than the patient should only be included in such a way as to safeguard privacy and prevent the disclosure of the other person's PHI.
6. A breach is defined as an unauthorized disclosure of PHI and must be reported to appropriate institutional and governmental agencies.

Evaluation and management (E/M) documentation and CPT codes

In 2013 major changes occurred in the psychiatry section of the American Medical Association's Current Procedural Terminology (CPT: the codes that must be used for billing and documentation for all insurers). Psychiatrists, in line with other medical professionals, now use E/M codes, employing a standardized set of practices established by the Centers for Medicare and Medicaid Services. Psychiatrists may also use add-on codes for psychotherapy performed as part of an E/M visit. For a description of the requirements for E/M documentation and the use of CPT codes please refer to the American Psychiatric Association guidelines: https://www.psychiatry.org/psychiatrists/practice/practice-management/coding-reimbursement-medicare-and-medicaid/coding-and-reimbursement.

Documentation of risk assessment

Assessment of risk to self or others is an integral component of any psychiatric assessment and requires careful, thorough consideration and documentation. Critical junctures for documentation of risk assessment may include:

- the first psychiatric assessment or admission;
- any occurrence of suicidal, aggressive, or violent thinking or behavior;
- any point in treatment when the patient's clinical presentation changes in a way that would suggest a change in risk;
- discharge from a setting of care, if risk is a factor.

A risk level may be summarily described in a categorical manner (e.g., low, moderate, high) or by a more qualitative description, and *the crux in documentation is to best describe how the clinician arrived at the particular risk designation, given the specific circumstances*. A clinician may prove to be wrong in her/his assessment, but thorough documentation of clinical decision-making provides a record attesting to a thoughtful and careful clinical assessment and may be protective in the case of legal action.

The elements comprising a risk assessment can be viewed in two domains:

- *Static elements* exist as a backdrop against which to view the current situation (e.g., past history).
- *Modifiable elements* give clinicians the opportunity to intervene (e.g., symptoms, attitude and response to treatment, access to weapons, family support).

Documentation creates a conspicuous record of one's clinical decision-making that takes into account relevant areas of these two domains, their interplay, and current clinical interventions.

The clinician should assemble a detailed portrait of factors that may have influenced risk in the past so as to best determine points of intervention in the present. Such factors may include substance use, non-adherence, and whether a past act was impulsive or premeditated, singular or recurrent, and if it was associated with any weapons. The setting of the act and any related ER or hospital admissions are also important to include.

The clinician should elaborate on the effect of current contextual circumstances and exacerbating and protective factors on the current clinical presentation.

A safety plan, developed collaboratively with the patient and documented in the record, may provide a tool for the patient to use when thoughts of suicide, self-injury, aggression, or violence occur. Recording triggers and exacerbating behaviors as well as coping strategies and names and numbers of supports (including the provider) are elements in many safety plans. For a more comprehensive discussion and an example template, refer to The Suicide Prevention Resource Center (http://www.sprc.org). Suicide prevention contracts must never be substituted for careful assessment and management; documenting such a contract is not only an inadequate strategy, it may also falsely suggest that risk has been lowered when in fact it has not.

In some states the presence of risk may oblige reporting to a central agency. The New York State SAFE Act requires that mental health professionals report patients who are "likely to engage in harm to self or others" with the intended purpose being to limit the licensing of firearms to the potentially dangerous. The decision-making around any such reporting should be thoroughly documented as part of the risk assessment.

Special considerations in inpatient settings

Thorough documentation on the inpatient unit encompasses a record of the daily clinical interactions with the patient, including evaluation and exam, relevant test results, clinical consultations, notable events, and the assessment and plan, with elaboration of clinical decision-making around the provision of care. This includes discussions with patients and/or family regarding proposed interventions, risks/benefits, and alternatives, as well as education and counseling. The time and date of the note and the time of the patient encounter are essential elements.

Documentation of treatment team conferences is essential and particularly relevant on an inpatient unit where multidisciplinary teams collaborate in the delivery of care; such documentation is a requirement of many regulatory and accrediting agencies.

Unanticipated events and incidents (e.g., patient self-injury, altercations among patients, attempted/completed elopements) should be documented in the medical record, including the following elements:

- time of the event, who informed you, and the time you were informed;
- summary description of the event, including quotations whenever possible;
- physical and/or mental status exam as indicated;
- with whom you discussed the event (e.g., other providers, the patient, the patient's family, other members of the care team);
- all relevant clinical information and plan of care.

The use of restraints and seclusion is a highly regulated area of care, and documentation helps record the event as a clinical intervention as well as a demonstration of compliance with institutional and governmental policies. Required documentation includes: (1) the rationale for the intervention, and (2) the procedure by which the intervention was implemented.

Other forms of documentation: process notes and personal notes

Process notes

Because of the sensitive nature of the material in psychiatric encounters, the U.S. Department of Health and Human Services (HHS), in compliance with the HIPAA, established a special category of protection for psychotherapy, or "process" notes, which are defined as "notes recorded (in any medium) by a health care provider who is a mental health professional, documenting or analyzing the contents of conversations during a private counseling session or a group, joint, or family counseling session." For example, details of fantasies, sensitive information about other individuals in the patient's life, and the psychiatrist's own reactions to the material could be documented in a process note format. Psychotherapy notes should be securely maintained, kept separate from the rest of the medical record, and used only by the clinician who created them.

Disclosure of psychotherapy notes requires specific authorization by the patient and is not covered by consent for release of the medical record. That said, patient authorization is not required in several instances of disclosure, including the following:

- use by students, trainees, or practitioners to learn under supervision;
- use by the practitioner to defend him or herself in legal action brought by the patient;
- necessary disclosures that may prevent or lessen a serious and imminent threat to any person or the public.

Psychiatrist's personal working notes

A psychiatrist may make personal working notes, unidentified and kept physically apart from the medical record. These may contain intimate details of the patient's mental phenomena, observations of others in the patient's life, reactions to the treatment, etc. Such notes may be used as a memory aide, as a guide for future work, training, supervision, or for research that would not identify the patient. Every effort should be made to exclude information in these notes that may identify the patient to others. Patient authorization should be obtained for the use of material contained in these notes. As long as these notes are not identifiable and are not part of the patient's medical record, they are not covered by HHS regulations. However, these notes might be subject to discovery during litigation; destroying such notes after a subpoena arrives is legally risky and should not be done. These notes should be destroyed as soon as their purpose is served and in a systematic, routine way.

Reading list

American Psychiatric Association. Assessing and Treating Suicidal Behaviors: A Quick Reference Guide. American Psychiatric Association Practice Guidelines: http://psychiatryonline.org/pb/assets/raw/sitewide/practice_guidelines/guidelines/suicide-guide.pdf

American Psychiatric Association; The Commission on Psychotherapy by Psychiatrists. Documentation of Psychotherapy by Psychiatrists: Resource Document. American Psychiatric Association, March 2002: http://www.americanmentalhealth.com/media/pdf/200202apaonnotes.pdf

Blumenthal D. Implementation of the Federal Health Information Technology Initiative. N Engl J Med 2011;365:2426–31.

Buchanan A, Binder R, Norko M, Swartz M. Psychiatric violence risk assessment. Am J Psychiatry 2012;169:340.

Mossman D. Tips to make documentation easier, faster and more satisfying. Current Psychiatry 2008;7(2):80, 84–6.

Sittig DF, Singh H. Electronic health records and national patient-safety goals. N Engl J Med 2012;367:1854–60.

Suggested website

U.S. Department of Health & Human Services. American Psychiatric Association Minimum Necessary Guidelines for Third Party Payers for Psychiatric Treatment: http://aspe.hhs.gov/datacncl/reports/MHPrivacy/appendix-g.htm

---

Additional material for this chapter can be found online at:
www.mountsinaiexpertguides.com/psychiatry

This includes multiple choice questions.

PART 2

Adult Disorders

CHAPTER 10

Depressive Disorders

Hiwot Woldu[1,2], James W. Murrough[1], and Dan V. Iosifescu[1]

[1] Icahn School of Medicine at Mount Sinai, New York, NY, USA
[2] New York University School of Medicine, New York, NY, USA

OVERALL BOTTOM LINE
- Depressive disorders are highly prevalent, with a significant burden of disease worldwide.
- Important contributors to etiology include genetic vulnerability, changes in neurotransmitter levels, neuroendocrine function, and psychosocial stressors.
- There are no specific tests to confirm a diagnosis of depression, but ruling out certain contributors to illness can help inform diagnosis and guide treatment.
- Treatments include pharmacotherapies, psychotherapies, other somatic treatments, and lifestyle changes.
- More than 60% of patients with major depressive disorders (MDD) are at risk for recurrence, and some may require lifelong antidepressant treatment.

Background
Definition of disease
Depressive disorders include a number of psychobiological syndromes that share the common feature of sad mood or anhedonia associated with somatic and cognitive disturbances that result in functional impairment. The DSM-5 diagnoses in this category are differentiated by duration, timing, or presumed etiology, and include:
- Major Depressive Disorder (including major depressive episode) (Table 10.1);
- Persistent Depressive Disorder (Dysthymia);
- Disruptive Mood Dysregulation Disorder;
- Premenstrual Dysphoric Disorder.
- See Table 10.2 for a complete list of diagnoses.

This chapter will focus on MDD as a representative example of this class of disorders.

Mount Sinai Expert Guides: Psychiatry, First Edition. Edited by Asher B. Simon, Antonia S. New, and Wayne K. Goodman.
© 2017 John Wiley & Sons, Ltd. Published 2017 by John Wiley & Sons, Ltd.
Companion website: www.mountsinaiexpertguides.com/psychiatry

Table 10.1 DSM-5 Diagnostic criteria for major depressive episode.

≥5 of the following symptoms must be simultaneously present for 2 weeks and represent a change from baseline functioning. At least one of the symptoms must be (1) depressed mood or (2) anhedonia.
- Depressed mood (or irritability in children/adolescents) most of the day, nearly every day
- Diminished interest or pleasure in activities (anhedonia)
- Change in appetite or weight
- Insomnia or hypersomnia
- Psychomotor agitation or retardation
- Fatigue or loss of energy
- Feelings of worthlessness or excessive/inappropriate guilt
- Decreased concentration or indecisiveness
- Recurrent thoughts of death and suicidal ideation with or without a specific plan

Symptoms should not be secondary to a substance (e.g., drug of abuse, medication, toxin) or another medical condition.

Disease classification

Table 10.2 Disorders classified under DSM-5 depressive disorders.

Diagnosis	DSM-5 core features
Major Depressive Disorder (including Major Depressive Episode)	Criteria (see Table 10.1) must be present most of the day, nearly every day for ≥2 weeks [with the exception of weight change and suicidal ideation]
Persistent Depressive Disorder (Dysthymia)	Depressed mood present more than 50% of days over a 2-year period. For individuals that met criteria for MDD during the last 2 years, one should specify persistent/intermittent major depressive episode
Disruptive Mood Dysregulation Disorder	Chronic, severe irritability in children with frequent episodes of extreme behavioral dyscontrol
Premenstrual Dysphoric Disorder (PMDD)	Significant dysphoria, anxiety, mood lability, and irritability during the 1–2 weeks before menses and resolving with menses
Substance/Medication-Induced Depressive Disorder	A substance (e.g. drug of abuse, medication, toxin) appears to be etiologically related to the mood disturbance. Symptoms persist beyond the expected length of physiological effects, intoxication, or withdrawal
Depressive Disorder Due to Another Medical Condition	Persistent and significant depressed mood, diminished interest and anhedonia thought to be the direct pathophysiological consequence of a specific medical condition (e.g., multiple sclerosis, stroke, hypothyroidism)
Other Specified Depressive Disorder	Presence of depressive symptoms with significant distress and impairment that do not meet full criteria for any disorder in the depressive disorders diagnostic class. Used when the clinician chooses to communicate the specific reason that the presentation does not meet criteria for specific disorder
Unspecified Depressive Disorder	Presence of depressive symptoms with significant distress and impairment that do not meet full criteria for any of the disorders in the depressive disorders diagnostic class. Used when clinician chooses not to communicate a specific reason or has insufficient information to determine why the presentation does not meet criteria for a specific disorder

Incidence/prevalence
- MDD is relatively common in the U.S.
  - Lifetime prevalence: 16.6%.
  - 12-month prevalence: 6.7%.
  - Prevalence in 18- to 29-year-olds is 3-fold greater than in those ≥60 years old.
- Female:male prevalence is approximately 2:1.

Economic impact
- Overall economic burden in the U.S. was estimated at ≥ $83 billion in 2000.
- Costs due to lost productivity exceed direct costs of treatment by a factor of 6–7.
- World Health Organization projections list unipolar depressive disorders as the second leading cause of burden of disease worldwide by 2030.

Etiology
- Genetic vulnerability: first-degree relatives have a 2- to 4-fold higher risk for MDD.
  - Complex pattern of inheritance: concordance rates of approximately 20% in dizygotic and 50% in monozygotic twins.
- Changes in neurotransmitter levels (e.g., catecholaminergic, serotonergic).
- Altered neuroendocrine function (e.g., adrenal axis, thyroid axis dysregulation).
- Psychosocial stressors or trauma.

Pathophysiology
- Not clearly defined.
- Current evidence points to complex interactions between various factors including neurotransmitter regulation and receptor sensitivity. Serotonin, norepinephrine, dopamine, glutamate, and brain-derived neurotrophic factor are the main neurotransmitters that have been linked to depressive disorders.

Prevention

> **BOTTOM LINE/CLINICAL PEARLS**
> - No intervention has proven effective to prevent the development of MDD.

Screening
- Screen those with significant risk factors as well as individuals who present with nonspecific symptoms suggestive of depression.
  - Quick Inventory of Depressive Symptomatology (QIDS-SR).
  - Beck Depression Inventory.
  - Patient Health Questionnaire-9 (PHQ-9) and shorter version (PHQ-2).

Secondary (and primary) prevention

> **BOTTOM LINE/CLINICAL PEARLS**
> - No intervention has proven effective for primary prevention.
> - Indefinite maintenance treatment with antidepressants and psychotherapy may help prevent relapse in patients at high risk (e.g., those with a history of ≥3 depressive episodes).

Diagnosis

> **BOTTOM LINE/CLINICAL PEARLS**
> - *History*. Ask about depressed mood and anhedonia. Include details of presentation, possible substance use, and impact of symptoms on daily functioning. Always assess for risk of harm to self or others.
> - *Exam findings*. There are no specific physical exam findings. On mental status exam, look for poor grooming, psychomotor retardation, depressed mood and affect. Suicidality and mood-congruent delusions or hallucinations may be present in severe depression and in MDD with psychotic features.
> - *Investigations*. There are no specific imaging or laboratory tests to confirm depression. Thyroid function, rapid plasma reagin (RPR), and vitamin B_{12} and folate levels can help rule out potentially reversible contributors to mood symptoms.

Differential diagnosis

Differential diagnosis	Features
Sadness	Short duration, fewer symptoms, no clinically significant distress or impairment
Adjustment Disorder with Depressed Mood	Response to an immediate psychosocial stressor; full criteria for major depressive episode (MDE) are not met
Bipolar Depression	Full criteria for an MDE are met, but past history is relevant for presence of manic or hypomanic episodes
Substance/Medication-Induced Depressive Disorder	Depressive episode results from a substance (including medications)
Mood Disorder Due to Another Medical Condition	Depressive symptoms are direct pathophysiological consequence of a specific medical condition (e.g., multiple sclerosis, stroke, hypothyroidism)
Manic Episode with Irritable Mood or Mixed Episode	Presence of manic symptoms
Attention-Deficit/Hyperactivity Disorder (in children)	Hyperactivity-impulsivity, inattention, and possibly irritability that significantly impair functioning
Seasonal Depression	Seasonal pattern of episodes with onset in fall or winter and often full remission by spring
Postpartum Depressive Disorder	Full depressive episode with onset a few months following delivery
Premenstrual Dysphoric Disorder (PMDD)	Symptoms present during the 1–2 weeks before menses and resolve with menses
Persistent Depressive Disorder (Dysthymia)	Depressed mood present more days than not over a 2-year period. Individuals that meet criteria for MDD during this time should be diagnosed with both MDD and persistent depressive disorder

(Continued)

Differential diagnosis	Features
Schizoaffective Disorder	Recurrent periods of at least 2 weeks of delusions or hallucinations occurring in the absence of prominent mood symptoms
Schizophrenia, Delusional Disorder, Unspecified Schizophrenia Spectrum and Other Psychotic Disorder	Depressive periods are brief relative to the total duration of the psychotic disturbance (e.g., delusions, hallucinations)
Post-Traumatic Stress Disorder (PTSD)	Onset within 6 months following traumatic event; characterized by hyperarousal, flashbacks, nightmares, detachment, and maladaptive coping responses
Dementia	Progressively declining cognitive function often precedes depressive symptoms; low scores (usually ≤23) on mini mental status examination (MMSE)

Typical presentation

In clinical practice patients often present with nonspecific symptoms that may include DSM-5 criteria of depressed mood, anhedonia, change in appetite and sleep, fatigue, distractibility, feelings of worthlessness and guilt, or recurrent thoughts of death and suicidal ideation. Depressed individuals may also present with anxiety, irritable mood, panic attacks, crying spells, somatic pain (e.g., back pain, headaches), and muscle tension.

Clinical diagnosis

History

- Assess for depressed mood and anhedonia. Include onset/duration/course of symptoms, accompanying psychological symptoms, and possible psychosocial stressors (precipitating factors). Assess impact of symptoms on patient's daily life. Knowledge about past depressive episodes and treatments, other psychiatric disorders (including mania), and possible use of alcohol and other substances can help inform assessment and guide treatment.
- Risk of suicide is 20-fold higher in patients with MDD than in the general population.
  - Always ask and document any thoughts of death, suicide, and homicide. Any affirmative responses must be further investigated for the content of thoughts (plans or intent), and efforts must be made to collaborate with patient and family to limit access to lethal means (e.g., firearms and large amounts of medications).

Changes from DSM-IV to DSM-5

- New diagnosis of Disruptive Mood Dysregulation Disorder (DMDD) is included for children under 18 who exhibit persistent irritability and frequent episodes of extreme behavioral dyscontrol, without meeting criteria for bipolar mood elevation.
- Omitted bereavement exclusion in depressive disorders (i.e., bereaved individuals can be diagnosed with a depressive disorder if they otherwise meet symptom and severity criteria).
- Chronic MDD and dysthymia combined into a single category of Persistent Depressive Disorder.
- Specifiers have been added for syndromes comprising mixed symptoms and anxiety.
- Greater guidance for clinician assessment of suicidality (risk factors, ideation, plans).

Rating scales
- Standardized rating scales can be useful in screening, quantifying symptoms, and monitoring treatment response.
  - Self/patient-administered scales can be quickly completed and scored, making them ideal for clinic settings: QIDS-SR, Beck Depression Inventory, PHQ-9 and its shorter version, PHQ-2.
    - Geriatric Depression Scale (GDS) and Zung Self-Rating Depression Scale are helpful in elderly patients who may have mild to moderate dementia.
  - Practitioner-administered scales [e.g., Hamilton Depression Rating Scale (HAM-D), Montgomery-Asberg Depression Rating Scale, and Raskin Depression Rating Scale] are more time-intensive and more often used in research settings or when a more in-depth evaluation is indicated (e.g., HAM-D may be necessary for cognitively impaired patients).
    - Standardized scales in evaluating children include Children's Depression Rating Scale-Revised (CDRS-R), Child Depression Inventory (CDI), and Center for Epidemiological Studies Depression Scale Modified for Children (CES-DC).

Physical and mental status exams
- While there are no specific physical findings in depressive disorders, a physical exam and a review of systems can help rule out the possibility of depressive disorders due to other medical conditions.
- On mental status exam, depressed individuals may exhibit poor grooming, psychomotor retardation, depressed or constricted affect, and report depressed mood. In severe forms, patients may have suicidality and mood-congruent delusions and/or hallucinations.

Laboratory diagnosis
List of diagnostic tests
- There is no confirmatory diagnostic test.
- Routine and specific laboratory tests (e.g., thyroid function, RPR, vitamin B_{12} and folate levels) can help rule out potentially reversible contributors to mood symptoms and detect abnormalities in a subset of patients who do not respond to standard antidepressant treatments.

Lists of imaging techniques
- Although various illnesses such as multiple sclerosis (seen on MRI) and strokes (seen on CT, MRI) are associated with depression, there are currently no imaging techniques that are specific to identifying or diagnosing depressive disorders.

Diagnostic algorithm (Algorithm 10.1)

Potential pitfalls/common errors made regarding diagnosis of disease
- Lack of suspicion. Depression is significantly under-recognized, with epidemiological studies indicating that fewer than half of all cases are accurately identified by physicians.
- Failure to screen for substance use (medications, drugs of abuse, alcohol) that may be causing or exacerbating depressive symptoms.

Algorithm 10.1 Diagnostic approach to MDD

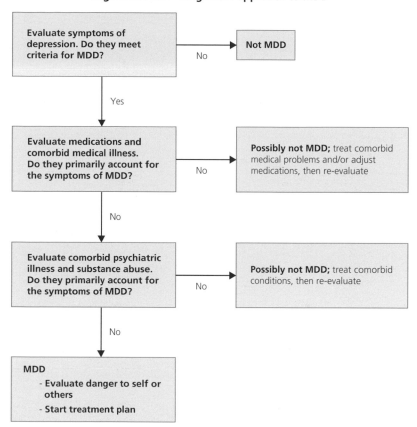

Treatment
Treatment rationale
- Pharmacotherapy, focused psychotherapies, other somatic treatments, and lifestyle changes.
- FDA-approved antidepressants differ in pharmacological and side effect profiles. None are clearly superior in efficacy, and for all the onset of efficacy may take up to several weeks.
- As a general rule, side effects can be minimized by going slowly when making dosage increases.

Table of treatment

Medical (FDA-approved)						
Pharmacologic class	Examples in the United States	Daily dose range (mg)	Starting dose (mg)	Notes	Common adverse effects	Serious adverse effects
Selective serotonin reuptake inhibitors (SSRIs)	Citalopram (Celexa)	20–40	10		Class effects: nausea, diarrhea, headache, insomnia, somnolence, sexual dysfunction, weight gain	Class effects: bleeding, seizure, serotonin syndrome, worsening depression or anxiety, suicidal thoughts
	Escitalopram (Lexapro)	10–20	5–10	Few drug–drug interactions		
	Fluoxetine (Prozac)	10–80	10	Few drug–drug interactions / Longest half-life		
	Paroxetine (Paxil)	20–50	10			
	Sertraline (Zoloft)	50–200	25			
	Vilazodone (Viibryd)	20–40	10			
+ serotonin modulation	Vortioxetine (Trintellix)	10–20	5–10			
Serotonin–norepinephrine reuptake inhibitors (SNRIs)	Desvenlafaxine (Pristiq)	50–100	50		Class effects: nausea, headache, dry mouth, diarrhea, constipation, dizziness, tremor, sweating, hypertension, blurred vision, sexual dysfunction, tachycardia, hyperlipidemia, urinary hesitancy, orthostatic syncope	Class effects: seizure, serotonin syndrome, suicidal thoughts, bleeding, hyponatremia, glaucoma, hypertension, hepatotoxicity (duloxetine), hyperglycemia
	Duloxetine (Cymbalta)	60–120	30–60			
	Venlafaxine (Effexor XR)	75–225	37.5			

Class	Drug	Dose range	Starting dose	Notes	Side effects	Class effects
Tricyclic antidepressants (TCAs)	Amoxapine (Asendin)	75–300	10–25		Class effects: dry mouth, constipation, urinary retention, somnolence, dizziness, weight gain, sexual dysfunction, orthostasis	Class effects: can be lethal in overdose, cardiac arrhythmia, hematological abnormalities, suicidal thoughts
	Amitriptyline (Elavil)	100–300	10–50			
	Clomipramine (Anafranil)	25–250	12.5–25			
	Desipramine (Norpramin)	75–300	10–25	Favorable tolerability		
	Imipramine (Tofranil)	100–200	10–25			
	Maprotiline (Ludiomil)	40–150	10–25			
	Nortriptyline (Pamelor)	15–60	12.5–25	Favorable safety, tolerability		
	Protriptyline (Vivactil)	75–300	5–10	Activating		
Monoamine oxidase inhibitors (MAOIs)	Isocarboxazid (Marplan)	20–60	10		Class effects: dry mouth, constipation, orthostasis, weight gain, sexual dysfunction, somnolence, dizziness, headache	Class effects: hypertensive crisis, serotonin syndrome, suicidal thoughts
	Phenelzine (Nardil)	45–90	15			
	Selegiline transdermal (Emsam)	6–12	6			
	Tranylcypromine (Parnate)	30–60	10			

(Continued)

Medical (FDA-approved)

Pharmacologic class	Examples in the United States	Daily dose range (mg)	Starting dose (mg)	Notes	Common adverse effects	Serious adverse effects
Atypical antidepressants	Bupropion (Wellbutrin)	300–450	100–150	Available as SR and XL	Agitation, dry mouth, insomnia, nausea, constipation, tremor, headache	Increased seizure risk, suicidal thoughts
	Mirtazapine (Remeron)	30–45	15		Sedation, increased appetite, weight gain, hypotension, dry mouth, constipation, dizziness	Suicidal thoughts
	Trazodone (Oleptro)	150–375	150		Sedation, orthostatic hypotension, dizziness, headache, dry mouth	Priapism, suicidal thoughts, arrhythmias

Device-based/somatic (FDA-approved)

Electroconvulsive therapy (ECT)
- Suitable for patients with treatment-resistant depression who have failed pharmacologic trials, those with psychotic depression, and those with acute suicidality
- Requires anesthesia and can cause cognitive side effects and transient amnesia in addition to hypertension and arrhythmias

Repetitive transcranial magnetic stimulation (rTMS)
- Approved for patients with unipolar depression who failed to respond to a single medication trial
- Common side effects include headache and scalp pain; rare (<0.5%) occurrence of seizures

Deep transcranial magnetic stimulation (dTMS)
- Approved for patients with unipolar major depression (no limitations re number of previous failed treatments)
- Different coil structure than rTMS; magnetic field penetrates deeper and may stimulate subcortical brain structures
- Similar side effects to rTMS

Vagus nerve stimulation (VNS)	• FDA approved for treatment of chronic treatment-resistant depression in patients who have failed to respond to at least four trials of antidepressants • Requires neurosurgery to implant device and to attach connector to ascending branch of left vagus nerve. Side effects include complications of surgery, neck or jaw pain, cough, and hoarseness

Psychological

Cognitive behavioral therapy (CBT) Interpersonal psychotherapy (IPT)	• Among psychotherapies, CBT and IPT have the most evidence for efficacy in randomized clinical trials • CBT provides durable benefits, and acute outcomes are comparable to psychopharmacological treatments • Combining CBT and pharmacological treatments may be most effective in moderate to severe depression

Complementary medicine

Currently, no complementary or "alternative" remedy has FDA approval for the treatment of depressive disorders. The best studied are St. John's Wort (hypericum), omega-3 fatty acids, S-adenosylmethionine (SAMe), and l-methyl-folate (Deplin). Physical exercise has been shown to have efficacy in mild to moderate depression

When to hospitalize
- Suicidality with plan and intent (i.e., imminent risk to self).
- Unable to care for self.
- Homicidality with plan and intent (i.e., imminent risk to others).

Prevention/management of complications
- *Suicidality*. All antidepressant classes have a black box warning for increased risk of suicidality in children, adolescents, and young adults (<24yo) with MDD or other psychiatric disorders. Close observation for clinical worsening and suicidality is required.
- *Serotonin syndrome*. A constellation of symptoms including autonomic signs, hypertonicity, tremor, and myoclonus resulting from excess serotonergic activity in the central nervous system. Could be life-threatening with rapid onset of hyperthermia, hypertension, tachycardia and shock. Can be caused by various medications, but MAOIs carry the highest risk due to their irreversible inhibition of MAO and resultant higher risk of interaction with sympathomimetic or serotonergic medications. Treatment is by supportive care and discontinuation of the offending medications/agents.
- *Hypertensive crisis*. A side effect in MAOIs that occurs with ingestion of tyramine-containing foods such as aged cheese and meats, fava bean pods, soy sauce, tap beer, and wine. Two weeks must pass post-MAOI discontinuation before stopping an MAOI diet or beginning a contraindicated medication. Hypertensive crisis is a medical emergency that requires hospitalization to stabilize blood pressure and prevent organ damage.
- *Increased seizure risk*. Various medications including TCAs, MAOIs, and bupropion lower seizure threshold. Avoid bupropion in patients with history of seizures or bulimia nervosa.

Management/treatment algorithm

TREATMENT OF AN ACUTE EPISODE OF MDD
First line:
- For mild–moderate depression: pharmacotherapy with SSRI, SNRI, mirtazapine, or bupropion and/or psychotherapy.
- For severe (non-psychotic) depression: pharmacotherapy as above plus psychotherapy, or ECT.
- For psychotic depression: pharmacotherapy (antidepressant + antipsychotic) and/or ECT.
Second line – for partial (insufficient) response or non-response:
- In patients treated with an antidepressant, consider increasing the dose (if well tolerated), changing to a different antidepressant, or using augmentation strategies*.
- In patients treated with psychotherapy, consider adding pharmacotherapy and/or switching psychotherapy modality.
Third line:
- Changing to a different antidepressant class (MAOI, TCAs); using augmentation strategies*.

* Select *evidence-based augmentation therapies* include atypical antipsychotics (e.g., aripiprazole, quetiapine, brexpiprazole), lithium, thyroid hormones, combining antidepressant from different classes, somatic therapies (rTMS, dTMS, ECT), and psychotherapy.

CONTINUATION AND MAINTENANCE PHASE TREATMENT
Continuation. Effective treatment should be continued unchanged for 4–9 months following successful acute phase treatment.

Maintenance. Patients who have had ≥3 prior major depressive episodes should receive indefinite maintenance treatment, given their high risk of relapse. Patients with significant risk factors for recurrence (e.g., presence of significant residual symptoms, ongoing psychosocial stressors, significant family history of mood disorders, very severe prior episodes) should consider ongoing maintenance treatment for relapse prevention.

CLINICAL PEARLS
- It takes 6–12 weeks to fully evaluate the efficacy of an antidepressant treatment.
- If no improvement in symptoms and functioning by 6–12 weeks, consider increasing dose to the most effective tolerable level.
- If dose escalation is not sufficient, consider switching to another medication within the same class or switching classes.
- In the case of partial response to medication, consider combining antidepressants from different classes (e.g., if on an SSRI, adding bupropion, low-dose TCA, or mirtazapine) or using augmentation strategies (e.g., atypical antipsychotics, lithium, psychostimulants, triiodothyronine, or dopaminergic agents).

Special populations
Pregnancy
In the old FDA classification, all antidepressants were listed in the pregnancy category C, except for maprotiline (B), paroxetine (D), and nortriptyline (D). The new FDA approved labeling for each antidepressant (listed since December 2014 in each medication Package Insert) presents more specific data regarding use in pregnancy and lactation, in narrative format. The decision to treat with antidepressants during pregnancy should be based on careful considerations of risks and benefits in the individual patient. Overall, SSRIs are well tolerated and the most frequently used pharmacologic class to treat depression during pregnancy. Of the SSRIs, fluoxetine and sertraline have the most data regarding use in pregnancy.

Others
- *Children.* All FDA-approved antidepressant classes carry a risk of increased suicidality in children and youths under 24. Careful monitoring for risk of self-harm and worsening of symptoms is required.
- *Elderly.* Use lower initial medication doses and go slower with titration.

Prognosis

BOTTOM LINE/CLINICAL PEARLS
- Only about 30–45% of patients with MDD who receive adequate pharmacotherapy achieve full remission.
- Comorbid anxiety disorders, substance use, and medical illness have been linked to lower rates of treatment response.

Reading list
American Psychiatric Association. Diagnostic and Statistical Manual of Mental Disorders, 5th edn. Arlington, VA: American Psychiatric Association, 2013.
American Psychiatric Association. Guidelines for the Treatment of Patients with Major Depressive Disorder, 3rd edn. DOI: 10.1176/appi.books.9780890423387.654001

Cassano P, Cassem NH, Papakostas GI, Fava M, Stern TA. Mood-disordered patients. In: Stern TA, Fricchione GL, Cassem NH, Jellinek MS, Rosenbaum JF (eds). Massachusetts General Hospital Handbook of General Hospital Psychiatry. Philadelphia, PA: Saunders Elsevier, 2010, pp. 73–92.

Schatzberg AF, Nemeroff CB. The American Psychiatric Publishing Textbook of Psychopharmacology, 4th edn. Washington, DC: American Psychiatric Publications, 2009.

Stahl SM. Depression and Bipolar Disorder: Stahl's Essential Psychopharmacology. Cambridge: Cambridge University Press, 2008.

Suggested websites

American Academy of Child & Adolescent Psychiatry. http://www.aacap.org

American Psychiatric Association. https://www.psychiatry.org

PsychiatryOnline. http://www.psychiatryonline.com

Guidelines

Title	Source	Weblink
Practice Guideline for the Treatment of Patients With Major Depressive Disorder, 3rd edn	American Psychiatric Association (APA), 2010	http://psychiatryonline.org/pb/assets/raw/sitewide/practice_guidelines/guidelines/mdd.pdf
Practice Parameter for the Assessment and Treatment of Children and Adolescents with Depressive Disorders	Journal of the American Academy of Child and Adolescent Psychiatry, 2007	http://www.ncbi.nlm.nih.gov/pubmed/18049300

Evidence

Type of evidence	Title and comment	Weblink
Meta-analysis	Atypical antipsychotic augmentation in major depressive disorder: A meta-analysis of placebo-controlled randomized trials. **Comment:** Atypical antipsychotic medications are effective augmentation agents in treating MDD. However, there is higher discontinuation rate due to side-effects compared to placebo augmentation.	http://www.ncbi.nlm.nih.gov/pubmed/19687129
Meta-analysis	Efficacy of bupropion and the selective serotonin reuptake inhibitors in the treatment of anxiety symptoms in major depressive disorder: a meta-analysis of individual patient data from 10 double-blind, randomized clinical trials. **Comment:** Bupropion and SSRIs have equal efficacy in treating anxiety symptoms in MDD.	http://www.ncbi.nlm.nih.gov/pubmed/17631898

(Continued)

(*Continued*)

Type of evidence	Title and comment	Weblink
Multisite, prospective, randomized, multistep clinical trial	The STAR*D Project results: a comprehensive review of findings. **Comment:** Patients with MDD who had initial treatment failure can obtain symptom relief through change in treatment strategies. However, the likelihood of response and illness remission decreases with increased number of additional treatment strategies needed.	http://www.ncbi.nlm.nih.gov/pubmed/18221624

Additional material for this chapter can be found online at: www.mountsinaiexpertguides.com/psychiatry

This includes advice for patients, ICD codes, and multiple choice questions.

CHAPTER 11

Bipolar Disorders

Le-Ben Wan[1], Joseph F. Goldberg[2], Katherine E. Burdick[2], and Dan V. Iosifescu[2]
[1]New York University School of Medicine, New York, NY, USA
[2]Icahn School of Medicine at Mount Sinai, New York, NY, USA

OVERALL BOTTOM LINE
- Bipolar disorders are associated with significant functional disability, morbidity, and mortality.
- Diagnosis relies primarily on clinical interview, with laboratory tests important for differential diagnosis.
- Pharmacotherapy with a mood stabilizer is recommended across the board for patients with bipolar disorder.
- Specific psychotherapies have shown efficacy during acute episodes and in relapse prevention.

Background
Definition of disease
Bipolar spectrum disorders are syndromes of altered behavior and mood characterized by discrete periods of mania, hypomania, and depression. Several subtypes are defined.

Disease classification
Mood disorder with specific classification based on the nature, duration, and severity of mood elevation (mania or hypomania).

Incidence/prevalence
- Lifetime prevalence in US: 4.5%.
  - Bipolar I: 1%.
  - Bipolar II: 1.1%.
  - Subthreshold bipolar disorder: 2.4%.
- Mean age of onset: 18.2 years (bipolar I) and 20.3 years (bipolar II).

Economic impact
- In the Global Burden of Disease, Injuries, and Risk Factors study (2010) bipolar disorder accounted for 14% of disability-adjusted life years (DALYs) associated with all mental health and substance use disorders. The 2009 total costs of bipolar I/II disorders were conservatively estimated at ~ $150 billion, with roughly 80% of that amount reflecting indirect costs.

Etiology
- Unknown etiology but may involve biological, psychosocial, and environmental factors.
- Polygenic and highly heritable.

Mount Sinai Expert Guides: Psychiatry, First Edition. Edited by Asher B. Simon, Antonia S. New, and Wayne K. Goodman.
© 2017 John Wiley & Sons, Ltd. Published 2017 by John Wiley & Sons, Ltd.
Companion website: www.mountsinaiexpertguides.com/psychiatry

- Several associated risk alleles, each of small effect.
- Structural genetic variation has been implicated in early-onset disease.

Pathophysiology
- Familial transmission is non-Mendelian.
  - Monozygotic concordance is 40–70%, implicating both non-genetic and genetic factors in pathophysiology.
  - First-degree relatives of affected individuals have a lifetime risk of 15–25%, compared to 2–4% for the general population.
  - Children of parents with bipolar disorder are more likely to have subthreshold mood disorder symptoms (e.g., day-to-day mood swings, irritability, high energy, fast thinking).
- Temporal association between multiple stressful life events and relapse/recurrence (may reflect kindling and behavioral sensitization).
- fMRI studies show limbic hyperactivity and frontal hypoactivity.
  - One hypothesis is that genetic and temperamental factors interact with psychosocial and other unknown environmental factors to disrupt brain networks that modulate emotional behavior.
  - Once established, the disease can be further exacerbated by psychosocial stress.

Predictive/risk factors
Risk factors
- Family history of bipolar or unipolar mood disorders.
- Cyclothymia and episodic/distinct mood symptoms.
- Early age at onset of mood symptoms.

Prevention

> **BOTTOM LINE/CLINICAL PEARLS**
> - To date, no intervention has been demonstrated to prevent the development of the disease.

Screening
- *Self-report screening tools* are validated for use in general populations, including primary care settings. While not a substitute for a careful clinical interview, these measures can provide initial clues about the possible presence of bipolar disorder:
  - Mood Disorders Questionnaire (MDQ; www.integration.samhsa.gov/images/res/MDQ.pdf);
  - Bipolar Inventory of Symptoms Scale (BISS);
  - Brief Bipolar Disorder Symptom Scale (BDSS).
- *Provider-completed rating scales* are often used not for diagnostic purposes but for assessing symptom severity and tracking changes in mood symptoms over time:
  - Young Mania Rating Scale (YMRS);
  - Montgomery-Asberg Depression Rating Scale (MADRS);
  - Hamilton Depression Rating Scale (HAM-D);
  - Inventory for Depressive Symptoms (IDS);
  - Clinical Global Impressions Scale (CGI).

Secondary (and primary) prevention

> **BOTTOM LINE/CLINICAL PEARLS**
> - Relapse prevention is crucial and includes long-term treatment with one or more mood stabilizers and possible adjunctive medications, with or without focused psychotherapies.
> - Proper sleep hygiene, avoidance of street drugs or excessive alcohol use, and effective strategies for stress management may help reduce the risk for relapse.

Diagnosis

> **BOTTOM LINE/CLINICAL PEARLS**
> - Bipolar disorders are diagnosed based on the presence or history of at least one manic or hypomanic episode. Depressive episodes are frequently present (and required to diagnose bipolar II).
> - On exam, manic and depressive symptoms are observable as changes in mood, energy, activity, and thought processes.
> - No imaging or lab test is diagnostic for bipolar disorder, although testing is used to rule out possible medical causes of symptoms.

Differential diagnosis

Differential diagnosis	Features
Major Depressive Disorder	Presence of one or more full major depressive episodes but no lifetime manic or hypomanic episodes. Per DSM-5, subthreshold manic/hypomanic symptoms may occur during depressive episodes ("with mixed features") but are too few in number or scope to count as syndromal
Borderline Personality Disorder	Ongoing affective instability (often daily, changing by minute or hour), self-mutilation, desperate attempts to avoid abandonment, chronic feelings of emptiness, and identity disturbance
Post-Traumatic Stress Disorder	Triggered by trauma-related stimuli; persistent anxiety; rare euphoria
Substance-Related Disorders	Time course matches intoxication/withdrawal/addiction pattern
Attention-Deficit/Hyperactivity Disorder	Symptoms are pervasive/persistent; present prior to age 12
Disruptive, Impulse-Control, and Conduct Disorders	Behavior is often deliberate and may be lacking in remorse, guilt, or empathy; chronic non-distinct episodes
Schizoaffective Disorder	Delusions or hallucinations for ≥2 weeks in the absence of a major mood episode
Depressive Disorders	Absent hypomania or mania
Anxiety Disorders	Absent hypomania or mania. Anxious mood may be present in bipolar disorder, but it is not the primary affect

Typical presentation

Individuals with bipolar disorder can present in a euthymic, manic/hypomanic, or depressed mood state. Subsyndromal or residual affective symptoms are common during the intervals between full manic, hypomanic, or depressive episodes. A depressive episode often precedes the first manic episode, and depressive symptoms are often more common than manic symptoms throughout the course of the illness. High levels of anxiety may accompany mood episodes (captured in DSM-5 by the course specifier "with anxious distress") and are associated with poorer outcomes. Psychotic symptoms, both mood-congruent and mood-incongruent, may also accompany mood episodes, and represent a mark of severity. Mood episodes are often mixed, with depressive symptoms accompanying a manic episode and vice versa. Some individuals may present with rapid cycling, defined as four or more distinct mood episodes in a 12-month period.

Clinical diagnosis

History

- Inquire about current/past manic or hypomanic and depressive symptoms.
  - Assess time course, precipitants, and functional consequences.
  - Make use of collateral historians.
  - DSM-5 criteria emphasize changes in activity, energy, and mood.
- Distinguish between bipolar subtypes.
  - Bipolar I: ≥1 manic episode (≥7 days).
  - Bipolar II: ≥1 hypomanic episode (≥4 days) and ≥1 depressive episode.
  - Cyclothymic disorder in adults: multiple subthreshold hypomanic and subthreshold depresive periods over the course of 2 years.
  - Others:
    - Substance/Medication-Induced Bipolar and Related Disorder;
    - Bipolar and Related Disorder Due to Another Medical Condition;
    - Other Specified Bipolar and Related Disorder and Unspecified Bipolar and Related Disorder replace DSM-IV's bipolar disorder not otherwise specified (NOS); e.g., individuals with a history of major depressive disorder who meet all criteria for hypomania except the duration criterion of ≥4 consecutive days.
  - DSM-IV mixed episode (simultaneously meeting full criteria for both mania and major depressive episode) is replaced in DSM-5 with a new specifier, "with mixed features," to be applied to episodes of mania/hypomania when depressive features are present and to episodes of depression when features of mania/hypomania are present (e.g., a major depressive episode with 3 manic symptoms is described in DSM-5 as "with mixed features").
    - A few hypomanic symptoms during a major depressive episode is no longer characterized as bipolar NOS.
- Psychiatric comorbidity is common; carefully evaluate medical, psychiatric, and substance use histories.
- In all, always assess for psychosis, anxiety, and suicidal ideation.

Physical and mental status exams

- Mania
  - Mood may be elevated (with excessive/expansive affect) or irritable (with impatience or hostility).
  - Pressured speech, flight of ideas, distractibility, psychomotor agitation.
  - Impaired insight, especially into need for treatment.
  - Poor judgment may lead to excessive involvement in risky activities.

- Depression
  - Mood may be sad/numb with relatively unreactive and/or blunted affect.
  - Slow thinking, soft speech.
  - Psychomotor retardation or psychomotor agitation (pacing/fidgeting).
  - May appear preoccupied or easily distracted.

Disease severity classification
- Severity of illness during a given episode is often captured categorically (e.g., in DSM-5 via fifth digit coding of a bipolar diagnosis as reflecting mild, moderate, or severe levels of illness).
- Symptom severity rating scales (e.g., MADRS, YMRS) provide continuous measures of severity of depression or mania, respectively, with scoring systems that by convention can be designated into categories of mild, moderate or severe symptomatology.
- Severity also can be measured using the 7-point Clinical Global Impressions-Severity (CGI-S) scale.

Laboratory diagnosis
List of diagnostic tests
- Toxicology screening to rule out intoxication or withdrawal.
- Thyroid stimulating hormone (TSH) to rule out thyroid conditions.
- Rapid plasma reagin (RPR) to rule out neurosyphilis.
- Folate/B$_{12}$ to rule out vitamin deficiency.
- Appropriate tests to rule out delirium, especially if the individual appears manic or with an altered mental status.

Lists of imaging techniques
- Brain MRI to rule out structural lesions, especially for first-episode mania or if the individual has focal neurologic signs.

Diagnostic algorithm (Algorithm 11.1)

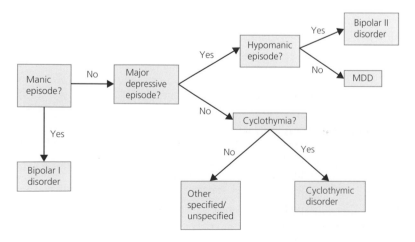

Algorithm 11.1 Diagnostic algorithm for bipolar spectrum disorders

Potential pitfalls/common errors made regarding diagnosis of disease

- Bipolar disorders can be difficult to differentiate from other psychiatric disorders with shared features, especially affective instability.
- Essential corroborative history from family, friends, and medical records is often overlooked.

Treatment
Treatment rationale

Fundamental treatment goals include ameliorating current affective symptoms and avoiding polarity switches. Mood stabilizers form the cornerstone of bipolar pharmacotherapy but vary in antimanic vs antidepressant, and acute vs prophylactic, properties.

- Lithium, divalproex, and carbamazepine remain "gold standard" acute antimanic mood stabilizers.
- Lithium more robustly prevents mania than depression.
- Divalproex and carbamazepine are commonly used off-label as preventative agents.
- Lamotrigine carries FDA approval for prevention of recurrent episodes in bipolar I disorder (although its effect is more robust against depression than mania, in contrast to lithium); its acute antidepressant properties are not well established from placebo-controlled trials.
- Second-generation antipsychotics (SGAs), long recognized as adjunctive therapies in acute mania, are increasingly regarded as first-line interventions either alone or in conjunction with mood stabilizers for acute manic or mixed episodes as well as relapse prevention. Some (but not all) SGAs have demonstrated efficacy and FDA approval for acute bipolar depression (notably, quetiapine, lurasidone, and olanzapine–fluoxetine combination).
- Other anticonvulsants (e.g., oxcarbazepine, gabapentin, topiramate) are not well established for treating bipolar mood symptoms but are sometimes used adjunctively for associated non-affective symptoms (e.g., anxiety, neuropathic pain, binge eating).
- Traditional antidepressants remain controversial for both short- and long-term use in bipolar depression.
  - Small (~10–15%) risk of inducing mania in a subgroup of bipolar patients (bipolar I > II; rapid cycling; past antidepressant-induced mania; recent mania; mixed features).
  - Efficacy appears no greater than that seen with adequately dosed mood stabilizers alone.
  - Antidepressants without antimanic mood stabilizers or SGA co-therapies are discouraged in bipolar I depression.
  - While none has shown robust efficacy for bipolar depression, bupropion and some SSRIs may be more benign than TCAs or SNRIs with respect to risk for inducing mania.
  - In treating bipolar depression, favor evidence-based treatments over medications with multiple negative randomized trials (e.g., paroxetine, aripiprazole, ziprasidone) or those with no controlled data (e.g., duloxetine, vilazodone, asenapine).

Approaches to complex patients with bipolar disorder

- *Anxiety:* Differentiate anxiety from hypomania, agitation, or akathisia. Favor SGAs with anxiolytic properties (e.g., quetiapine). Consider anxiolytic anticonvulsants (e.g., gabapentin, pregabalin). Use benzodiazepines judiciously. Anxiolytic antidepressants (e.g., SSRIs) may be of value but are relatively unstudied in this setting.
- *Substance abuse:* Assess need for independent treatment of substance use disorder and extent to which current affective symptoms may be substance-induced.
- *Personality disorders:* Longitudinal history should help reveal the nature of affective disturbance, interpersonal conflicts, and coping styles in the absence of an index episode. Comorbid personality disorders can impair medication adherence, undermine the therapeutic alliance, and mimic symptoms of a primary mood disorder (e.g., affective instability governed by

interpersonal sensitivities). Consider the role for psychotherapy in the setting of prominent features of a comorbid significant personality disorder.

- *Suicide risk*. May be highest in those with a history of past attempts; more common if depressed episode or mixed features than pure mania. Lithium may confer ~6-fold decreased risk for suicidal behavior.
- *Cognitive symptoms*. May be inherent to bipolar, independent of current affective symptoms (i.e., continue during inter-episode intervals). Consider adverse medication effects (e.g., anticholinergic, sedative-hypnotic) on cognitive function and longitudinal history to assess likely etiology. Neuropsychological testing may be of value.

When to hospitalize

- When patients pose an imminent risk for self-harm or harm to others.
- When symptoms markedly impede functioning (e.g., manic patients who gravely jeopardize their professional, financial, or social welfare due to reckless decision-making).
- Depressed patients who may be unable to care for themselves due to progressive debilitation, regardless of suicidal or psychotic features.

Managing the hospitalized patient

- Assess risk for suicidal or violent behavior and need for 1:1 monitoring.
- First-episode presentations of mania or psychosis may warrant medical-neurologic evaluation if atypical features are present (e.g., localizing neurological signs, unusual longitudinal course of illness).
- Resist the temptation to change or increase medication doses faster than pharmacokinetic and pharmacodynamic principles indicate (e.g., steady-state drug levels require at least five half-lives; adequate trials to determine drug efficacy may not be feasible during short hospital admissions; excessively frequent drug changes may obscure adverse effects and clinical symptoms).
- Monitor for and ensure the absence of withdrawal from illicit substances.
- Consider reasons for treatment non-adherence that may have contributed to relapse.
- Consider electroconvulsive therapy (ECT) in patients who have had treatment-resistant symptoms, are urgently ill (actively suicidal or psychotic), or are pregnant.

Table of treatment

Medical	Comments
Mood stabilizers	
Lithium carbonate: start at 300–900 mg/day in mania; increase usually by 300 mg every few days; target blood level 0.6–1.2 mEq/L	Favored in euphoric/non-mixed, non-rapid-cycling, non-substance-abusing manic patients in first few episodes; responsivity may be familial. Monitor renal function and TSH at least semi-annually
Divalproex: start at 750 mg/day or orally load at 20–30 mg/kg in divided doses in acute mania; increase usually by 250–500 mg every few days if necessary, targeting a blood valproate level of 50–120 μg/dL	Favored over lithium in setting of mixed features, multi-episode presentations, comorbid substance use. Divalproex + lithium may yield better prophylaxis than divalproex alone. Monitor LFTs, valproic acid level, and platelets semi-annually
Carbamazepine: start at 400 mg/day in divided doses; increase by 200 mg every few days; target dose of 600–1600 mg/day; blood levels not established for psychotropic purposes	Weight-neutral; possibly better efficacy than lithium in mixed episodes; can be used synergistically with lithium, divalproex, and/or lamotrigine; autoinduces its own metabolism and that of other cytochrome P450 substrates

(Continued)

Lamotrigine: start at 25 mg/day for 2 weeks, then 50 mg/day for 2 weeks, then 100 mg/day for 1 week, then to target dose of 200 mg/day; dosing must be halved with divalproex co-therapy and doubled with carbamazepine co-therapy; target blood levels not established for psychotropic purposes	Experimental for acute bipolar depression; established efficacy in relapse prevention in bipolar I disorder (depression > mania)
Second-generation antipsychotics Aripiprazole: start at 15–30 mg/day in mania	Demonstrated efficacy in mania but not bipolar depression; dose-related akathisia may be common; risk for weight gain may stratify by baseline weight
Asenapine: 5–10 mg twice daily in manic or mixed episodes	Established efficacy in manic or mixed episode; novel sublingual route of administration; possibly less metabolic liability than older SGAs
Lurasidone: 20–120 mg/day for bipolar I depression	No data in manic episodes or manic episodes with mixed features. Preliminary favorable placebo-controlled data in bipolar depression with mixed features or major depressive disorder with mixed features
Olanzapine: start at 10–15 mg/day; maximum 20 mg/day though some practitioners may dose to 30–60 mg/day if indicated in manic or mixed episodes	Often perceived as reliable acute agent but with potentially substantial metabolic adverse effect burden
Olanzapine–fluoxetine combination: proprietary formulation for acute bipolar depression dosed as 6–12 mg/day of olanzapine plus 25–50 mg/day of fluoxetine	Risk for treatment-emergent affective switch no greater than with placebo; efficacy may be apparent within one week of initiation; long-term efficacy and safety not established
Quetiapine: for manic/mixed episodes, start at 300 mg/day with a target dose of 400–800 mg/day in adults (400–600 mg/day in children and adolescents)	Randomized trial database supports efficacy in all phases of bipolar disorder; common soporific adverse effects may not be dose-related but nevertheless can pose obstacles in non-psychotic, non-agitated patients
Risperidone: for manic/mixed episodes, target dose 1–6 mg/day in adults	FDA-approved for short-term treatment in bipolar I disorder; prophylactic efficacy has not been demonstrated except for prevention of mania with long-acting injectable formulation
Ziprasidone: for manic/mixed episodes, start at 40 mg twice daily; maximum 80 mg twice daily, though some practitioners advocate 240 mg/day	Heightened risk for QTc prolongation (additive with other QTc-prolonging drugs); relatively weight-neutral; no demonstrated efficacy for bipolar depression
Cariprazine: Start at 1.5 mg/day on Day 1 and increase to 3 mg/day on Day 2; may then increase by 1.5 or 3 mg/day increments to maximum of 6 mg/day	Established efficacy in manic or mixed episodes; preliminary favorable data in bipolar depression. Long half-life of parent drug and active metabolites (2–5 days) leads to prolonged time until steady state pharmacokinetics
Clozapine: off-label in treatment resistant bipolar disorder, dose approximately 50–400 mg/day	May be of value in rapid cycling or persistent mania; efficacy for depressive symptoms not well-demonstrated; unknown if recognized value for suicide prevention in schizophrenia may also pertain to those with bipolar disorder; substantial metabolic burden and hematologic risks require close monitoring

(Continued)

(Continued)

Device-based	
Electroconvulsive therapy (ECT): may be of value in any phase of bipolar disorder	Right unilateral ECT may be more sparing of adverse cognitive effects although efficacy may require a greater number of treatments; treatment of choice in severe/psychotic bipolar depression or during pregnancy
Psychological	
Reducing vulnerability to mood episodes by fostering greater ability to manage stressful life events is a central goal of several effective psychosocial treatments for bipolar disorder <ul><li>Cognitive behavioral therapy (CBT): focuses on challenging and restructuring thought patterns associated with depression</li><li>Interpersonal/social rhythm therapy (IPSRT): addresses regularity of sleep-wake cycle and patterns of interpersonal experiences related to mood</li><li>Family focused therapy (FFT): addresses negative expressed emotion within family unit and its impact on relapse</li></ul>	Adjunctive psychotherapy may hasten response to antidepressant regimen and reinforce role for medications and foster adherence; no significant differences in efficacy have been reported among evidence-based forms of psychotherapy (intensive psychoeducation, CBT, IPSRT, FFT). Can help patients recognize early mood decompensations and need for early additional treatment
Complementary	
Omega-3 fatty acids: 2–6 g/day; modest value for bipolar depression or relapse prevention	Limited data support value for relapse prevention; acute efficacy less well established
N-acetylcysteine: 1000 mg twice daily	Preliminary data support value in prevention of bipolar depression
S-adenosylmethionine: 400–800 mg twice daily	Preliminary data support value in major depression; less well studied in bipolar depression; has been associated with induction of mania in some reports
Inositol: 2–18 g/day	Theoretical value based on mechanism of action involving second messenger systems; modest demonstrated efficacy in bipolar depression

Prevention/management of complications

- Lamotrigine: serious skin rashes or hypersensitivity reactions: most common with rapid dose escalations and in first few weeks of treatment; discontinue therapy if occurs.
- Divalproex:
  - Pancreatitis: consider in differential diagnosis of abdominal pain.
  - Thrombocytopenia: usually indicates dose-related toxicity.
  - Periodically monitor CBC.
  - Transaminitis or hepatic failure: periodically monitor hepatic function.
- Lithium:
  - Renal insufficiency: monitor renal function at least semi-annually.
  - Secondary hypothyroidism: monitor thyroid function at least semi-annually.
- Carbamazepine: rare aplastic anemia; monitor CBC at least semi-annually.
- SGAs:
  - Metabolic dysregulation (weight gain, dyslipidemias, hyperglycemia): monitor for clinical signs regularly and laboratory parameters (e.g., serum lipids, fasting glucose) at baseline and at least annually thereafter.

- Ziprasidone: cardiac arrhythmias (e.g., QTc prolongation); periodically monitor ECG and recognize co-therapies that may also cause QTc prolongation (e.g., trazodone, cyclobenzaprine, fluoroquinolone antibiotics).
- Clozapine: agranulocytosis (monitor CBC weekly for 6 months, then biweekly for 6 months, then monthly or per manufacturer's guidelines); myocarditis (consider in differential diagnosis of fever and chest pain).
- Movement disorders (e.g., akathisia, extrapyramidal signs, tardive dyskinesia): clinically monitor regularly.

Management/treatment algorithm

TREATMENT OF ACUTE MANIC/MIXED EPISODES
First line: lithium, divalproex, or carbamazepine as cornerstone treatments.
- Divalproex or carbamazepine may be preferable to lithium when mixed features are present.
- May augment with atypical antipsychotic if severe/psychotic.
- Adjunctive sedative-hypnotics may help treat sleeplessness and agitation.
- SGA may be appropriate alternative monotherapy.
- Eliminate antidepressants if present.
- ECT if severe psychosis/mixed features, "urgency," pregnancy.
Second line: if inadequate response to a first-line treatment after 2–4 weeks:
- Combinations of two or more antimanic mood stabilizers, with or without SGA.
Third line: ECT; clozapine.
- Experimental anticonvulsants (e.g., oxcarbazepine) first generation antipsychotics; TMS; tamoxifen adjunctive dihydropyridone L-type calcium channel blockers (e.g., nimodipine, isradipine).

TREATMENT OF BIPOLAR DEPRESSION
First line*:
- Quetiapine[†], olanzapine–fluoxetine combination[†], lurasidone[†]; lamotrigine–lithium combination; ECT if severe/"urgent" presentation (e.g., psychosis, high suicide risk) or pregnant.
Second line:**
- Lithium, divalproex, carbamazepine, lamotrigine; augmentation with SSRI or bupropion if unresponsive to mood stabilizer alone.
Third line:**
- Antimanic drug plus one of the following: adjunctive pramipexole, modafinil or armodafinil, N-acetylcysteine, tranylcypromine, tricyclics, inositol, venlafaxine, riluzole.
Fourth line:
- Adjunctive thyroid hormone, stimulants, omega-3 fatty acids, TMS.

* All agents with at least one positive large-scale placebo-controlled trial.
** All agents with at least one positive proof-of-concept randomized (active comparator) or placebo-controlled trial.
[†] FDA-approved for acute bipolar depression.

MAINTENANCE TREATMENT OF BIPOLAR DISORDER

First line:

- Lithium or divalproex; combination may be synergistic and superior to divalproex alone.
- Lamotrigine prevents depressions more robustly than manias and in bipolar I disorder may provide better prophylaxis when paired with an antimanic drug.
- Olanzapine, adjunctive quetiapine, risperidone long-acting injectable, and adjunctive ziprasidone are evidence-based; aripiprazole has been shown to prevent recurrent manias but not depressions.
- Maintenance treatment with an adjunctive antidepressant after an acute depressive episode may be appropriate in the absence of rapid cycling if there has been a robust acute response so long as manic or hypomanic symptoms remain absent.

Second line:

- Carbamazepine.
- Combination of ≥2 mood stabilizers (lithium, divalproex, carbamazepine, lamotrigine) if monotherapies are ineffective.
- Maintenance ECT if there has been robust and unique efficacy for an acute episode in treatment-resistant patients.
- Long-acting injectable depot formulations of SGAs in setting of poor adherence.
- Adjunctive omega-3 fatty acids; adjunctive N-acetylcysteine.

Third line:

- Clozapine.
- Other anticonvulsants (e.g., oxcarbazepine, gabapentin).

CLINICAL PEARLS

- Avoid antidepressants in manic or mixed episodes; favor their long-term use only when robust acute efficacy has been evident and there are no signs of rapid cycling.
- Favor lithium particularly during the first few illness episodes, in euphoric/non-mixed presentations.
- Rapid cycling rarely responds to a single mood stabilizer and may be best treated using combinations, with or without an SGA, and generally with no antidepressants.
- Recognize that not all anticonvulsants have demonstrated antimanic efficacy.
- Combination regimens are common in bipolar disorder; optimal treatments involve synergistic/non-redundant mechanisms that aim to optimize doses of primary agents in order to minimize "cluttered" treatments with unnecessary burden of cumulative adverse effects.

Special populations

Pregnancy

- High risk of relapse, particularly if pharmacotherapy is discontinued.
- Significant risk for teratogenicity with divalproex or carbamazepine.
- The potential for cardiac teratogenicity with lithium appears to be lower than once thought but still higher than base rate in the general population; first trimester lithium exposure may also increase risk for miscarriage or preterm delivery. Nevertheless, potential benefits of lithium during pregnancy may outweigh possible risks in individual cases.

- The decision to maintain, switch, or discontinue existing medications during pregnancy depends on illness severity, risk of teratogenicity, efforts to minimize additional agents, and patient preference.
- Monitor psychiatric status and mood episodes in collaboration with other medical care providers.

Others

- Comorbid psychiatric disorders can worsen overall treatment outcome and generally require their own independent treatments. For example, prioritized treatment of comorbid borderline personality disorder may facilitate subsequent pharmacotherapy of mood episodes in bipolar disorder. Similarly, active alcohol or substance use disorders can aggravate or mimic mood symptoms associated with bipolar disorder and render pharmacotherapies for bipolar disorder less effective, usually making acute stabilization of substance use disorders a prerequisite for effective treatment of comorbid bipolar disorder.

Prognosis

Natural history of untreated disease

> **BOTTOM LINE/CLINICAL PEARLS**
> - Despite treatment, mood episodes recur in 85–95% of individuals with bipolar disorder.
> - The average individual with bipolar disorder is symptomatically ill almost 50% of the time, with depressive symptoms predominating over manic symptoms.
> - Subsyndromal symptoms and functional impairment are common between mood episodes.
> - 30% lifetime risk of suicide attempts.
> - Lithium maintenance treatment can reduce the number of episodes and time spent ill by an average of >50%.

- Progressively increasing frequency of manic and depressive episodes (e.g., a patient with illness onset at age 18 may experience, in the absence of treatment, ~10 severe mood episodes by age 30, with severe impairment in professional and social development).
- Increased suicide risk.

Prognosis for treated patients

- Reduction in number and frequency of relapses.
- Improved functional status.

Follow-up tests and monitoring

- During acute episodes, outpatients should be monitored at least weekly, with regular reassessment of appropriate level of care.
- Symptoms can be monitored by rating scales (e.g., YMRS, MADRS, IDS) alongside improvement measures (e.g., CGI severity and improvement scales).
- Laboratory monitoring includes semi-annual routine measurement of serum lithium or valproate levels, thyroid and renal functioning during lithium treatment, and hepatic function and complete blood counts during divalproex or carbamazepine treatment.
- In patients taking second-generation antipsychotics, weight/blood pressure/waist circumference should be monitored periodically, and lab-based metabolic parameters (fasting glucose, hemoglobin A1c, lipids) monitored at baseline and annually thereafter.

- ECG monitoring is advisable in patients with risk factors for QTc prolongation during treatment with antipsychotics, and with other potentially arrhythmogenic medications (e.g., tricyclics, some SSRIs) depending on individual risk factors.

Reading list

Goodwin FK, Jamison KR. Manic-Depressive Illness: Bipolar Disorders and Recurrent Depression, 2nd edn. New York: Oxford University Press, 2007.

Hales RE, Yudofsky SC, Roberts LW (eds). The American Psychiatric Publishing Textbook of Psychiatry, 6th edn. Washington, DC: American Psychiatric Publishing, 2014.

Ketter TA (ed). Handbook of Diagnosis and Treatment of Bipolar Disorder. Washington, DC: American Psychiatric Publishing, 2010.

Schatzberg AF, DeBattista C. Manual of Clinical Psychopharmacology, 8th edn. Washington, DC: American Psychiatric Publishing, 2014.

Suggested websites

APA Treatment Guidelines. http://psychiatryonline.org/guidelines.aspx

National Institute of Mental Health: Bipolar Disorders. http://www.nimh.nih.gov/health/publications/bipolar-disorder/index.shtml

Guidelines
National society guidelines

Title	Source	Weblink
APA's Practice Guideline for the Treatment of Patients With Bipolar Disorder, 2nd edn	American Psychiatric Association (APA), 2002	http://psychiatryonline.org/pb/assets/raw/sitewide/practice_guidelines/guidelines/bipolar.pdf
Guideline Watch (November 2005): Practice Guideline for the Treatment of Patients with Bipolar Disorder, 2nd Edition	Hirschfeld RMA, Focus 2007; 5: 34–39	http://focus.psychiatryonline.org/doi/10.1176/foc.5.1.34?trendmd-shared=0
Texas Medication Algorithm Project (TMAP)	JPS Health Network, 2007	https://www.jpshealthnet.org/sites/default/files/tmap_bipolar_2007.pdf
US Veterans Administration/Department of Defense	US Department of Veterans Affairs, 2010	http://www.healthquality.va.gov/bipolar/bd_306_sum.pdf

International society guidelines

Title	Source	Weblink
Collaborative Update of CANMAT Guidelines for the Management of Patients with Bipolar Disorder	Canadian Network for Mood and Anxiety Treatments (CANMAT) and International Society for Bipolar Disorders (ISBD), 2013	http://canmat.org/resources/CANMAT%20Bipolar%20Disorder%20Guidelines%20-2013%20Update.pdf
Bipolar Disorder: assessment and management. NICE Clinical Guideline 185	UK National Institute for Health and Care Excellence (NICE), 2014	http://www.nice.org.uk/Guidance/CG185

Evidence

Type of evidence	Title and comment	Weblink
Prospective RCT	Effectiveness of adjunctive antidepressant treatment for bipolar depression. **Comment:** Antidepressants added to a mood stabilizer for acute bipolar depression provided neither greater benefit nor higher risk for inducing mania as compared to placebo.	http://www.nejm.org/doi/full/10.1056/NEJMoa064135
Prospective RCT	Lithium plus valproate combination therapy versus monotherapy for relapse prevention in bipolar I disorder (BALANCE): a randomized open label trial. **Comment:** Divalproex + lithium superior to divalproex monotherapy for relapse prevention of either polarity.	http://www.ncbi.nlm.nih.gov/pubmed/20092882
Prospective RCT	A 20-month, double-blind, maintenance trial of lithium versus divalproex in rapid-cycling bipolar disorder. **Comment:** Only 24% of rapid cyclers stabilized on open label lithium + divalproex; half of those remained stable on either monotherapy over 20 months.	http://www.ncbi.nlm.nih.gov/pubmed/16263857
Meta-analysis	Comparative efficacy and acceptability of antimanic drugs in acute mania: a multiple-treatments meta-analysis. **Comment:** Gabapentin, lamotrigine, and topiramate no better than placebo; lithium, divalproex. and all second-generation antipsychotics superior to placebo though overlapping confidence intervals suggest no clear differences in relative efficacies; haloperidol showed greatest magnitude of improvement.	http://www.ncbi.nlm.nih.gov/pubmed/21851976
Meta-analysis	Antidepressants for the acute treatment of bipolar depression: a systematic review and meta-analysis. **Comment:** Across 15 studies with 2373 total subjects, antidepressants did not differ significantly from placebo in response, remission, or affective switch.	http://www.ncbi.nlm.nih.gov/pubmed/21034686

Additional material for this chapter can be found online at:
www.mountsinaiexpertguides.com/psychiatry

This includes advice for patients, a case study, ICD codes, and multiple choice questions.

CHAPTER 12

Anxiety Disorders

Marc S. Lener[1], Dennis S. Charney[2], and Adriana Feder[2]
[1] National Institute of Mental Health, Bethesda, MD, USA
[2] Icahn School of Medicine at Mount Sinai, New York, NY, USA

OVERALL BOTTOM LINE

- Anxiety is an emotion characterized by worry or tension that may become greater than warranted by the situation and associated with physiological changes and anticipation of negative outcomes.
- Anxiety may be caused or exacerbated by non-psychiatric medical conditions or medication side effects.
- The anxiety disorders, grouped by contextual domains, are characterized by excessive and severe anxiety that interferes with daily activities and relationships.
- In primary care settings, patients with anxiety disorders commonly present with somatic symptoms or more frequent visits.
- The development of anxiety disorders is mediated by genetic, environmental, psychological, and neurobiological mechanisms.
- Treatment with pharmacological and psychological interventions is aimed at attenuating dysregulated psychological and physical responses.

Background

- Anxiety disorders are the most common mental disorders. Behavioral avoidance is a frequent cause of resulting impairment.
  - Panic disorder (PD): panic attacks + consequent worry/avoidance.
  - Specific phobia (SP): excessive fear + avoidance of object.
  - Social anxiety disorder (SAD): excessive fear of embarrassment + avoidance of social situations.
  - Generalized anxiety disorder (GAD): excessive worry/anxiety about multiple things.
- Lifetime prevalence in community = 25%.
- Average age of onset = 11 years.
- Female:male = 1.6:1.
- Interacting genetic and non-genetic factors confer risk.
- Treatments for anxiety disorders are some of the most effective in psychiatry.

Definition of disease

Anxiety disorders are a category of mental disorders characterized by fear and anxiety that cause marked distress in the individual. Whereas fear is a physiological response to perceived threat, anxiety is a more persistent physiological response to anticipated threat and can cause significant impairment in functioning.

Mount Sinai Expert Guides: Psychiatry, First Edition. Edited by Asher B. Simon, Antonia S. New, and Wayne K. Goodman.
© 2017 John Wiley & Sons, Ltd. Published 2017 by John Wiley & Sons, Ltd.
Companion website: www.mountsinaiexpertguides.com/psychiatry

Incidence/prevalence

	Lifetime prevalence	Female:male	Age of onset (years)
PD	4.7%	2.5:1	Bimodal; peaks in late adolescence and young adulthood
SP	12.5%	2:1	5–9: natural environmental (e.g., heights) and blood/injection/injury types Mid-20s: situational phobias (e.g., flying)
SAD	12.1%	Unknown	5–35, peak in adolescence
GAD	5.7%	2:1	Usually <25

Economic impact
- Overall costs > $42 billion annually due to psychiatric treatment, unnecessary medical treatments, work impairment, and mortality.
- SAD: given high comorbidity with alcohol and substance use, indirect health care costs may be significant.

Etiology
- Genes (e.g., serotonin transporter, catechol-O-methyltransferase) contribute risk.
- Temperamental behavioral inhibition.
- Environment (e.g., parental style marked by alternating overprotection and rejection) may enhance genetic predispositions and further reinforce anxious traits.

	Increased risk in first degree relatives	Heritability	Genetics
PD	7×; 17× if PD develops by age 20	0.28–0.43	Locus on chromosome 13q associated with risk for PD, mitral valve prolapse, serious headaches, thyroid problems
SP	2–3×	Unknown	Chromosome 16, in a region proximal to norepinephrine transporter
SAD	6×	0.10	Unknown
GAD		0.15–0.20	Possible shared liability with major depressive disorder (MDD) via genetic variant of serotonin transporter

Pathophysiology
Fear-conditioning models have been widely used in research and involve pairing an aversive event with a neutral stimulus, which leads to the subject's anxious response to the latter. Such physiological responses involve autonomic (sympathetic nervous system), neuroendocrine [hypothalamic-pituitary-adrenal (HPA) axis], and behavioral components. Current evidence suggests that in individuals prone to anxiety, alterations in the way the amygdala and hippocampus process non-harmful information lead to exaggerated fear responses, including a generalization of fear to non-harmful stimuli. The regulation of fear is mediated by areas such as the medial prefrontal

cortex and anterior cingulate cortex, and an imbalance of top-down control (e.g., frontal hypoactivity in the setting of amygdala hyperactivity) has been associated with anxiety states.

Panic disorder
- Associated with hyperactivity of noradrenergic neurons in the locus coeruleus, dysfunction in parvocellular neurons within the paraventricular nucleus, and elevated hypothalamic cortico-tropin-releasing hormone (CRH) within the HPA axis.
- Unusually frequent harm-related cognitive interpretations of stimuli, inappropriate activation of the fear network, and increased CO_2 sensitivity.

Specific phobia
- Biological tendency to develop a nonspecific fear forms a vulnerability background for abnormal fear conditioning in which an aversive experience connects a neutral object with a fearful response; this connection may be further reinforced by psychosocial factors and behavioral avoidance.
- Dysregulation in neurotransmitter systems (e.g., monoaminergic) involved in fear.
- Dysregulation in anterior cingulate may be more prominent in SP than in other anxiety disorders.

Social anxiety disorder
- Hypothesized as an amalgam of inhibited temperament, heightened alertness/arousal, and abnormal fear-conditioning in the setting of low self-esteem, interpersonal sensitivity, and/or limited social skills.
- Impaired recognition/identification of others' emotional expressions may limit socially appropriate responses and fulfill negative expectations.

Generalized anxiety disorder
- Shared biological underpinnings with MDD.
- Exposure to persistent psychosocial stressors induces long-term changes in brain structure/function.
- Altered levels of brain-derived neurotrophic factor (BDNF) and cyclic adenosine monophosphate (cAMP) response element-binding protein (CREB); reversed by antidepressants.

Predictive/risk factors
PD:
- Family history
- Psychosocial stressors (e.g., death/illness of loved one, major life changes)
- Caffeine or nicotine
- History of sexual/physical trauma
- Childhood separation anxiety

SP:
- Family history of SP or other anxiety disorders
- Experience or observation of a traumatic event

SAD:
- Behavioral inhibition/shyness
- Separation anxiety
- Parental figures who are more rejecting or overprotective

GAD:
- Family history

- Increased psychosocial stressors
- History of emotional, physical, or sexual trauma

Prevention

> **BOTTOM LINE/CLINICAL PEARLS**
> - **PD**: with treatment, full remission occurs in 10–35%; distinguishing features of treatment responders are still unknown.
> - **SP**: early childhood intervention through CBT may facilitate extinction of the fear and prevent progression to chronic course.
> - **SAD**: pharmacological and psychotherapeutic interventions prevent worsening.
> - **GAD**: patients with early signs may warrant psychiatric evaluation.

Screening

- **PD**: given high rates of psychiatric comorbidity, screen for panic attacks or avoidance behaviors in most patients with pre-existing or newly-diagnosed psychiatric conditions.
- **SP**: early childhood screening for extreme fear or avoidance of specific objects or situations identifies early warning signs.
- **SAD**: facilitated in school setting where interpersonal behaviors are closely observed; entails a team approach (school, parents, clinician).
- **GAD**: consider if persistent worry, emotional tension, or anxiety.
  - General questions about work, finances, family, or relationship stressors may lead patients to talk about their excessive worries. Asking about how they have been able to manage or cope with stressors may identify maladaptive coping (e.g., substance abuse).

Secondary (and primary) prevention

- Stress reduction and psychotherapy are beneficial for all anxiety disorders for primary and secondary prevention.
- Medications are used for secondary prevention for PD and GAD.

Diagnosis

> **BOTTOM LINE/CLINICAL PEARLS**
> - **PD**: panic attacks are the primary focus of the patient's anxiety.
>   - Diagnosis of exclusion after thorough medical history, substance use history, psychiatric review of symptoms, and physical exam.
> - **SP**: different objects/situations.
>   - Fainting in response to blood or injuries in 75% of individuals with SP.
>   - Determine circumstances that immediately precede fear or extreme avoidance (in history of present illness and childhood).
> - **SAD**: childhood history is important to differentiate from social withdrawal due to other causes (MDD, personality disorders, schizophrenia, PTSD).
>   - The content of the anxiety helps differentiate from other anxiety disorders.
> - **GAD**: typically no defining boundaries of the patient's anxiety, so requires thorough history to determine the presence/absence of triggers.
>   - High comorbidity (62% with MDD, 39.5% with dysthymia, 37.6% with alcoholism, 34.4% with SAD) confers greater functional impairment.

(Continued)

Differential diagnosis

Differential diagnosis of anxiety due to a non-psychiatric medical condition

Condition	Features
Angina and myocardial infarction (MI)	Dyspnea, chest pain, palpitations, diaphoresis, hypertension, diabetes mellitus, hyperlipidemia, obesity, possible history of MI
Asthma	Dyspnea, wheezing
Cardiac dysrhythmias	Palpitations, dyspnea, syncope
Hyperthyroidism	Palpitations, diaphoresis, tachycardia, heat intolerance
Hypoglycemia	Random glucose <70 mg/dL
Hypoparathyroidism	Muscle cramps, paresthesias
Pheochromocytoma	Headache, diaphoresis, hypertension
Pulmonary embolus	Dyspnea, hyperpnea, chest pain
Seizure disorder	Unilateral or bilateral convulsions, abrupt change in behavior or personality that resolves after an episode
Substance/medication-induced anxiety disorder	Positive urine toxicology; history of substance use/abuse
Transient ischemic attacks	Unilateral or bilateral weakness or change in sensation, speech, vision

Differential diagnosis of anxiety among psychiatric conditions

Condition	Features
Fear or normal shyness	Fear response is appropriate and does not impair work, school, or interpersonal functioning
Separation anxiety disorder	Excessive anxiety about physical separation from a loved one
Panic disorder	Recurrent and unprovoked panic attacks with consequent anticipatory anxiety
Agoraphobia	Avoidance of certain places (e.g., bridges, crowds) due to fear of having a panic attack; may avoid leaving home; often comorbid with panic disorder
Specific phobia	Intense anxiety (possibly panic) provoked by exposure to specific object, animal, or situation
Social anxiety disorder	Excessive fear of embarrassment/humiliation in social situations; may trigger panic attack
Generalized anxiety disorder	Sustained anxiety/worry about multiple things (e.g., work, school performance, finances) and accompanied by persistent physiological symptoms; anxiety is not limited to a specific object or scrutiny in social situations
Post-traumatic stress disorder	Re-experiencing of past traumatic event with associated fear response (intrusive memories, nightmares, flashbacks) may occur spontaneously or be triggered by trauma reminders
Obsessive-compulsive disorder	Repetitive obsessive thoughts and/or ritualistic behaviors; anxiety may be temporarily relieved by compulsions; preventing compulsions may trigger panic attack

Differential diagnosis of anxiety among psychiatric conditions	
Condition	Features
Major depressive disorder	Depressed mood and/or lack of interest, associated with changes in sleep and appetite and other symptoms, including possible suicidal ideation; anxiety disorders often comorbid
Illness anxiety disorder	Fear of developing a serious illness; may seek medical attention repeatedly
Avoidant personality disorder	Pervasive social inhibition, feelings of inadequacy, extreme sensitivity to negative evaluation; diminished capacity for intimacy and omnipresence of symptoms differentiates from those with SAD

Typical presentation

- **PD:** young adult patient with recent life stressor presents (1) with impairing anxiety about having spontaneous panic attacks, or (2) to primary care or ER for evaluation of terrifying physical symptoms (of panic attack).
- **SP:** fearful avoidance of specific activities; usually begins in childhood but may be more impairing in adulthood.
- **SAD:** patient who was shy as a child presents for treatment in early adulthood. Describes problems during school transitions when s/he had to interact with new peers, and has a history of avoiding school-related activities. Longs for interpersonal relationships, though either avoids important social situations (e.g., misses good friend's wedding) or attends by using excessive alcohol.
- **GAD:** young adult patient has always been a "worrier;" has trouble sleeping, feels on edge, tense, and cannot relax; finances, family, and work are focus of worry.

Clinical diagnosis

History

Panic disorder

- Spontaneous and recurrent panic attacks followed by ≥1 month of persistent concerns about additional attacks, and/or a clear change in behavior related to the attacks (e.g., avoidance of activities).
- *Panic attacks are necessary but not sufficient.*
  - Panic attack = intense fear and physical symptoms of anxiety that rapidly increase (~10 minutes) and usually last 20–30 minutes.
  - Palpitations, sweating, trembling, choking sensation, chest pain, nausea, dizziness, paresthesias, chills or hot flashes, dyspnea, derealization/depersonalization, fear of losing control or "going crazy," fear of dying or imminent doom.
  - Can occur in multiple psychiatric conditions or with emotional excitement, physical exertion, sexual activity, emotional trauma, or substances (e.g., caffeine, nicotine, cocaine).
- Differential must rule out medical causes of panic attacks, especially if patient is beyond young adulthood.

Specific phobia

- Changes from DSM-IV to DSM-5:
  - Same core features, including behavioral avoidance and/or excessive fear that interferes with psychosocial functioning.

- Removed requirement that adults must recognize that their fear is excessive or unreasonable.
  - ≥6 month duration requirement now applies to all ages.
- Fears are common in childhood, but SP represents fears that extend beyond age-appropriate period. Specific types:
  - Animal; natural environmental (e.g., heights, storms, water); blood/injection/injury; situational (e.g., airplanes, elevators, enclosed spaces); other (e.g., avoidance of situations that may lead to choking, vomiting, or contracting an illness; in children, avoidance of loud sounds or costumed characters).

Social anxiety disorder

- Determine whether social avoidance is persistent/pervasive, unrelated to an altered mood or cognitive state, and contextually linked to embarrassment/humiliation.
- Assess reasons for social anxiety/avoidance.
- Assess for symptoms in childhood; delineate course and chronicity.
- Evaluate for impairment (school, work, presence/absence of relationships).
- Obtain corroborative information from family (and teachers if patient is school-aged).
- Screen for substance abuse.

Generalized anxiety disorder

- Excessive anxiety/worry about multiple activities for more days than not over 6 months.
- ≥3 of 6 symptoms:
  1. restlessness or feeling on edge;
  2. easily fatigued;
  3. difficulty concentrating or mind going blank;
  4. irritability;
  5. muscle tension;
  6. sleep disturbance.
- Known as a "worrier" for a significant time prior to onset of the disorder.
- Always screen for depressive symptoms and substance use; with comorbidity, anxiety usually develops first.
- Medical comorbidities may predispose to or may exacerbate existing GAD.
  - Physical symptoms are common (e.g., headache, abdominal pain, intermittent diarrhea).

Physical and mental status exams

- Diagnosis for all is based on history.
- In SAD, behavior during clinical interview (e.g., inhibition, poor eye contact, soft/paucity of speech) may provide initial data (although some may perform well in intimate environments).

Disease severity classification

- Panic Disorder Severity Scale.
  - Proposed as standard rating scale to assess severity and response to treatment; score of ≤5 may indicate remission.
- Hamilton Anxiety Rating Scale (HAM-A): 14 items to assess GAD severity and response to treatment.

Laboratory diagnosis

List of diagnostic tests

- All tests are to rule out non-primary-psychiatric conditions.

- **PD**: CBC, metabolic panel, EKG, and chest x-ray (CXR) as initial work-up for cardiac, metabolic, pulmonary, and infectious etiologies.
  - Thyroid panel.
  - If risk factors and high suspicion of myocardial infarction, consider troponins × 3.
  - If hemoptysis and high suspicion of pulmonary disease, consider chest CT with contrast to rule out pulmonary embolus.
- Urine toxicology if comorbid substance abuse is suspected.

Diagnostic algorithm

- **PD**: history of recurrent, unprovoked panic attacks for which medical causes were ruled out by laboratory and imaging tests, and substances or medications that may activate the sympathetic nervous system are absent.

Potential pitfalls/common errors made regarding diagnosis of disease

- **PD**: rule out non-psychiatric etiologies first.
- **SP**: avoidance of situations may mask fear symptoms.
- **SAD**: may be masked by depressive disorders or alcohol use.
- **GAD**: rule out non-psychiatric etiologies first.
  - Patients may feel pervasive worry is warranted.
  - Always assess for comorbid MDD.

Treatment
Treatment rationale

- The goal of treatment is full remission.
- The first step should consist of educating the patient about the disorder.
  - Include supportive counseling about sleep hygiene, minimizing caffeine consumption, incorporating an exercise routine, and coping with stress.
  - Education is especially important in PD, as many patients benefit from knowing that their symptoms have a medical explanation.
- Referral for psychotherapy or psychiatric evaluation should be guided by patient preference, symptom severity, and potential drug–drug interactions and side effects.
- Psychotherapies:
  - Moderate evidence for efficacy, either alone or in combination with medications.
  - Therapists range in degrees (e.g., MD, PhD, LCSW) as well as modality; matching modality to disorder aids in effective referrals.
- Medications:
  - First line for all except SP is generally a serotonin-selective reuptake inhibitor (SSRI) or serotonin–norepinephrine reuptake inhibitor (SNRI) ± short-term benzodiazepine.
    - Start antidepressants at low dose and follow with slow titration; may want to inform patients that panic symptoms may initially get worse before improving.
    - Conservative approach: SSRI without benzodiazepine.
    - If high frequency or severe panic attacks and/or significant impairment in daily functioning, may include short course (4–8 weeks) of benzodiazepine alongside SSRI.
  - For performance-based SA (e.g., playing an instrument, giving a speech), prn beta-adrenergic receptor antagonists (e.g., propranolol, atenolol) have demonstrated moderate success.

- Benzodiazepines are very useful, with choice of agent determined by target symptom and method of use.
  - Panic attacks may be treated with prn lorazepam or alprazolam, but short half-lives and high addiction potential may make use problematic in vulnerable patients.
  - Clonazepam is longer-acting and may have lower addiction potential; perhaps the best choice when used for immediate relief as SSRI takes effect.
- Tricyclic antidepressants (TCAs) and monoamine oxidase inhibitors (MAOIs) are third- and fourth-line treatments, due to their significant side effects, dietary restrictions, and drug–drug interactions.
  - Among TCAs, clomipramine and imipramine have largest evidence base. Avoid TCAs in patients at increased risk for suicide.
  - MAOIs may have greater efficacy for SAD.
- If >1 antidepressant in a class (e.g., SSRI) is not tolerated or effective, consider switching to a different class (e.g., SNRI), or augmenting with a benzodiazepine (GAD, PD), bupropion, buspirone (GAD), tricyclic (GAD, PD), or an anticonvulsant (SAD).
- Use caution when combining an SSRI with a TCA, as increased TCA blood levels can result.
- Continue medications for ≥8–12 months in all anxiety disorders.
  - Due to often chronic course, may need to continue for longer, or indefinitely.

When to hospitalize
- Hospitalization for an isolated anxiety disorder is uncommon, but admission for further work-up may be necessary for a first presentation.

Managing the hospitalized patient
- Benzodiazepines atop an SSRI or SNRI may be warranted in order to abate intense symptoms. Patients may also benefit from brief supportive psychotherapy in this setting.

Table of treatment

Medical Antidepressants	

SSRI
• Citalopram, fluoxetine, and paroxetine
  • Start 10 mg/day; increase by 10 mg every week; target dose 10–40 mg (60 mg max with fluoxetine)
• Escitalopram (½ dosing of citalopram)
  • Start 5 mg/day; increase by 5 mg every week; target dose 10–20 mg
• Sertraline
  • Start 25 mg/day; increase by 25 mg every 3–5 days; target dose 50–200 mg
• Fluvoxamine ER
  • Start 100 mg/day; increase by 50 mg every week; target dose 100–300 mg
	• Target: PD, GAD, SAD
	• May hold at low target dose for 3–4 weeks and assess for effect
	• Side effects: nausea, vomiting, dry mouth, headache, somnolence, insomnia, sweating, tremor, diarrhea, sexual dysfunction, syndrome of inappropriate antidiuretic hormone (especially in elderly), CYP 2D6 inhibition (paroxetine; less for citalopram and escitalopram), withdrawal/discontinuation effects (fatigue, dysphoria, psychomotor changes)

(Continued)

(Continued)

SNRI
• Venlafaxine XR
  • Start 37.5 mg/day; increase by 37.5 mg every 4–7 days; target dose 75–225 mg
• Duloxetine
  • Start 20 mg/day; increase by 20–30 mg every 4–7 days; target dose 60–120 mg
	• Target: PD, GAD, SAD
	• Side effects: nausea, somnolence, dizziness, dry mouth, nervousness, tremor, insomnia, constipation, sexual dysfunction, sweating, anorexia, blood pressure elevation, orthostasis, conduction defects, ventricular arrhythmias, discontinuation effects; half usual dose used in moderate hepatic or renal impairment (not applicable for duloxetine)

Noradrenergic and specific serotonergic antidepressant (NASSA) • Mirtazapine • Start 7.5–15 mg/day at bedtime; increase by 7.5–15 mg every week; target dose 15–45 mg **TCA and MAOI** • Recommend referral to experienced psychiatrist	• Target: GAD • Side effects: increased appetite, weight gain, headache, drowsiness, dizziness, nausea, vomiting, diarrhea, increased heart rate, overactive reflexes, loss of coordination

Benzodiazepines
Longer-acting
• Clonazepam
  • 0.25 mg twice daily; increase by 0.25–0.5 mg every 4 days; target 0.5–2 mg/day
Shorter-acting
• Alprazolam
  • 0.5 mg every 6–8 hours; increase by 0.5 mg every 3 days; target 1–4 mg/day
	• Target: PD, GAD, SAD, SP
	• Side effects: sedation, ataxia, hypotonia, paradoxical agitation, memory changes, withdrawal syndrome, dependence, interaction with alcohol

5-HT$_{1A}$ agonist
• Buspirone
  • 5 mg twice daily; increase by 5 mg every 2–3 days; target 10–60 mg/day
Beta-adrenergic antagonist
• Propranolol
  • 20–40 mg 1 hour before performance
	• Target: GAD
	• Side effects: dizziness, headache, drowsiness, light-headedness, fatigue, nausea, insomnia, restlessness
	• Target: off-label use for SP or SAD related to public speaking or performance
	• Ensure no history of asthma; caution in patients with diabetes as it can mask hypoglycemia; caution if low blood pressure
	• Side effects: fatigue, vomiting, diarrhea, constipation, rash, dizziness, irregular heartbeat, low blood pressure, shortness of breath

Anticonvulsant (GABAergic) • Gabapentin • 100 mg 2–3 times daily; increase by 100 mg every 3 days; target dose 100–1800 mg/day	• Target: off-label use for SAD, GAD, or SP • May be used instead of benzodiazepines in patients at risk for addiction • Side effects: somnolence, dizziness, ataxia, fatigue, nystagmus, nausea, dry mouth, constipation, peripheral edema, rhinitis, pharyngitis, visual changes, myalgia
Psychological • PD → CBT, focused psychodynamic therapy • SP → behavior therapy, exposure therapy • SAD → CBT, focused psychodynamic therapy • GAD → CBT	Begin with brief therapies (≤3 months)

(Continued)

Complementary	Meditation and mindfulness exercise have been
• Mindfulness exercises • Meditation • Herbals and extracts (limited efficacy)	shown to have most benefit; no evidence for efficacy of herbals or extracts
Other	Have been shown to reduce anxiety and stress
• Exercise • Sleep hygiene	and to aid in preventing relapse

Prevention/management of complications

Complication	Management
Potential psychopharmacologic complications	
Activating psychological and behavioral effects (e.g., fluoxetine) or sedating effects (e.g., paroxetine) may occur during the initial 1–2 weeks of treatment	• Small initial doses and slow titration may prevent activation effects • For activation effects, consider short-term use of prn benzodiazepines • For intolerable sedating effects, consider change to different SSRI
Tolerance and potential dependence may occur with long-term use of benzodiazepines	Consider cross-tapering to a different adjunctive medication
Increased blood pressure may occur with SNRI (e.g., venlafaxine)	• Measure blood pressure at initial and subsequent visits • If hypertension persists or worsens, try switching to an SSRI, or consult with primary care physician if patient prefers to remain on SNRI
Potential psychotherapy complications	
Heightened anxiety and increased frequency of panic attacks may emerge in initial phase of treatment, particularly with exposure therapy	• Consider initiating a short-term course of a potent anxiolytic (e.g., alprazolam)

Management/treatment algorithm (Algorithm 12.1)

CLINICAL PEARLS
- For medication initiation, "start low and go slow," particularly in patients with prominent autonomic hyperactivity.
  - Medication and psychotherapy treatments require continual supportive communication with the patient, as both are associated with heightened anxiety symptoms in the initial phases.
  - Work with the patient to set reasonable and reachable goals to avoid early drop-out from treatment.

Special populations
Pregnancy
- Consider referral for new or additional psychotherapy in pregnant patients with anxiety disorders.

Algorithm 12.1 Proposed treatment algorithm for anxiety disorder

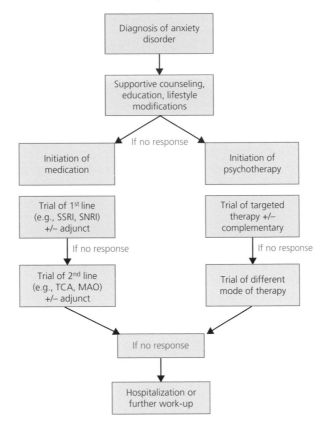

(Note: adequate duration of medication trials ranges from 3 to 6 months. Adequate duration of brief psychotherapy trials should not exceed 3 months. If initial onset of anxiety symptoms is sudden and not consistent with patient's temperament, consider further medical work-up.)

- Increased risk for GAD onset or worsening during pregnancy and post partum.
- Evaluate risk/benefit of remaining on medications.
  - Exposure to TCAs and SSRIs during the first trimester was not associated with a statistically significant increased risk of congenital anomalies.
  - No conclusive evidence of teratogenicity with benzodiazepine use, although possible 2-fold increased risk of orofacial clefts. Perinatal use has been linked to neonatal hypotonia, apnea, hypothermia, and feeding problems.
  - If patient becomes pregnant while taking an SSRI, benzodiazepine, or TCA, consider a safely scheduled taper, especially in patients with less severe anxiety.
    - Requires increased vigilance and symptom monitoring.

Others
- In patients with a history of addiction, limit/avoid use of benzodiazepines.

Prognosis

> **BOTTOM LINE/CLINICAL PEARLS**
> - **PD**: chronic disorder that may abate with treatment but often recurs.
> - **SP**: relapse is expected; non-adherence and treatment drop-out are common.
> - **SAD**: fluctuating course based on life stressors; unknown prognosis but psychotherapy may ameliorate impairment.
> - **GAD**: if medical comorbidities exist, prognosis is considered poor.

Natural history of untreated disease
- **PD**: may result in agoraphobia, comorbid substance use disorders, increased anger outbursts.
- **SP**: worsening avoidant behaviors. Increased likelihood of encountering the situation if the object is a necessary part of functioning (e.g., dentist). The majority of untreated phobias may not limit daily functioning.
- **SAD**: possible isolation from supportive networks from avoidance of school or work; increased risk for development of comorbidity (e.g., agoraphobia, substance use). If symptoms are severe and onset is during childhood, may lead to impairment of educational attainment and subsequently higher unemployment and financial dependency.
- **GAD**: typical course is chronic with a low rate of remission and a moderate recurrence rate; increased risk for comorbid substance use and MDD.

Prognosis for treated patients
- **PD**:
  - SSRI: 50–70% response.
  - CBT: 50–70% response.
  - Combined treatment is more effective.
- **SP**: despite a low rate of seeking treatment (~8%), patients experience a high response rate to exposure therapy (~90%).
- **SAD**:
  - SSRI: 15–35% response.
  - CBT, psychodynamic therapy: 70% response; 40% remission.
- **GAD**:
  - SSRI: 60–70% response; 50% remission.
  - Placebo: 30–50% response; 25% remission.
  - CBT: 33% response.
  - Not yet shown if combined treatment has greater benefit.

Reading list
Culpepper L. Use of algorithms to treat anxiety disorders in primary care. J Clin Psychiatry 2003;64(suppl 2):30–33.

Fricchione G. Clinical practice. Generalized anxiety disorder. N Engl J Med 2004; 351(7):675–82.

Goodwin RD, Fegusson DM, Horwood LJ. Early anxious/withdrawn behaviours predict later internalizing disorders. J Child Psychol Psychiatry 2004;45:874–83.

Hettema JM, Neale MC, Kendler KS. A review and meta-analysis of the genetic epidemiology of anxiety disorders. Am J Psychiatry 2001;158(10):1568–78.

Hettema JM, Prescott CA, Myers JM, Neale MC, Kendler KS. The structure of genetic and environmental risk factors for anxiety disorders in men and women. Arch Gen Psychiatry 2005;62(2):182–9.

Kessler RC, Chiu WT, Jin R, Ruscio AM, Shear K, Walters EE. The epidemiology of panic attacks, panic disorder, and agoraphobia in the National Comorbidity Survey Replication. Arch Gen Psychiatry 2006;63(4):415–24.

Leichsenring F, Salzer S, Beutel ME, et al. Long-term outcome of psychodynamic therapy and cognitive-behavioral therapy in social anxiety disorder. Am J Psychiatry 2014;171(10):1074–82.

Lieb R, Wittchen HU, Höfler M, Fuetsch M, Stein MB, Merikangas KR. Parental psychopathology, parenting styles, and the risk of social phobia in offspring: a prospective-longitudinal community study. Arch Gen Psychiatry 2002;57:859–66.

Martin EI, Ressler KJ, Binder E, Nemeroff CB. The neurobiology of anxiety disorders: brain imaging, genetics, and psychoneuroendocrinology. Psychiatr Clin North Am 2009;32:549–75.

Suggested websites

Anxiety and Depression Association of America. http://www.adaa.org

National Alliance on Mental Illness. https://www.nami.org/Learn-More/Mental-Health-Conditions/Anxiety-Disorders

National Institute of Mental Health. http://www.nimh.nih.gov/health/topics/anxiety-disorders/index.shtml

TeensHealth. http://teenshealth.org/teen/your_mind/mental_health/anxiety.html

Guidelines
National society guidelines

Title	Source	Weblink
Treatment (Anxiety)	Anxiety and Depression Association of America (ADAA), 2015	http://www.adaa.org/resources-professionals/practice-guidelines-gadandhttp://www.adaa.org/resources-professionals/clinical-practice-review-social-anxiety
Anxiety Disorders	American Family Physician (AFP), 2015	http://www.aafp.org/afp/topicModules/viewTopicModule.htm?topicModuleId=85

Evidence

Type of evidence	Title and comment	Weblink
Review and meta-analysis	A review and meta-analysis of the genetic epidemiology of anxiety disorders. **Comment:** Genetic risk of anxiety disorders.	http://www.ncbi.nlm.nih.gov/pubmed/11578982
Review and meta-analysis	A review and meta-analysis of the heritability of specific phobia subtypes and corresponding fears. **Comment:** A review of heritability of specific phobia.	http://www.ncbi.nlm.nih.gov/pubmed/23774007
Review and meta-analysis	Newer antidepressants and panic disorder: a meta-analysis. **Comment:** A meta-analysis of SSRI and SNRI for treatment of anxiety and panic disorders.	http://www.ncbi.nlm.nih.gov/pubmed/23111544

(Continued)

(*Continued*)

Type of evidence	Title and comment	Weblink
Epidemiologic study	The epidemiology of panic attacks, panic disorder, and agoraphobia in the National Comorbidity Survey Replication. **Comment:** Epidemiological data on panic attacks, panic disorder, and agoraphobia.	http://www.ncbi.nlm.nih.gov/pmc/articles/PMC1958997/
Review	The structure of genetic and environmental risk factors for anxiety disorders in men and women. **Comment:** Genetic and environmental risk factors for anxiety disorders.	http://www.ncbi.nlm.nih.gov/pubmed/15699295
Review	Contributions of the amygdala to emotion processing: from animal models to human behavior. **Comment:** Emotion processing and role of amygdala.	http://www.ncbi.nlm.nih.gov/pubmed/16242399
Review	Neuronal signaling of fear memory. **Comment:** Key brain structures involved in establishing and consolidating fear memory.	http://www.ncbi.nlm.nih.gov/pubmed/15496862
Review	Neuroanatomical hypothesis of panic disorder, revised. **Comment:** Neuroanatomical aspects of panic disorder.	http://www.ncbi.nlm.nih.gov/pubmed/10739407

Additional material for this chapter can be found online at: www.mountsinaiexpertguides.com/psychiatry

This includes advice for patients, a case study, ICD codes, and multiple choice questions.

CHAPTER 13

Trauma- and Stressor-Related Disorders

Rachel Yehuda, Amy Lehrner, and Laura C. Pratchett

Icahn School of Medicine at Mount Sinai, New York; and, James J. Peters VA Medical Center, Bronx, NY, USA

OVERALL BOTTOM LINE
- Trauma exposure is common in the population, but only a small percentage of those exposed develop posttraumatic stress disorder (PTSD).
- Risk factors for the development of PTSD include nature and severity of the stressor, prior traumatization, personal and family psychiatric history, lack of social support, recent life stressors, female gender, and low education.
- Effective treatments, such as trauma focused and other psychotherapeutic options and medications, are available; in many, there is spontaneous remission as natural recovery resources are mobilized.
- When trauma exposure involves traumatic brain or other physical injury, and/or when there is a history of prior trauma exposures, and/or when posttraumatic symptoms present with comorbidities such as substance use disorders, depression, or suicidality, PTSD symptoms are particularly intractable and may not abate even with treatment.

Background
- The essential feature of PTSD and other stressor-related disorders (e.g., acute stress disorder, adjustment disorder) is that they reflect psychological reactions attributed to exposure to environmental events.
- Disorders primarily related to trauma in childhood have been added to DSM-5 (e.g., Reactive Attachment Disorder, Disinhibited Social Engagement Disorder).
- The multiple conditions and subtypes acknowledge individual differences in expressions of clinical distress, which may include anxiety- or fear-based reactions, dysphoric/anhedonic symptoms, angry/aggressive behaviors, or dissociative symptoms.

Definition of disease
- PTSD develops following exposure to actual or threatened death, serious injury, or sexual violence, and includes symptoms across four clusters:
  1. intrusions (e.g., unwanted and intrusive memories or images);
  2. avoidance (e.g., avoidance of people, places, or things that serve as reminders of the trauma);

Mount Sinai Expert Guides: Psychiatry, First Edition. Edited by Asher B. Simon, Antonia S. New, and Wayne K. Goodman.
© 2017 John Wiley & Sons, Ltd. Published 2017 by John Wiley & Sons, Ltd.
Companion website: www.mountsinaiexpertguides.com/psychiatry

3. alterations in cognitions or mood (e.g., anhedonia, numbness, exaggerated negative beliefs about oneself, others, or the world);
4. arousal (e.g., hypervigilance, irritable/angry behavior).

- The symptoms co-occur for at least a month and cause significant distress and/or impairment in social, interpersonal, and occupational function.

Disease classification

PTSD and other stressor-related disorders (e.g., acute stress disorder, adjustment disorder) are now classified in their own category – Trauma- and Stressor-Related Disorders – in recognition of the common etiological factor of exposure to trauma or a stressful event. PTSD and acute stress disorder had been classified as anxiety disorders since 1980 (DSM-III).

Incidence/prevalence

- Projected lifetime risk for PTSD is close to 9% (DSM-5); 12-month prevalence rate among adults is 3.5% (DSM-5), with women showing twice the prevalence of men.
- Among those exposed to traumatic events that can elicit PTSD, approximately 15–25% develop the disorder, but the conditional probability varies as a function of specific population, individual risk factors, and trauma type.
- Higher prevalence rates (1/3 to 1/2) are found in those exposed to rape, combat, and genocide.

Economic impact

- PTSD patients have high healthcare utilization and great loss of productivity as a result of unemployment, disability, and sick leave.
- Additional costs to society occur due to frequently comorbid medical conditions such as cardiovascular disease, diabetes, metabolic syndrome, immune-related conditions, and pain disorders.
- Estimates of the cost of PTSD among military personnel due to medical care, lost productivity, and suicide range from $4 to 6 billion over 2 years.

Etiology

- PTSD cannot occur in the absence of trauma exposure, but it is now clear that PTSD results from a complex interplay of genetic, developmental, endocrine, neurobiological, cognitive, and environmental factors.
- No specific gene has been identified to date as universally applicable to PTSD risk, but promising genes have been identified that may increase susceptibility to PTSD, including genes involved in regulation of the neuroendocrine stress response. More research is needed.

Pathophysiology

- Alterations in stress-related systems in the brain and periphery have been observed, leading to heightened reactivity to environmental stimuli.
- PTSD is associated with:
  - enhanced glucocorticoid sensitivity and increased sympathetic nervous system activation;
  - resultant hormonal imbalances (e.g., lower peripheral cortisol levels and elevated catecholamines);
  - altered inflammatory processes;
  - elevated baseline heart rate, blood pressure, and startle responses.
- Brain alterations in PTSD suggest a dysregulation of the neural circuit controlling amygdala inhibition by the anterior cingulate cortex, which likely amplifies fear signals and concomitant behavioral responses. The size of the hippocampus is smaller and that of the amygdala larger, compared to non-trauma-exposed controls, perhaps related to cognitive complaints frequent in PTSD.

Predictive/risk factors

Pre-traumatic risk factors:

- Individual and/or family psychiatric history, particularly prior PTSD.
- Female gender.
- Childhood abuse or adversity, or prior trauma exposure in adulthood.
- Low socioeconomic status, education.
- Younger age.

Peri-traumatic risk factors:

- Severity and duration of trauma.
- Biological dysregulation: increased glucocorticoid sensitivity, low cortisol signaling, elevated heart rate and catecholamines.
- Extreme distress, anxiety, or dissociation.

Post-traumatic risk factors:

- Lack of social support.
- Ongoing/new life stress and continued adverse events.
- Comorbid physical conditions (traumatic brain injury, loss of limb, pain).
- Poor behavioral coping strategies, e.g., drug abuse, poor sleep hygiene.

Prevention

> **BOTTOM LINE/CLINICAL PEARLS**
> - No primary or secondary prevention intervention has been demonstrated to prevent the development of the disease.
> - Preliminary findings suggest that early specialized psychosocial interventions with children and families may enhance recovery following trauma exposure.
> - Current investigations examine interventions that target distress (e.g., cortisol administration, noradrenergic blockers). There is also interest in resilience training as a prophylactic.

Screening

- The goal of screening those with recent trauma exposure is to identify extreme reactions – either extreme distress or extreme disconnection (which can be manifested as lack of normal distress).
- Acute distress that seems appropriate to the event will most likely lead to natural recovery as most post-trauma symptoms resolve within 1–3 months.
- When screening for PTSD several months or years after an event, it is important to establish the range of traumatic events and then identify the nature and severity of posttraumatic symptoms to the specific event(s).
- Symptoms can be identified using several checklists.
  - For patients with a known history of trauma:
    - Impact of Event Scale – Revised (IES-R; Weiss DS, Marmar CR. In: Wilson J, Keane TM (eds). Assessing Psychological Trauma and PTSD. New York: Guilford Press, 1996, pp. 399–411);
    - Trauma Screening Questionnaire (TSQ; Brewin CR, Rose S, Andrews B, et al. Brief screening instrument for post-traumatic stress disorder. Br J Psychiatry 2002;181:158–162);
    - The Peritraumatic Dissociative Experiences Questionnaire (PDEQ; Marmar CR, Weiss DS, Metzler TJ. In: Wilson JP, Keane TM (eds). Assessing Psychological Trauma and PTSD. New York: Guilford Press, 1997, pp. 412–28) can assess peri-traumatic dissociation.

Diagnosis

> **BOTTOM LINE/CLINICAL PEARLS**
> - Ask directly about trauma exposure because patients may not spontaneously report trauma history. Ask about *childhood abuse, sexual assault, intimate partner violence, serious accidents, and criminal victimization*.
> - Then ask about the impact these events have had in terms of distress and functional impairment in the immediate aftermath of their occurrence and in the present. Patients do not experience such inquiries as intrusive.
> - Essentially, in PTSD, the memory of trauma is re-experienced in an intrusive manner and results in distress. Attempts are made to avoid reminders and shifts occur in the way a person feels about the world or his/her personal safety. These disrupt relationships and functioning. Physiological manifestations such as anger and irritability, reckless or self-destructive behavior, hypervigilance, exaggerated startle, and problems with concentration and sleep also occur.

Differential diagnosis

Differential diagnosis	Features
Bipolar disorder	- Major depressive episodes may occur in the aftermath of trauma but do not specifically include re-experiencing symptoms such as nightmares and intrusive memories, or efforts to avoid reminders of the trauma - The irritability, reduced sleep, and impulsiveness associated with PTSD differ from symptoms of (hypo)mania in that they are more variable and reactive (rather than pervasive and consistent as in mania, for example) - Sleep problems in PTSD do not reflect a reduced need for sleep (although nightmares may drive reduced desire for sleep), and the impulsiveness is not linked specifically to periods of mood elevation/irritability
Obsessive-compulsive disorder	In PTSD, apparently compulsive behaviors such as repeated checking of doors and windows may be one aspect of the exaggerated concerns for safety and hypervigilance characteristic of the disorder. Other behaviors such as repeated washing may reflect the experience of being physically violated, rather than a delusional concern with cleanliness. Unwanted intrusive thoughts are distinguished from obsessions in that they are related to the trauma and are not irrational in content
Phobia	Avoidance of trauma reminders is common in PTSD and can mirror phobic avoidance. However, in PTSD the object is avoided in order to minimize the intense distress triggered by reminders of the trauma, rather than because the object itself is feared
Generalized anxiety disorder (GAD)	While individuals with PTSD often report frequent worry and anxiety, GAD should not be diagnosed when the worry occurs in the context of PTSD
Personality disorders (especially borderline personality disorder and antisocial personality disorder)	Without knowledge of trauma exposure, some of the behaviors and symptoms of PTSD might be seen as reflecting chronic emotional dysregulation or interpersonal and behavioral problems. In personality disorder these occur without a specific antecedent, although personality disorder patients frequently report childhood trauma. In PTSD, trauma-related changes in world view and sense of self are thought to underlie personality changes

Typical presentation

- Patients often present with mood swings (including anger, anxiety, numbness, guilt, and shame), poor sleep, emotional detachment from others, and diminished sense of safety.
- The identification of a trauma may be complicated by the intense desire to avoid talking about the experience.
- The defining features for diagnosis are the re-experiencing symptoms of nightmares (focused on either the content or emotional themes of the trauma), involuntary and intrusive recollections, intense emotional and physiological reactivity to reminders and, less frequently, dissociative flashbacks to the trauma.
- Interpersonal problems, substance use, and suicidality are common.

Clinical diagnosis

History

The diagnosis of PTSD requires that an individual has experienced or witnessed a traumatic event, or learned of trauma to a loved one. DSM-5 has slightly expanded on the type of events that qualify – actual or threatened death, serious injury, or sexual injury – and more clearly stipulates that the death of a loved one must occur in a violent or accidental way to be a precipitant of PTSD. DSM-5 removed the requirement for a specific peri-traumatic emotional response.

There are two new specifiers that more clearly delineate dissociative subtypes: depersonalization and derealization. Indeed, persons who have histories of chronic trauma or adverse childhood antecedents may have responded using dissociative mechanisms. These present quite differently and may have treatment implications. Dissociation may imply a host of other problems with emotion regulation and self-damaging behaviors.

A PTSD diagnosis requires that symptoms are present for at least one month. Classically, these symptoms have been thought to occur immediately following trauma exposure, but delayed onset is now recognized by a subtype.

Physical and mental status exams

- No physical exam is necessary, but it should be noted that trauma survivors with PTSD often have somatic complaints and physical consequences of traumatic events due to physical injury.
- Cognitive problems due to brain injury should be considered depending on the nature of the trauma.
- A mental status exam should pay close attention to *suicidality,* particularly in patients who have experienced extreme childhood trauma or atrocities. Dissociative flashbacks may include sensory experiences that can be differentiated from psychotic hallucinations by their focus on details of the trauma. PTSD flashbacks may also include amnesia for the experience or a sense of lost time. A chronic and exaggerated state of guilt or shame, intense hypervigilance, and fears for safety, or extreme mistrust of others could ostensibly appear paranoid or delusional, but when considered in the context of trauma reflect altered cognitions and hypervigilance.

Diagnostic algorithm (Algorithm 13.1)

Algorithm 13.1 Diagnostic algorithm for PTSD

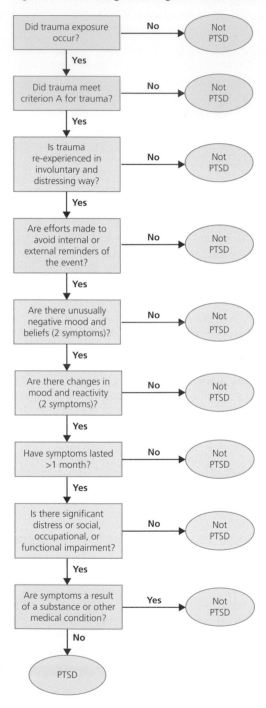

Potential pitfalls/common errors made regarding diagnosis of disease

• PTSD should not be diagnosed in response to events below the threshold specified in the diagnostic criteria, nor in response to the presence of one or two intrusive symptoms in the absence of the other required symptoms.

Treatment
Treatment rationale

• Psychotherapy is first-line treatment and much research supports cognitive behavioral and exposure based therapies such as cognitive processing therapy (CPT), prolonged exposure (PE), and eye movement desensitization and reprocessing (EMDR). Psychopharmacology is often used for stabilization, sleep, or comorbid depression, or as an alternative to psychotherapy for those unable or unwilling to engage in such treatment.
  • Sertraline and paroxetine have FDA approval for treating PTSD and should be considered first.
  • Preliminary support for the SNRI venlafaxine, and for atypical antipsychotics such as risperidone and quetiapine for sleep, re-experiencing symptoms, and irritability/anger, and for prazosin for nightmares.
  • Sleep medications such as trazodone and zolpidem are commonly prescribed. There is no evidence for the effectiveness of benzodiazepines.

When to hospitalize

• Suicidality, uncontrolled expressions of anger, or substance-related illness are the likely cause of hospitalization in this population.
• Residential PTSD treatment programs provide structure and supervision for patients to engage in intensive trauma-focused psychotherapy in a safe, substance-free environment.

Managing the hospitalized patient

• The goal of hospitalization is most commonly stabilization in these patients, and as such exploration of the trauma or related material is usually unhelpful.

Table of treatment

Medical	Comments
• Sertraline titrated to maximum response with tolerable side effects (max. 200 mg/day) • Paroxetine titrated to maximum response with tolerable side effects (max. 40–60 mg/day)	• Most common side effect complaints are sexual dysfunction and fatigue/drowsiness • Paroxetine is more sedating, whereas sertraline is more activating. These side effects can be used therapeutically and may guide medication choice. For example, paroxetine may help with insomnia and agitation; sertraline may be used with more depressive presentations
Psychological • CPT • PE • EMDR	• These treatments are all supported by efficacy studies • There is insufficient research to demonstrate whether cognitive behavioral therapies for trauma can be safely and effectively provided to patients with comorbid substance abuse disorders, although there is some evidence supporting congruent, rather than staggered, treatment • Patients with acute suicidality may not be appropriate for these intensive therapies in an outpatient setting

> **CLINICAL PEARLS**
> - Psychotherapy is the first-line treatment for PTSD.
> - Pharmacotherapy targeting specific symptoms such as nightmares may also help with symptom reduction.
> - Patients often complain that sleep is impossible without medication.

Special populations

- 80% of patients with PTSD have another comorbid disorder, most frequently MDD or substance abuse.
- Clinical symptoms may vary across cultures, and cultural concepts of distress should be evaluated with immigrant, refugee, or minority populations.

Prognosis

> **BOTTOM LINE/CLINICAL PEARLS**
> - PTSD trajectories include natural recovery, delayed onset, and chronic PTSD.
> - Symptoms can wax and wane; anniversary reactions are common.
> - Clinical studies indicate that over 80% of patients improve after specialized trauma-focused psychotherapy, although response rates are lower for combat veterans. Roughly 60% of patients respond to medication.
> - Many patients continue to report symptoms following brief interventions and require ongoing treatment.

Natural history of untreated disease

- While some patients experience recovery without treatment (1/2 of adults within 3 months), for others PTSD can be chronic and debilitating, lasting years and even decades.
- Symptoms usually begin within 3 months of the trauma, but there is evidence for a "delayed expression" course in which full criteria are not met for months or years.

Follow-up tests and monitoring

- Self-report measures, such as the PTSD Checklist (PCL), Davidson Trauma Scale (DTS), or IES-R can be used for symptom monitoring.

Reading list

Brady K, Pearlstein T, Asnis GM, et al. Efficacy and safety of sertraline treatment of posttraumatic stress disorder: a randomized controlled trial. JAMA 2000;283(14):1837–44.

Davidson J, Baldwin D, Stein DJ, et al. Treatment of posttraumatic stress disorder with venlafaxine extended release: a 6-month randomized controlled trial. Arch Gen Psychiatry 2006;63(10):1158–65.

Foa EB, Keane TM, Friedman MJ, Cohen JA (eds). Effective treatments for PTSD: practice guidelines from the International Society for Traumatic Stress Studies. New York: Guilford Press, 2008.

Institute of Medicine. Treatment of Posttraumatic Stress Disorder: An Assessment of the Evidence. Washington, DC: The National Academies Press, 2008.

Ipser JC, Stein DJ. Evidence-based pharmacotherapy of post-traumatic stress disorder (PTSD). Int J Neuropsychopharmacol 2012;15(6):825–40.

Marshall RD, Beebe KL, Oldham M, Zaninelli R. Efficacy and safety of paroxetine treatment for chronic PTSD: a fixed-dose, placebo-controlled study. Am J Psychiatry 2001;158(12):1982–8.

Watts BV, Schnurr PP, Mayo L, Young-Xu Y, Weeks WB, Friedman MJ. Meta-analysis of the efficacy of treatments for posttraumatic stress disorder. J Clin Psychiatry 2013;74(6):e541–50.

Zoladz PR, Diamond DM. Current status on behavioral and biological markers of PTSD: a search for clarity in a conflicting literature. Neurosci Biobehav Rev 2013;37(5):860–95.

Suggested websites

International Society for Traumatic Stress Studies. http://www.istss.org

National Center for PTSD. http://www.ptsd.va.gov/index.asp

National Institute of Mental Health. http://www.nimh.nih.gov/health/topics/post-traumatic-stress-disorder-ptsd

Guidelines
National guidelines

Title	Source	Weblink
VA/DoD Clinical Practice Guidelines	Veterans Affairs/Department of Defense, 2010	http://www.healthquality.va.gov/guidelines/MH/ptsd/
Practice Guideline for the Treatment of Patients with Acute Stress Disorder and Posttraumatic Stress Disorder	American Psychiatric Association, 2009	http://psychiatryonline.org/pb/assets/raw/sitewide/practice_guidelines/guidelines/acutestressdisorderptsd-watch.pdf
A guide to guidelines for the treatment of PTSD and related conditions	Journal of Traumatic Stress, 2010	http://www.ncbi.nlm.nih.gov/pubmed/20839310

International guidelines

Title	Source	Weblink
ISTSS Treatment Guidelines	International Society for Traumatic Stress Studies, 2nd edn, 2008	http://www.istss.org/treating-trauma/effective-treatments-for-ptsd,-2nd-edition.aspx

Evidence

Type of evidence	Title and comment	Website
Meta-analysis	Meta-analysis of the efficacy of treatments for posttraumatic stress disorder. **Comment:** Effective psychotherapies include: cognitive therapy, exposure therapy, and eye movement desensitization and reprocessing. Effective pharmacotherapies include: paroxetine, sertraline, fluoxetine, risperidone, topiramate, and venlafaxine.	http://www.ncbi.nlm.nih.gov/pubmed/23842024

(Continued)

(*Continued*)

Type of evidence	Title and comment	Website
RCT	Efficacy and safety of sertraline treatment of posttraumatic stress disorder: a randomized controlled trial. **Comment:** Double-blind, placebo-controlled trial demonstrating efficacy of sertraline in PTSD in flexible daily dosages of 50–200 mg/d, following 1 week at 25 mg/d vs placebo.	http://www.ncbi.nlm.nih.gov/pubmed/10770145
RCT	Efficacy and safety of paroxetine treatment for chronic PTSD: a fixed-dose, placebo-controlled study. **Comment:** Randomized, placebo-controlled study demonstrating efficacy of 20 and 40 mg paroxetine for PTSD.	http://www.ncbi.nlm.nih.gov/pubmed/11729013
RCT	Multicenter, double-blind comparison of sertraline and placebo in the treatment of posttraumatic stress disorder. **Comment:** Double-blind, placebo-controlled study demonstrating efficacy of sertraline in flexible daily doses ranging from 50 to 200 mg.	http://www.ncbi.nlm.nih.gov/pubmed/11343529

Additional material for this chapter can be found online at: www.mountsinaiexpertguides.com/psychiatry

This includes advice for patients, a case study, ICD codes, and multiple choice questions.

CHAPTER 14

Obsessive-Compulsive and Related Disorders

Dorothy E. Grice, Timothy Rice, and Wayne K. Goodman

Icahn School of Medicine at Mount Sinai, New York, NY, USA

OVERALL BOTTOM LINE
- Obsessive-compulsive disorder (OCD) is a common, often persistent illness marked by intrusive and disturbing thoughts, images, or urges (obsessions) and repetitive behaviors (compulsions). Typical obsessional themes include fears of illness/contamination, unwanted aggressive or sexual thoughts, fear of failed responsibilities, and need for symmetry/exactness. Compulsions such as excessive cleaning, repetitive checking, reassurance-seeking, and rearranging serve to neutralize the distress of obsessions. OCD presents with a wide range of symptoms and severity. The two mainstays of treatment are specialized psychotherapy and psychopharmacology.
- Body dysmorphic disorder (BDD) is characterized by significant chronic preoccupations and negative assessments regarding one's physical features, not related to an eating disorder.
- The core feature of hoarding disorder (HD) is persistent difficulty or distress discarding accumulated possessions such that the accrued items impede functional and safe use of living space.
- Trichotillomania (TTM) is defined by compulsive hair-pulling.

Background
Definition of disease
- **OCD:** intrusive, recurrent, and disturbing thoughts (obsessions) and repetitive behaviors (compulsions) that the individual feels driven to perform.
  - Obsessions (e.g., fear of illness, contamination, or death) trigger high levels of distress, and compulsions (e.g., excessive washing or checking) often serve to diminish or neutralize that distress.
- **BDD:** functionally impairing preoccupation with a perceived physical defect(s) that is not observable or appears slight to others.
  - Can lead to serial dermatological or surgical interventions that are medically unnecessary but of utmost importance to the patient.
- **HD:** persistent difficulty parting with possessions, regardless of their actual value.
  - Strong urge to collect and save items, and/or distress associated with letting go of possessions, leading to chronic patterns of excess acquisition.
- **TTM:** significant chronic hair-pulling.
  - Two phenomenologic subtypes. Individuals with automatic subtype report little or no awareness of their pulling, while individuals with targeted subtype report tension that is relieved through pulling.

Mount Sinai Expert Guides: Psychiatry, First Edition. Edited by Asher B. Simon, Antonia S. New, and Wayne K. Goodman.
© 2017 John Wiley & Sons, Ltd. Published 2017 by John Wiley & Sons, Ltd.
Companion website: www.mountsinaiexpertguides.com/psychiatry

Disease classification

OCD is in the new DSM-5 category "Obsessive-Compulsive and Related Disorders" that also includes BDD, HD, TTM, and Excoriation (skin-picking) Disorder. The common feature of these disorders is a preoccupation that is persistent, interfering, and accompanied by repetitive behaviors.

Incidence/prevalence

- OCD, BDD, and HD each have a general prevalence of 2–3%.
  - 20% of individuals with HD also have OCD.
  - BDD affects ~12% of dermatology and 50% of cosmetic surgery patients.
- TTM has a general prevalence of 1% and is more common in females.

Economic impact

The World Health Organization places OCD as one of the top 10 leading causes of disability in the developed world.

Etiology

- Research implicates both overlapping and unique genetic and environmental factors in the etiologies of OCD, BDD, HD, and TTM.
- Genetics accounts for nearly 50% of the variance of each disorder.
  - Early-onset OCD and tic-related OCD seem to have especially strong genetic risks.

Pathophysiology

- The observation that serotonin reuptake inhibitors (SRIs) are effective in OCD led to the serotonin hypothesis. However, direct support for a role of serotonin in OCD pathophysiology remains elusive.
- A role of the glutamatergic system in OCD is emerging from imaging studies and animal models.
- In OCD and BDD, functional brain imaging studies show increased activity in cortico-striato-thalamo-cortical circuitry that normalizes after successful treatment, whether with SRIs or cognitive behavioral therapy (CBT). TTM may be related to dysfunction in similar pathways.
- In HD, neuroimaging studies suggest the involvement of fronto-limbic circuits, including the ventromedial prefrontal and cingulate cortices.

Predictive/risk factors
OCD

Risk factor	
Temperament	Greater internalizing, negative emotionality, and behavioral inhibition in childhood
Environment	Traumatic events, perinatal complications
Genetics	First-degree relatives of those with early-onset OCD have 10-fold increased risk

Prevention

> **BOTTOM LINE/CLINICAL PEARLS**
> - Clinical experience suggests that early recognition and treatment of OCD may improve prognosis. However, there are no studies of prevention of OCD, BDD, HD, or TTM.

Screening

Patients are often reluctant to disclose unwanted obsessions and compulsive behaviors, and children may lack insight regarding their symptoms. Therefore, clinicians should probe for OCD symptoms in patients or parents of children presenting with mood or anxiety complaints (e.g., "Sometimes people are bothered by unwanted or repetitive thoughts or sudden, strong urges to check, wash, or count things. Does this ever happen to you?"). Some with OCD or BDD may present at dermatology practices due to sequelae from harsh washing rituals or with complaints and distress about body features. With HD, initial presentation may be in medical clinics or emergency departments from accidents in an unsafe and congested home. The scalp is the most common pulling site in TTM, although individuals may attempt to cover up signs of pulling with hats, wigs, makeup, etc.

Diagnosis

> **BOTTOM LINE/CLINICAL PEARLS**
> - Clinical history is paramount in diagnosis:
>   - OCD: typically both obsessions and compulsions;
>   - BDD: preoccupation and distress about perceived bodily flaws;
>   - HD: distress and difficulty when confronted with discarding accumulated possessions and a perceived need for ongoing accrual of items;
>   - TTM: pervasive hair-pulling aimed at relieving an urge or inner tension.
> - Insight can range from good to poor to absent at times.
> - The Yale–Brown Obsessive Compulsive Scale (Y-BOCS) is a clinician-administered scale that rates OCD severity and thus guides treatment recommendations.
> - Co-occurring depression should be considered.

Differential diagnosis

OCD

Differential diagnosis	Features that distinguish it from OCD
Delusions or psychosis	Themes tend to be more bizarre or paranoid; insight is less common
Generalized anxiety disorder	Excessive worries about real-life events; rituals usually absent
Obsessive-compulsive personality disorder	Excessive perfectionism and rigid control; obsessions and compulsions are absent
Complex motor tics	Tics typically have no meaning and are associated with other tics
Social anxiety	Withdrawal, avoidance, and isolation not due to specific obsessions

Typical presentation

Patients may not seek treatment until impairment (i.e., social, work, school) is significant, comorbid depressive symptoms have developed, or family members have urged evaluation. Childhood OCD is often recognized by parents or teachers who become aware of ritualized behaviors or reassurance-seeking that interferes with functioning. In HD, falls or other medical complications may be an unmasking event, particularly in the elderly. Individuals with BDD frequently present in cosmetic clinical settings seeking multiple procedures; self-injurious or self-mutilative behavior may also precipitate psychiatric contact. TTM may present concurrently with anxiety, depression, or OCD.

Clinical diagnosis

History

OCD

- Assess for obsessions and compulsions by asking about common themes (worries about contamination; cleaning/ordering; feared aggression/checking; unwanted sexual thoughts; need to ask, tell, or confess; reassurance-seeking).
- Full assessment for comorbid mood, anxiety, and OCD-related disorders is important.
- OCD with comorbid tic disorder is a new DSM-5 subtype.
- With an abrupt, explosive onset of OCD symptoms in a child, inquire about recent exposure to infectious agents, such as streptococcus.

BDD

- Elicit somatic preoccupations; common areas of concern include skin, hair, and nose.
- Preoccupation with muscle mass is denoted through a unique specifier in DSM-5.

HD

- Screen during routine exams, as symptoms are typically not volunteered.
- Difficulty parting with items, regardless of their value, helps establish accurate diagnosis. Up to 40% may accumulate an excessive number of pets.
- Ask if loved ones have ever expressed concerns about his/her accumulation of possessions.

TTM

- Elicit history of hair-pulling.
- Most common site is the scalp; the face, arms, legs, or other areas may be involved.

Physical and mental status exams

- In OCD, contamination obsessions and excessive washing compulsions can lead to abraded and damaged skin while other symptoms related to hygiene can cause avoidance of cleaning (to avoid activating time-consuming rituals) and thus an unkempt and unclean presentation. Contamination fears may lead to avoidance of appointments or difficulty shaking hands. Significant distress and anxiety is usually present. Patients with insight may fear for their mental health ("I know it sounds crazy but I have to…").
- In BDD, physical exam may be negative or discordant, despite the patient's concerns about flaws or imperfections. Scarring, skin lesions, or use of makeup to camouflage scars or perceived flaws is common. Significant anxiety and emotional dysregulation may emerge when discussing the clinical history. Suicidality, poor self-esteem, and limited insight frequently occur.
- In HD, individuals endorse feelings of distress, sadness, or grief when confronted with parting from their accrued possessions. Thoughts associated with hoarding are egosyntonic and not experienced as intrusive or unwanted.
- In TTM, individuals may be ashamed and actively attempt to mask or hide signs of hair-pulling.

Useful clinical decision rules and calculators

The Y-BOCS is the gold standard to assess OCD severity. As a rule of thumb, mild to moderate scores indicate that CBT and specifically exposure and response-prevention (ERP) may be appropriate as the first treatment intervention. Moderate, severe, or extreme scores indicate that both medication and CBT/ERP are warranted.

Disease severity classification

The Y-BOCS and children's Y-BOCS (CY-BOCS) aid in severity classification for OCD, can guide treatment choices, and can be used to assess response to treatment.

Laboratory diagnosis

List of diagnostic tests

There is no diagnostic laboratory test.

Lists of imaging techniques

Imaging tests are not indicated for a typical OCD, BDD, HD, or TTM presentation.

Diagnostic algorithm (Algorithm 14.1)

Algorithm 14.1 Diagnosis of OCD

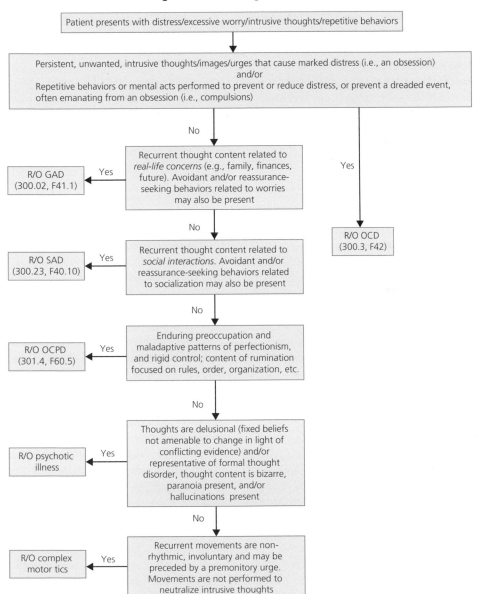

Potential pitfalls/common errors made regarding diagnosis of disease

- Mislabeling "compulsive" eating, gambling, or sexual behavior as OCD. OCD compulsions are not inherently pleasurable – at best, they relieve anxiety and distress generated by obsessions.
- In adults, the presence of insight distinguishes OCD from a psychotic illness. For children and adults, obsessions typically involve unrealistic fears; unlike delusions, obsessions are not fixed false beliefs.
- Distinguishing complex tics, as seen in Tourette syndrome and tic-related OCD, from compulsions may be difficult. There is often an urge to perform a tic but there is no meaning associated with involuntary tic behavior. Compulsions are typically done to prevent a feared consequence or reduce distress from an obsession.
- Always assess for suicide risk. Nearly two-thirds of those with BDD experience suicidal ideation, and almost one-third have attempted suicide.
- Providers in non-psychiatric medical settings should have a reasonable index of suspicion for HD in individuals who present with falls, injury, or fire at their congested or dangerously cluttered homes.
- Consider dementia and physical impairment in elders who present with falls and cluttered homes. Falls are common in the elderly and the causes need to be identified accurately. Cognitive impairment can lead to lack of attention to mail, bills, and cleaning.
- HD or BDD co-occurring with OCD may be difficult to identify.
- If an individual denies hair-pulling, the differential diagnosis includes medical etiologies for hair loss (e.g., infectious, hormonal, autoimmune).

Treatment
Treatment rationale
Established evidence-based treatments for OCD are CBT with ERP and psychopharmacology with SRIs (either the selective serotonin reuptake inhibitors or the non-selective tricyclic antidepressant clomipramine). Research demonstrates a larger effect size for ERP compared to medication. Regardless of age, patients with moderate to extreme OCD are best treated with combination treatment (ERP+SRI). For children presenting with mild to moderate severity, CBT is first-line treatment. The Y-BOCS and CY-BOCS can aid in determining severity.

An adequate SRI trial is at least 10–12 weeks (longer than in the treatment of depression and anxiety disorders). In general, SRI doses for optimal control of OCD are higher than those for depression. "Responders" to SRI treatment usually continue to have some residual obsessive and compulsive symptoms. No data suggest that one SRI is superior to another; selection is based on side effect profile.

The augmentation strategy with the most favorable evidence is the addition of an antipsychotic (e.g., risperidone) to an SRI. This appears to work best in OCD patients with tics.

Although no medication is FDA-approved for BDD, SRIs are considered first-line pharmacotherapy. Evidence suggests antipsychotics are not helpful, even in delusional BDD. For HD, harm reduction through environmental management is first-line treatment, and some evidence supports the use of SRIs. Cognitive restructuring and ERP are also appropriate treatments for both BDD and HD. For TTM, habit reversal training (HRT) is the first line intervention. SRIs may be used but evidence for their utility is limited.

When to hospitalize
- Hospitalization is generally not recommended unless the patient is suicidal or gravely disabled. Specialized residential or intensive outpatient OCD treatment programs may be indicated for severe or treatment-refractory patients.

Table of treatment

Psychotherapy	OCD: 12–16 sessions of ERP followed by ERP booster sessions as needed BDD: ERP, cognitive restructuring HD: cognitive restructuring, ERP, decision-making training TTM: HRT
Pharmacotherapy	OCD: SRIs (SSRIs and clomipramine) See Table 14.1
Multidisciplinary	HD: risk reduction through environmental management
Device-based	OCD: deep brain stimulation (DBS); reserved for severe intractable adult cases

Prevention/management of complications
- Titrate SRI medications to the final target dose to minimize medication-induced agitation and other adverse reactions.
- In BDD, suicide risk assessment and close follow-up are indicated before and during treatment.
- In HD, extreme environmental manipulation without ongoing clinical treatment to minimize re-acquisition of items may increase distress and lead to relapse.
- In TTM, symptoms will often improve when co-occurring disorders are treated.

Management/treatment algorithm
- For OCD, see Algorithm 14.2.
- For BDD, HD, and TTM:
  - Establish an accurate diagnosis and assess for co-occurring disorders.
  - Treatment planning should include CBT-based interventions and pharmacotherapy can be considered.
  - For HD, determine if the conditions at home compromise safety and intervene as indicated.

CLINICAL PEARLS
- Experienced CBT and ERP therapists are important for effective treatment. Family accommodation of OCD rituals or related behaviors may be an impediment to good treatment response.
- Although the final dose of SRI may be higher than usually prescribed for depression, dosing should start low and be titrated slowly to maximize tolerability.

Special populations
Pregnancy
- Deciding whether to start or discontinue medications during pregnancy or breast-feeding requires a careful weighing of risks and benefits, preferably in consultation with an obstetrician.

Others
- If an elder patient presents with hoarding symptoms, cognitive impairment and dementia should be considered, and if indicated a neurological work-up should be completed.

Table 14.1 OCD medications, dosages, and adverse effects*.

Drug generic name (trade name)	Starting dose range (mg/day) Children and adolescents^	Starting dose range (mg/day) Adults	Target dose range (mg/day) Children and adolescents^	Target dose range (mg/day) Adults	Adverse effects Common	Adverse effects Rare
First-line OCD agents						
SSRIs					Insomnia, anxiety, GI upset, sedation, sexual, behavioral activation	Rash, headache, suicidality (citalopram: QT prolongation risk @ >40 mg/day)
• Citalopram (Celexa)	2.5–10	20	10–20	20–40		
• Escitalopram (Lexapro)	5	10	5–10	10–20		
• Fluoxetine (Prozac)§	2.5–10	20	20–60	20–80		
• Fluvoxamine (Luvox)**§	12.5–25	50	50–200	100–300		
• Paroxetine (Paxil)	2.5–10	10	10–40	20–60		
• Sertraline (Zoloft)§	12.5–25	25–50	50–150	100–200		
Tricyclics					Dry mouth, constipation, postural hypotension, sexual (including erectile dysfunction), weight gain, tremor, sedation, sweating	ECG changes, seizures, suicidality
• Clomipramine (Anafranil)**§	6.25–25		75–200	100–250		
Second-line augmenting agents						
Atypical antipsychotics					Weight gain, sedation, sexual	Metabolic syndrome, elevated prolactin, extrapyramidal symptoms, ECG changes (ziprasidone)
• Risperidone (Risperdal)§	0.25–0.5		0.5–3	1–5		
• Quetiapine (Seroquel)	25		25–200	50–400		
• Aripiprazole (Abilify)	2		2–10	10–15		

* Adapted from Stewart SE, Hezel D, Stachon AC. Assessment and medication management of paediatric obsessive-compulsive disorder. Drugs 2012;72(7):881–93. With kind permission from Springer Science and Business Media.

** Combining clomipramine with doses of fluvoxamine as low as 50 mg/d can result in toxic levels of clomipramine because fluvoxamine is a potent inhibitor of clomipramine metabolism.

^ Dosing for adolescents is intermediate between children and adults and depends upon age and weight.

§ Medications with the most published efficacy data.

Algorithm 14.2 Pharmacologic treatment algorithm for OCD

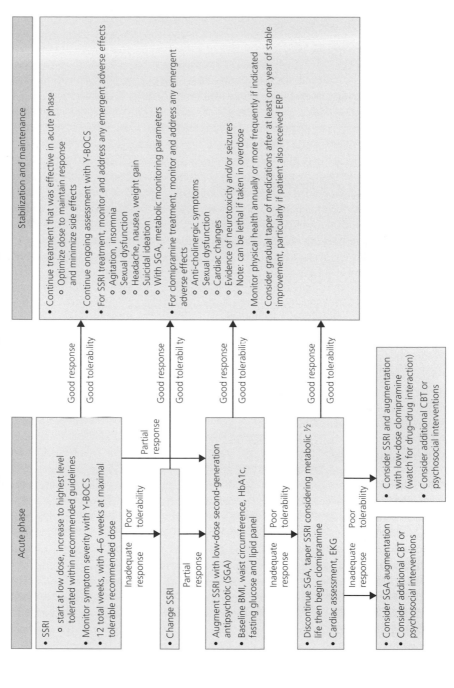

Acute phase	Stabilization and maintenance

Acute phase

- SSRI
  - ○ start at low dose, increase to highest level tolerated within recommended guidelines
  - Monitor symptom severity with Y-BOCS
  - 12 total weeks, with 4–6 weeks at maximal tolerable recommended dose

Inadequate response / Poor tolerability

- Change SSRI

Partial response

- Augment SSRI with low-dose second-generation antipsychotic (SGA)
- Baseline BMI, waist circumference, HbA1c, fasting glucose and lipid panel

Inadequate response / Poor tolerability

- Discontinue SGA, taper SSRI considering metabolic ½ life then begin clomipramine
- Cardiac assessment, EKG

Inadequate response / Poor tolerability

- Consider SGA augmentation
- Consider additional CBT or psychosocial interventions

- Consider SSRI and augmentation with low-dose clomipramine (watch for drug–drug interaction)
- Consider additional CBT or psychosocial interventions

Good response / Good tolerability

Partial response

Good response / Good tolerability

Good response / Good tolerability

Good response / Good tolerability

Stabilization and maintenance

- Continue treatment that was effective in acute phase
  - ○ Optimize dose to maintain response and minimize side effects
- Continue ongoing assessment with Y-BOCS
- For SSRI treatment, monitor and address any emergent adverse effects
  - ○ Agitation, insomnia
  - ○ Sexual dysfunction
  - ○ Headache, nausea, weight gain
  - ○ Suicidal ideation
  - ○ With SGA, metabolic monitoring parameters
- For clomipramine treatment, monitor and address any emergent adverse effects
  - ○ Anti-cholinergic symptoms
  - ○ Sexual dysfunction
  - ○ Cardiac changes
  - ○ Evidence of neurotoxicity and/or seizures
  - ○ Note: can be lethal if taken in overdose
- Monitor physical health annually or more frequently if indicated
- Consider gradual taper of medications after at least one year of stable improvement, particularly if patient also received ERP

Prognosis

> **BOTTOM LINE/CLINICAL PEARLS**
> - In OCD, >50% of patients show clinically meaningful responses to treatment. About one-third of patients require sequential treatment trials to achieve adequate symptom control. Once initial ERP treatment is complete, booster sessions help to maintain gains.
> - In the vast majority of treated individuals with BDD, cosmetic interventions do not yield improvements.
> - In HD, longitudinal care, including non-pharmacologic and pharmacologic management, is crucial to prevent relapse. The presence of comorbid OCD portends a greater response rate to pharmacotherapy.
> - Symptoms in TTM are often secondary to other psychiatric disorders and may improve when comorbidities are treated.

Natural history of untreated disease
- If untreated, OCD is usually chronic and follows a waxing and waning course.
  - 5–10% experience spontaneous remission.
  - 5–10% experience progressive deterioration.

Prognosis for treated patients
- About half of patients with OCD will respond to treatment. Conceptualizing the illness as chronic and remitting supports the use of ERP booster sessions and ongoing pharmacotherapy. Few studies have been done on medication discontinuation. If a patient has well-controlled mild symptoms and is motivated to continue to use the ERP and CBT skills, cautious titration off medication can be approached with close clinical oversight. If relapse occurs, medications should be increased to an effective level.

Follow-up tests and monitoring
- Y-BOCS and CY-BOCS, in conjunction with clinical assessment, can be used to assess response to both ERP and medication therapies.

Reading list
American Psychiatric Association. Guideline Watch: Practice Guideline for the Treatment of Patients With Obsessive-Compulsive Disorder. Washington, DC: American Psychiatric Association, 2013. Available at: http://psychiatryonline.org/guidelines. Accessed Sept 2015.

Fang A, Matheny NL, Wilhelm S. Body dysmorphic disorder. Psychiatr Clin North Am 2014;37(3):287–300.

Frost RO, Steketee G, Tolin DF. Diagnosis and assessment of hoarding disorder. Annu Rev Clin Psychol 2012;8:219–42.

Geller DA, March J. Practice parameter for the assessment and treatment of children and adolescents with obsessive-compulsive disorder. J Am Acad Child Adolesc Psychiatry 2012;51(1):98–113.

Koran LM, Hanna GL, Hollander E, Nestadt G, Simpson HB, American Psychiatric Association. Practice guideline for the treatment of patients with obsessive-compulsive disorder. Am J Psychiatry 2007;164(7 Suppl):5–53.

Pittenger C, Bloch MH. Pharmacological treatment of obsessive-compulsive disorder. Psychiatr Clin North Am 2014;37:375–91.

Woods DW, Houghton DC. Diagnosis, evaluation, and management of trichotillomania. Psychiatr Clin North Am 2014;37(3):301–17.

Suggested websites
International OCD Foundation. https://iocdf.org/
Trichotillomania Learning Center. http://www.trich.org

Guidelines
National society guidelines

Title	Source	Weblink
Practice Parameter for the Assessment and Treatment of Children and Adolescents with Obsessive-Compulsive Disorder	American Academy of Child & Adolescent Psychiatry (AACAP), 2012	www.aacap.org http://www.jaacap.com/article/S0890-8567(11)00882-3/pdf
Practice Guideline for the Treatment of Patients with Obsessive-Compulsive Disorder	American Psychiatric Association (APA), 2007	www.psychiatry.org http://psychiatryonline.org/pb/assets/raw/sitewide/practice_guidelines/guidelines/ocd.pdf
Guideline Watch (March 2013): Practice Guideline for the Treatment of Patients with Obsessive-Compulsive Disorder	APA, 2013	http://psychiatryonline.org/pb/assets/raw/sitewide/practice_guidelines/guidelines/ocd-watch.pdf
Treating Obsessive-Compulsive Disorder: A Quick Reference Guide	APA, 2007	http://psychiatryonline.org/pb/assets/raw/sitewide/practice_guidelines/guidelines/ocd-guide.pdf

International society guidelines

Title	Source	Weblink
	International OCD Foundation	https://iocdf.org/

Evidence
OCD

Type of evidence	Title and comment	Weblink
Meta-analysis	Atypical antipsychotic augmentation in SSRI treatment refractory obsessive-compulsive disorder: a systematic review and meta-analysis. **Comment:** Low-dose atypical antipsychotics may be effective as augmentation of SSRIs.	http://www.ncbi.nlm.nih.gov/pubmed/25432131
Meta-analysis	Selective serotonin re-uptake inhibitors (SSRIs) versus placebo for obsessive compulsive disorder (OCD). **Comment:** SSRI > placebo.	http://www.ncbi.nlm.nih.gov/pubmed/18253995
Randomized controlled trial (RCT)	Randomized, placebo-controlled trial of exposure and ritual prevention, clomipramine, and their combination in the treatment of obsessive-compulsive disorder. **Comment:** ERP = combination > clomipramine > placebo.	http://www.ncbi.nlm.nih.gov/pubmed/15625214
RCT	Cognitive-behavior therapy, sertraline, and their combination for children and adolescents with obsessive-compulsive disorder: the Pediatric OCD Treatment Study (POTS) randomized controlled trial. **Comment:** In patients age 7–17, combination > CBT = sertraline > placebo.	http://www.ncbi.nlm.nih.gov/pubmed/15507582

BDD

Type of evidence	Title and comment	Weblink
RCT	A randomized placebo-controlled trial of fluoxetine in body dysmorphic disorder. **Comment:** First and only RCT to examine SSRI in BDD.	http://www.ncbi. nlm.nih.gov/ pubmed/11926939
Large case series	Surgical and non-psychiatric medical treatment of patients with body dysmorphic disorder. **Comment:** Dermatological and surgical treatments rarely improve BDD symptoms.	http://www.ncbi. nlm.nih.gov/ pubmed/11815686
RCT	Clomipramine vs desipramine crossover trial in body dysmorphic disorder: selective efficacy of a serotonin reuptake inhibitor in imagined ugliness. **Comment:** Provided evidence that agents with high serotonergic reuptake activity correlate with efficacy.	http://www.ncbi. nlm.nih.gov/ pubmed/10565503
RCT	Cognitive-behavioral body image therapy for body dysmorphic disorder. **Comment:** CBT is efficacious in BDD.	http://www.ncbi. nlm.nih.gov/ pubmed/7751487

HD

Type of evidence	Title and comment	Weblink
Open-label trial	Neurobiology and treatment of compulsive hoarding. **Comment:** Efficacy of paroxetine and venlafaxine in treating OCD and non-OCD hoarding.	http://www.ncbi.nlm.nih.gov/ pubmed/18849909
Open-label trial	Paroxetine treatment of compulsive hoarding. **Comment:** In an open trial, hoarding and OCD (n = 79) showed similar positive responses to paroxetine.	http://www.journalofpsychiatricresearch. com/article/S0022-3956(06)00086-0/pdf
Open-label trial	An open trial of cognitive-behavioral therapy for compulsive hoarding. **Comment:** Manualized treatment approaches are efficacious in HD.	http://www.ncbi.nlm.nih.gov/ pubmed/17306221
Open-label trial	Group cognitive-behavioral therapy for HD: an open trial. **Comment:** Group CBT for hoarding may be an effective treatment option with greater accessibility and reduced cost.	http://www.ncbi.nlm.nih.gov/ pubmed/21925643

**Additional material for this chapter can be found online at:
www.mountsinaiexpertguides.com/psychiatry**

This includes advice for patients, a case study, ICD codes, and multiple choice questions.

CHAPTER 15

Schizophrenia Spectrum and Other Psychotic Disorders

Rachel Moster[1], Larry J. Siever[2], and Sophia Frangou[3]

[1] Columbia University Medical Center, New York, NY, USA
[2] James J. Peters VA Medical Center, Bronx, NY, USA
[3] Icahn School of Medicine at Mount Sinai, New York, NY, USA

OVERALL BOTTOM LINE
- Schizophrenia is a brain disorder.
- Delusions, hallucinations, and disorganized speech and behavior are core diagnostic symptoms.
- Treatment involves antipsychotic medication, psychological therapies, and social support.

Background

Definition of disease

Schizophrenia is a severe brain disorder diagnosed on the basis of psychotic (delusions, hallucinations, disorganized speech and behavior) and negative symptoms (avolition, affective flattening, and difficulties in initiating and sustaining activities).

Incidence/prevalence

- Median point, period, and lifetime prevalence per 1000 persons are estimated at 4.6, 3.3, and 4; higher in immigrants and in developed countries.
- Median incidence is estimated at 15.2 per 100,000; higher in men, immigrants, and urban settings; peaks in the teens and 20s.

Economic impact

- The World Health Organization has ranked schizophrenia the fifth most disabling disorder globally (www.who.int/healthinfo/global_burden_disease).

Etiology

- Heritability is approximately 65%.
- Urbanicity, migration, cannabis abuse, childhood abuse, as well as pregnancy, birth complications, and advanced paternal age are the most significant non-genetic factors.

Mount Sinai Expert Guides: Psychiatry, First Edition. Edited by Asher B. Simon, Antonia S. New, and Wayne K. Goodman.
© 2017 John Wiley & Sons, Ltd. Published 2017 by John Wiley & Sons, Ltd.
Companion website: www.mountsinaiexpertguides.com/psychiatry

Pathophysiology

- Schizophrenia is associated with (Figure 15.1):
  - increased ventricular volume;
  - reduced gray matter volume in the frontal cortex, temporal cortex, hippocampus/amygdala, and thalamus;
- widespread abnormalities in white matter tracts.
- Abnormalities in neurotransmitter systems implicate mostly dopamine and glutamate.
- Subcortical dopamine release is increased during acute psychotic episodes.

Predictive/risk factors

- Family history.
- Genetic risk alleles, increased genetic insertions/deletions, increased copy number variation.
- Substance abuse, particularly cannabis.

Prevention

> **BOTTOM LINE/CLINICAL PEARLS**
> - A variety of cognitive and pharmacological approaches have been used to delay the onset of psychosis.
> - Continued antipsychotic treatment is the most effective intervention in minimizing the risk of relapse.

Screening

- There is no general population screening for schizophrenia.
- Screening is available for help-seeking individuals at high risk for psychosis within the context of early intervention services.
- The most commonly used screening instruments are the Comprehensive Assessment of At-Risk Mental States (CAARMS) and the Structured Interview for Prodromal Syndromes (SIPS).

Secondary (and primary) prevention

- Primary prevention aims to lower the risk in asymptomatic individuals.
  - Frequent cannabis use in early adolescence carries a population-attributable risk of approximately 10% and represents a key target for primary prevention.
- Secondary prevention aims to stop or delay the progress of schizophrenia.
  - Early intervention services shorten duration of untreated psychosis (DUP), and may improve outcome and delay transition to worsened disease.
- Tertiary prevention aims to reduce disability and emergent physical or mental comorbidity through the following targets:
  - medication non-adherence (through case management and long-acting antipsychotic agents);
  - cognitive impairment (through cognitive remediation);
  - maladaptive cognitive styles (through cognitive behavioral therapy);
  - physical wellbeing (through medical care).

Diagnosis

- A particular challenge relates to patients' poor insight, which often prevents them from reporting psychotic experiences as symptomatic of an illness. A multisource approach to corroborate information is necessary.

- Patients with schizophrenia usually present with a history of:
  - poor academic achievement and difficulties in peer relationships;
  - increasing social withdrawal and progressive impairment in social function;
  - increasingly disorganized behavior and bizarre ideas or experiences.
- The mental state examination is used to elicit symptoms and evaluate their significance against operational diagnostic criteria for schizophrenia.
- Physical investigations are used to exclude other disorders known to present with psychosis.

Differential diagnosis

Differential diagnosis (alphabetical order)	Features
Medical conditions	
Acute intermittent porphyria	Test: urine porphobilinogen Clinical features: abdominal pain, vomiting, neuropathy, purple discoloration of feces and urine when exposed to light
Central nervous system (CNS) neoplasm (esp. frontal or limbic)	Test: brain magnetic resonance imaging (MRI) Clinical features: cognitive and behavioral disturbances, impaired smell or vision, ataxia, muscle weakness, headaches, seizures, increased intracranial pressure
CNS trauma	Test: brain MRI Clinical features: unequal, dilated and unresponsive pupils, persistent headache, vomiting, seizures, confusion
CNS metal toxicity	Test: urine or blood levels of suspected metal Clinical features: variable depending on agent and way of exposure; most commonly involve occupational exposure
Cerebrovascular accidents	Test: brain MRI Clinical features: focal neurological signs; psychosis is only seen post-stroke
Chromosomal syndromes	Test: genetic testing Clinical features: variable depending on the specific chromosome abnormality but may involve dysmorphic features
Epilepsy (esp. simple and complex partial seizures)	Test: abnormal electroencephalogram (EEG); Clinical features: amnestic sensations (e.g., déjà vu), sudden dysphoric or euphoric feelings, absence, automatic hand and mouth movements; short duration followed by recovery
Herpes encephalitis	Test: lumbar puncture Clinical features: fever, seizures, dysphasia, ataxia, history of immunosuppressant disorder or treatment
Human immunodeficiency virus (HIV) with CNS involvement	Test: HIV antibodies Clinical features: cognitive impairment, neuropathy
Huntington's disease	Test: genetic testing Clinical features: family history, chorea, abnormal posturing and writhing, dysphagia and dysphasia, cognitive impairment
Lyme disease	Test: serology Clinical features: erythema migrans, facial palsy, arthritis

(Continued)

(Continued)

Differential diagnosis (alphabetical order)	Features
Metachromatic leukodystrophy	Test: blood arylsulfatase A and urine sulfatide Clinical features: late childhood and adolescence; poor concentration, ataxia, seizures, optic nerve atrophy, dementia, abnormal tendon reflexes, tremor
Neuropsychiatric systemic lupus erythematosus	Test: antinuclear antibody Clinical features: malar (butterfly) rash, small joint arthritis, anemia, glomerulonephritis
Neurosyphilis	Test: rapid plasma reagin Clinical features: Argyll Robertson pupils, abnormal gait and tendon reflexes, muscle atrophy, cognitive impairment
Wilson's disease	Test: ceruloplasmin Clinical features: Kayser–Fleischer rings, chronic liver disease, parkinsonism, ataxia, seizures
Psychiatric conditions	
Autism spectrum disorder	Social and communication deficits and restricted/idiosyncratic preoccupations may be misidentified as psychosis; an individual must meet the full criteria of schizophrenia for at least one month before it can be considered as a comorbid diagnosis
Brief psychotic disorder	Duration of psychotic symptoms of less than a month followed by recovery; no negative symptoms at any point
Delusional disorder	Clinical features: delusions; minimal or no hallucinations; no abnormalities in behavior or function (unless directly linked to delusional beliefs)
Drug-induced psychosis	Positive toxicology; signs and symptoms of acute intoxication or chronic use; psychotic symptoms should resolve with abstinence
Schizotypal personality disorder	Psychotic symptoms are attenuated and present mostly during periods of crisis
Mood disorders with psychotic features	Core psychotic symptoms should occur exclusively during the mood episodes
Obsessive-compulsive disorder and body dysmorphic disorder	Severe obsessions may be misidentified for delusions, especially in the absence of insight; the content is usually restricted to themes of hoarding, counting, contamination, or body image
Posttraumatic stress disorder	Flashbacks and hypervigilance may be misidentified as hallucinations and paranoid delusions; history of traumatic event is necessary
Schizophreniform disorder	Psychotic symptoms, with or without negative symptoms, lasting from 1 to 6 months followed by recovery
Schizoaffective disorder	A major depressive or manic episode should occur concurrently with core psychotic symptoms and last for the majority of the total duration of psychotic periods

NB: The lists of tests and clinical features presented are illustrative and not exhaustive.

Typical presentation

- The clinical presentation varies between individuals and within the same individual at different stages of the illness (Figure 15.2).

- During acute episodes, psychotic symptoms (delusions, hallucinations, disorganization) are prominent and often associated with heightened arousal and agitation.
- Inter-episode periods vary greatly with respect to duration and level of psychopathology.
- The majority of patients continue to experience negative symptoms as well as cognitive, social, and occupational dysfunction.

Clinical diagnosis
History
- Determine symptoms, precipitating circumstances, timing, and psychiatric and medical history.
- DSM-5 requires ≥1 core psychotic symptom (delusions, hallucinations, disorganized speech) and either disorganized behavior or negative symptoms lasting for ≥6 months (unless treated), in the absence of a concurrent mood episode or significant substance use.
- Changes from DSM-IV to DSM-5.
  - The requirement that delusions be bizarre has been eliminated.
  - Most subtypes (paranoid, disorganized, catatonic, undifferentiated, and residual types) have been removed; catatonia may still be used as a specifier.
  - A new 8-item scale has been introduced for rating disease severity: Clinician-Rated Dimensions of Psychosis Symptom Severity Scale.

Physical and mental status exams
- The purpose of the physical examination is two-fold:
  1. to identify signs and symptoms of substance abuse, neurological disorder, or systemic disorder that may be causally linked to psychosis;
  2. to define a baseline against which to judge possible side effects of treatment.
- The purpose of the mental state examination is to elicit and record all psychiatric symptoms and to assess the level of risk to self and/or others.

Disease severity classification
- No formal staging classification.
- Measures of disease severity over the preceding 7 days can be captured using the Clinician-Rated Dimensions of Psychosis Symptom Severity Scale.
- Illness chronicity is measured by number of episodes.

Laboratory diagnosis
List of diagnostic tests
- No specific laboratory findings.
- Toxicology screening for drugs of abuse is recommended at presentation and as indicated thereafter.
- A pregnancy test should be carried out in women of childbearing potential to inform pharmacological choices and care planning.
- Additional tests may be indicated for differential diagnosis (see Differential diagnosis table).

Lists of imaging techniques
- No characteristic gross brain imaging findings.
- Brain MRI is recommended at onset and indicated when an underlying neurological disorder is suspected on clinical grounds.

Diagnostic algorithm (Algorithm 15.1)

Algorithm 15.1 Diagnostic algorithm for schizophrenia

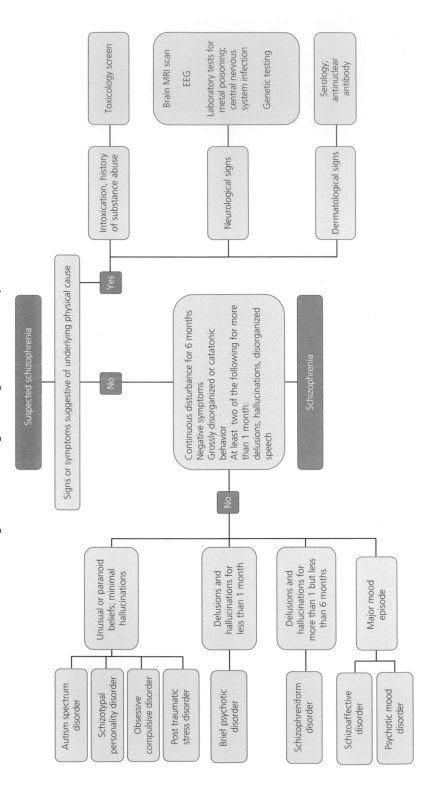

Potential pitfalls/common errors made regarding diagnosis of disease

- Regular substance abuse may be misdiagnosed as schizophrenia and, conversely, psychotic symptoms may be misattributed to substance abuse. Drug-induced psychosis should resolve within 2–3 weeks of abstinence, so a drug-free period of observation is clinically indicated prior to diagnosis.
- Concurrent affective symptoms and psychosis require careful evaluation to differentiate between schizophrenia, schizoaffective disorder, and severe mood disorders. Detailed longitudinal observation is usually the most informative approach.
- General medical conditions (e.g., delirium) are the most likely underlying cause of very rapid onset of psychosis.
- In young children (<10) schizophrenia is very rare; new-onset psychosis should trigger investigation for chromosomal disorders and degenerative neurological syndromes.
- In the elderly, new-onset psychotic symptoms are usually associated with dementia or other neurological disorders.

Treatment
Treatment rationale

- Symptomatic control:
  - Antipsychotic medication is currently the most effective intervention for symptom control and relapse prevention.
  - Adjunct psychological treatments can be used at any point to improve patients' coping skills or cognitive function.
- Maintenance of physical wellbeing:
  - Requires vigilance, advice about diet and healthy lifestyle choices, and regular general medical follow-up.
- Minimization of psychosocial disability:
  - A recovery approach using behavioral and vocational interventions can assist patients in re-engaging with social roles, thus reducing disability.

When to hospitalize

- During acute exacerbations of psychotic symptoms associated with distress and/or significant behavior disturbances.
- When suicide risk is high.
- When there is aggression and threatened or actual violence.

Table of treatment

Medical	
Antipsychotic medication (usual daily oral dose range)	
First-generation antipsychotics (FGA) • Chlorpromazine (300–1000 mg) • Fluphenazine (5–20 mg) • Haloperidol (5–20 mg) • Perphenazine (16–64 mg) • Trifluoperazine (15–50 mg)	• Baseline EKG and laboratory tests (including lipid profile and blood glucose) should be obtained before treatment initiation, at 3 months, and annually thereafter unless more frequent monitoring is clinically indicated

(Continued)

(Continued)

Medical	
Second-generation antipsychotics (SGA) • Aripiprazole (10–30 mg) • Asenapine (5–10 mg) • Clozapine (250–450 mg) • Olanzapine (10–20 mg) • Quetiapine (400–800 mg) • Risperidone (2–6 mg) • Ziprasidone (80–160 mg) • Lurasidone (40–160 mg) • Paliperidone (3–12 mg) • Iloperidone (6–12 mg)	• Extrapyramidal side effects (dystonic reactions, parkinsonism, akathisia) may occur with any antipsychotic but are more common with FGAs • Endocrine side effects, particularly hyperprolactinemia, may occur with most FGAs and some SGAs, but not with clozapine • Weight gain, glucose, and lipid dysregulation may occur with any antipsychotic but are most common with SGAs • Antipsychotics should start at the lowest effective dose and be titrated depending on response and tolerability • Efficacy should be assessed when patients have been on adequate dose for ≥2 weeks
Device-based	
Electroconvulsive therapy (ECT)	Rarely used in schizophrenia but can be considered in patients with severe symptoms, catatonia, or poor response to medication
Psychological	
Supportive care, including medication management and motivational interventions	Can be a variety of formats; targets adherence
Cognitive behavioral therapy	Structured sessions to develop cognitive and behavioral strategies to improve coping with symptoms
Cognitive remediation	Structured sessions target cognitive impairment
Psychoeducation	To promote acceptance and problem-solving; can be offered in individual or group and usually involves patient and family
Complementary	
Omega-3 fatty acids	Eicosapentaenoic acid may be of some benefit as adjunctive medication

NB: Medications are listed with their generic names in alphabetical order within each class.

Prevention/management of complications
• Extrapyramidal side effects: dose reduction; switch to antipsychotics with lower dopamine receptor potency; adjunct use of anticholinergics.
• Hyperprolactinemia: if patients are symptomatic (amenorrhea, galactorrhea) switch to antipsychotics with lower dopamine receptor potency; adjunctive low-dose aripiprazole may also be considered.
• Weight gain and metabolic side effects: advice about diet and exercise; switch to antipsychotics least likely to cause such side effects (aripiprazole, ziprasidone, lurasidone).
• Adjunctive metformin may be helpful for elevated glucose.

Management/treatment algorithm (Algorithm 15.2)

Algorithm 15.2 Pharmacological treatment algorithm for schizophrenia

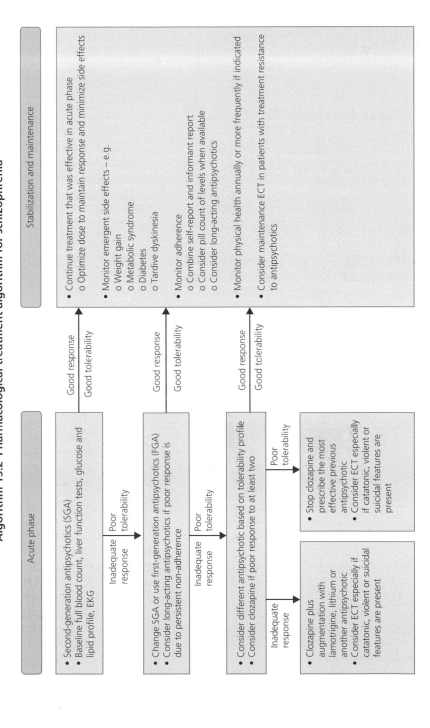

CLINICAL PEARLS
- Antipsychotic medication is the most effective intervention for acute treatment and relapse prevention.
- Side effects should be minimized by judicious medication choice, dosing, and regular monitoring.
- A range of psychological and vocational approaches can be used to improve patients' quality of life.

Special populations
Pregnancy
- FGAs are the preferred antipsychotics, as risk to the fetus is considered small. Psychotropic medications with teratogenic potential (e.g., certain anticonvulsants) should be discontinued.
- Engaging the mother in prenatal care and formulating a plan for the birth and postnatal period is essential to minimize obstetric risks and ensure safety and wellbeing of the infant.

Prognosis

BOTTOM LINE/CLINICAL PEARLS
- Chronic course in the majority of patients, with multiple relapses and variable, usually incomplete, inter-episode recovery; core psychotic symptoms become less prominent with increasing age.
- Suicide risk is high: ~20% of patients make ≥1 attempt; 5–6% commit suicide.
- Life expectancy is reduced, although mortality per cause of death does not differ from the general population. Poor lifestyle and poor engagement in health services are thought to contribute.

Reading list
Lieberman J, Murray RM. Comprehensive Care of Schizophrenia: A Textbook of Clinical Management, 2nd edn. New York: Oxford University Press, 2012.

Miller TJ, McGlashan TH, Rosen JL, et al. Prodromal assessment with the structured interview for prodromal syndromes and the scale of prodromal symptoms: predictive validity, interrater reliability, and training to reliability. Schizophr Bull 2003;29:703–15.

Yung AR, Yuen HP, McGorry PD, et al. Mapping the onset of psychosis: the Comprehensive Assessment of At-Risk Mental States. Aust N Z J Psychiatry 2005;39:964–71.

Suggested websites
National Institute of Mental Health. http://www.nimh.nih.gov/health/topics/schizophrenia/index.shtml

American Psychological Association. http://www.apa.org/topics/schiz/

National Alliance on Mental Illness. http://www.nami.org/Template.cfm?Section=schizophrenia9

Royal College of Psychiatrists. http://www.rcpsych.ac.uk/expertadvice/problemsdisorders/schizophrenia.aspx

Guidelines
National society guidelines

Title	Source	Weblink
Practice Guideline for the Treatment of Patients with Schizophrenia	American Psychiatric Association (APA), 2004 and 2009 update	http://www.psychiatryonline.com

International guidelines

Title	Source	Weblink
Psychosis and schizophrenia in adults: prevention and management	National Institute for Health and Care Excellence (NICE), 2014	http://www.nice.org.uk/cg178

Evidence

Type of evidence	Title and comment	Weblink
Meta-analysis	Neuroanatomical abnormalities in schizophrenia: a multimodal voxelwise meta-analysis and meta-regression analysis. **Comment:** The study found that schizophrenia is characterized by changes in bilateral prefrontal cortical, limbic and subcortical gray matter regions, and in the white matter tracts that connect affected structures.	http://www.ncbi.nlm.nih.gov/pubmed/21300524
Meta-analysis	Predicting psychosis: meta-analysis of transition outcomes in individuals at high clinical risk. **Comment:** Individuals at clinical high risk of psychosis are likely to convert to full blown disease within the first 3 years. Conversion rates are influenced by age, clinical symptoms, and treatment provided.	http://www.ncbi.nlm.nih.gov/pubmed/22393215
Systematic review	Schizophrenia and suicide: systematic review of risk factors. **Comment:** Prevention of suicide in schizophrenia is improved by treatment of affective symptoms, monitoring adherence to treatment, and close assessment of patients with risk factors.	http://www.ncbi.nlm.nih.gov/pubmed/15994566
Meta-analysis	Relapse prevention in schizophrenia: a systematic review and meta-analysis of second-generation antipsychotics versus first-generation antipsychotics. **Comment:** Second-generation antipsychotics show modest superiority to first-generation agents in relapse prevention.	http://www.ncbi.nlm.nih.gov/pubmed/22124274
Systematic review	Increased dopamine transmission in schizophrenia: relationship to illness phases. **Comment:** Increased dopaminergic neurotransmission is present in schizophrenia during acute episodes, but not during remission.	http://www.ncbi.nlm.nih.gov/pubmed/10394474
Population-based study	Common genetic determinants of schizophrenia and bipolar disorder in Swedish families: a population-based study. **Comment:** Analysis of genetic and environmental contributions to liability for schizophrenia, bipolar disorder showed evidence of genetic overlap.	http://www.ncbi.nlm.nih.gov/pubmed/19150704
Systematic review	Schizophrenia: a concise overview of incidence, prevalence, and mortality. **Comment:** Urbanicity, economic status, and migration adversely affect prevalence and mortality in schizophrenia.	http://www.ncbi.nlm.nih.gov/pubmed/18480098

(Continued)

(Continued)

Type of evidence	Title and comment	Weblink
Systematic review	Cannabis use and risk of psychotic or affective mental health outcomes: a systematic review. **Comment:** Cannabis increases the risk of psychosis but probably not of affective disorders.	http://www.ncbi.nlm.nih.gov/pubmed/17662880
Systematic review	The environment and schizophrenia. **Comment:** Genetic risk for psychosis interacts with environmental factors mainly adversity, urbanicity, minority group status, and cannabis use.	http://www.ncbi.nlm.nih.gov/pubmed/21068828
Systematic review	Neurochemical imaging in schizophrenia. **Comment:** Schizophrenia is associated with neurotransmitter changes affecting monoamines, GABA, and glutamate.	http://www.ncbi.nlm.nih.gov/pubmed/21312402

Images

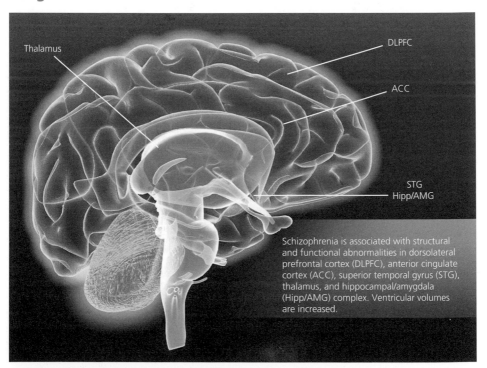

Figure 15.1 Brain abnormalities in schizophrenia.

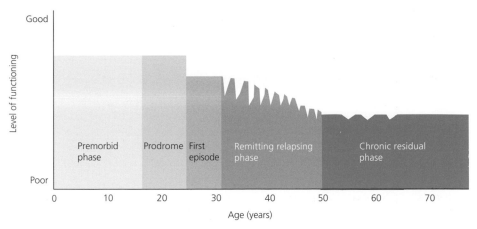

Figure 15.2 Natural history of schizophrenia, with level of functioning. Source: Sheitman BB, Lieberman JA. J Psychiatr Res 1998;32(3-4):143–50.

Additional material for this chapter can be found online at: www.mountsinaiexpertguides.com/psychiatry

This includes advice for patients, a case study, ICD codes, and multiple choice questions.

CHAPTER 16

Substance Use and Addictive Disorders

Allison K. Ungar[1], Anna B. Konova[2], Alkesh Patel[1], Rita Z. Goldstein[1], and Yasmin L. Hurd[1]

[1] Icahn School of Medicine at Mount Sinai, New York, NY, USA
[2] NYU Langone School of Medicine, and VA NY Harbor Healthcare System, New York, NY, USA

OVERALL BOTTOM LINE

- Substance use disorder (SUD) is a chronic, relapsing condition characterized by compulsions to use a substance, loss of control in limiting intake, and the emergence of a negative emotional state when access to the substance is denied. The phenomena of disease progression can be explained by neurobiological mechanisms of change and adaptation.
- SUDs have roots in both impulsivity and compulsivity, whereby the drive for substance use shifts from positive to negative reinforcement, respectively.
- Given the growing economic impact and increased morbidity and mortality seen with SUD, screening, diagnosis, and treatment efforts continue to be pursued among public and private sectors and across national, state, and local fronts.
- Treatment of SUD should involve a multidisciplinary approach considering pharmacotherapy, psychotherapy, self-help facilitation, and ongoing relapse prevention strategies.
- Prognosis and treatment outcomes can be improved by approaching individuals with SUD in a non-judgmental way that incorporates a team approach.

Background
Definition of disease
SUD is a chronic, relapsing condition characterized by the following progression of states:

1. initial binge/intoxication
2. negative emotionality
3. preoccupation/anticipation with intense craving
4. compulsive drug use.

Disease classification

- DSM-5 substance related disorders encompass 10 classes of drugs and associated syndromes (e.g., Opioid Use Disorder; Opioid Intoxication; Opioid Withdrawal; Opioid-Induced Disorders).
- ICD-10 classifies SUD under F10–F19 "Mental and Behavioral Disorders Due to Use of Psychoactive Substances."

Mount Sinai Expert Guides: Psychiatry, First Edition. Edited by Asher B. Simon, Antonia S. New, and Wayne K. Goodman.
© 2017 John Wiley & Sons, Ltd. Published 2017 by John Wiley & Sons, Ltd.
Companion website: www.mountsinaiexpertguides.com/psychiatry

Incidence/prevalence
- A 2013 nationwide survey of the past month in people over 11 years old found:
  - 22.9% (60.1 million) engaged in binge drinking of alcohol;
  - 25.5% (66.9 million) used tobacco;
  - 9.4% (24.6 million) used illicit drugs or abused a prescription;
  - 8.2% (21.6 million) were classified as having substance dependence or abuse.
- In a 2013 nationwide survey of middle and high school students, marijuana smoking surpassed tobacco with 1%, 4%, and 6.5% of 8th, 10th, and 12th graders, respectively, reporting daily marijuana use.

Economic impact
- SUDs cost the US over $600 billion annually due to related crimes, loss of productivity, and healthcare.

Etiology
- What specifically causes an individual person to develop SUD is not yet known.
- The interaction of genetic and environmental factors influences brain substrates that increase the propensity to develop drug addiction.
- SUDs are highly heritable with an estimated 30–80%, depending on the drug, attributed to variation in addiction liability.
  - Specific genes related to the dopamine, GABA, acetylcholine, opioid, and cannabinoid neurotransmitter systems have been implicated.

Pathophysiology
- The three stages of the addiction cycle include altered neurochemical adaptations in brain reward and motivational drive systems that often accompany compulsive drug use over time:
  1. **Binge and intoxication stage**: **activation** of neurotransmitter systems in basal forebrain (dopamine, opioid peptides, GABA, serotonin, and endocannabinoids).
  2. **Withdrawal stage:** (1) **dysregulation** of basal forebrain systems; (2) **recruitment** of brain stress systems (corticotropin-releasing factor, dynorphin, and norepinephrine); and (3) **dysregulation** of brain anti-stress systems (neuropeptide Y). All contribute to the negative emotional state often seen in protracted abstinence.
  3. **Preoccupation/anticipation stage: glutamatergic** and other projections from the frontal cortex and basolateral amygdala to the nucleus accumbens reward center contribute to relapse.
- With chronic substance use, changes in both the reward and stress systems are hypothesized to maintain an "altered reward set point," which furthers vulnerability for SUDs. Systems implicated in self-control and attribution of value/salience are also impacted.

Predictive/risk factors
- Personal or family history of SUD.
- Personality traits (impulsivity, novelty-seeking, and antisocial behavior).
- Early alcohol, drug, or nicotine use, including *in utero* exposure.
- History of mood/stress disorders [posttraumatic stress disorder (PTSD), bipolar disorder].
- History of chronic pain.
- History of childhood trauma and sexual abuse.
- History of *parental* psychopathology.
- Poor coping skills.

- Interpersonal conflicts.
- History of criminality.
- Low socioeconomic status.

Prevention

> **BOTTOM LINE/CLINICAL PEARLS**
> - Most evidence-based interventions are aimed at reducing the initiation or prevalence of youth drug use.

Screening
- For alcohol use:
  - Michigan Alcohol Screening Test (MAST and its short form, SMAST) (Selzer, 1971)
  - Alcohol Use Disorder Identification Test (AUDIT) (Saunders et al., 1993; WHO Collaborative Project).
- For alcohol, nicotine, and other drug use:
  - CAGE-Adapted to Include Drugs (CAGE-AID) questionnaire (Brown et al., 1998)
  - Alcohol, Smoking, and Substance Involvement Screening Test (ASSIST) (Humeniuk et al., 2010; WHO).
- For alcohol and drug use in adolescents:
  - CRAFFT Screening Tool (Knight et al., 1999; Children's Hospital Boston)
  - Drug Use Screening Tool (DUST) (Kent & Medway Drug Action Team).

Secondary (and primary) prevention
- Primary prevention aims to reduce the initiation and prevalence of youth drug use through community-based programs (e.g., campaigns to change social norms), family-based programs (e.g., improving communication), school-based programs (e.g., increasing knowledge of consequences of drug use and providing self-management and social skills training), regulatory approaches (e.g., age-of-purchase laws, drug-free zones), and public health initiatives (e.g., mass media campaigns).
- Secondary prevention efforts – to minimize the transition from occasional drug use to misuse, abuse, and addiction – are similar to the above.

Diagnosis

> **BOTTOM LINE/CLINICAL PEARLS**
> - Relevant clinical history includes the onset of drug use, time of last use, frequency and amounts used, route of drug administration, stressful triggers, protective factors aiding in relapse prevention, and whether the individual or friends and family have noticed any *impairment* at home or in the workplace.
> - Comprehensive physical, neurological, and mental status exams can reveal *acute* states of intoxication and withdrawal, as well as identify if there is a history of *chronic* substance use.
> - Toxicological laboratory tests are a routine part of the work-up.
> - There is no specific chemistry or imaging test that can confirm the presence or absence of SUD, although certain hematological markers could suggest chronic substance use (e.g., reduced liver function with alcohol use disorder).

Differential diagnosis

Differential diagnosis	Features
Primary psychiatric illness (major depression, bipolar disorder, psychotic disorder) or medical condition	Psychiatric or physical symptoms precede the onset of SUD, or occur in the absence of active substance use

Typical presentation

Depending on level of insight, a patient may or may not report experiencing any of the following signs and symptoms suggesting SUD: (1) needing more substance to obtain effects; (2) compulsive use despite adverse consequences; (3) intense drug craving; (4) excessive amount of time spent using or obtaining the substance; and, depending on the substance used, (5) the development of a characteristic *intoxication* or *withdrawal/abstinence syndrome*. The patient may have appetite and skin changes, or altered mental status with accompanying agitation, depression, or delirium.

Clinical diagnosis

History

- DSM-5 replaces both "Abuse" and "Dependence" with "[Specific Substance] Use Disorder" defined by the drug of choice. A "Craving" criterion has been added, and "Problems with law enforcement" has been removed.
  - These changes are intended, in part, to correct the misinterpretation of "Dependence" as implying addiction. Features of DSM-IV "Dependence" (e.g., tolerance, withdrawal) can be normal responses to prescribed medications and need to be differentiated from addiction.
- Assess for DSM-5 SUD criteria, subsumed under the following overall groupings:
  - Impaired control:
    - Substance taken in larger amounts than intended.
    - Unsuccessful efforts to cut down use.
    - Excessive time to obtain, use, or recover from substance.
    - Craving: ask if the patient has such strong urges to use that s/he could not think of anything else.
  - Social impairment:
    - Failure to fulfill major role obligations and/or reduction of important social activities.
    - Continued use despite social or interpersonal problems.
  - Risky use:
    - Ongoing use despite difficulty (e.g., physical hazards, psychological/physical problems).
  - Pharmacological changes:
    - Tolerance (i.e., larger doses needed to achieve effect, reduced effect at usual dose).
    - Withdrawal criteria depend on specific substance.
- Determine the onset of drug use, time of last use, frequency and amounts used, route of drug administration, stressful triggers, protective factors to prevent relapse, whether the individual or friends and family have noticed any impairment at home or in the workplace, and they perceive the substance use to be problematic.
- Assess for potentially *life-threatening comorbid medical conditions or withdrawal symptoms.*
  - Rating scales to assess clinical withdrawal (in addition to DSM-5 description of specific symptoms) include the Clinical Institute Withdrawal Assessment for Alcohol, Revised (CIWA-Ar, see Table 16.1) and the Clinical Opiate Withdrawal Scale (COWS, see https://www.drugabuse.gov/sites/default/files/files/ClinicalOpiateWithdrawalScale.pdf).

Table 16.1 Clinical Institute Withdrawal Assessment for Alcohol, Revised (CIWA-Ar).

NAUSEA & VOMITING: Ask "Do you feel sick to your stomach? Have you vomited?" Observation. 0 no nausea/vomiting 1 2 3 4 intermittent nausea with dry heaves 5 6 7 constant nausea, frequent dry heaves & vomiting	**TACTILE DISTURBANCES**: Ask: "Have you any itching, pins and needles sensations, any burning, any numbness or do you feel bugs crawling on or under your skin?" Observation. 0 none 1 very mild itching, pins and needles, burning or numbness 2 mild itching, pins and needles, burning or numbness 3 moderate pins and needles, burning or numbness 4 moderately severe hallucinations 5 severe hallucinations 6 extremely severe hallucinations 7 continuous hallucinations
TREMOR: Arms extended and fingers spread apart. Observation. 0 no tremor 1 not visible, but can be felt fingertip to fingertip 2 3 4 moderate, with patient's arms extended 5 6 7 severe, even with arms not extended	**AUDITORY DISTURBANCES**: Ask: "Are you more aware of sounds around you? Are they harsh? Do they frighten you? Are you hearing anything that is disturbing you? Are you hearing things you know are not there?" Observation. 0 not present 1 very mild harshness or ability to frighten 2 mild harshness or ability to frighten 3 moderate harshness or ability to frighten 4 moderately severe hallucinations 5 severe hallucinations 6 extremely severe hallucinations. 7 continuous hallucinations
PAROXYSMAL SWEATS 0 no sweat visible 1 barely perceptible sweating, palms moist 2 3 4 beads of sweat obvious on forehead 5 6 7 drenching sweats	**VISUAL DISTURBANCES**: Ask: "Does the light appear to be too bright? Is its color different? Does it hurt your eyes? Are you seeing anything that is disturbing to you? Are you seeing things you know are not there?" Observation. 0 not present 1 very mild sensitivity 2 mild sensitivity 3 moderate sensitivity 4 moderately severe hallucinations 5 severe hallucinations 6 extremely severe hallucinations 7 continuous hallucinations
ANXIETY: Ask: "Do you feel nervous?" Observation. 0 no anxiety, at ease 1 mildly anxious 2 3 4 moderately anxious, or guarded, so anxiety is inferred 5 6 7 equivalent to acute panic as seen in severe delirium or acute schizophrenic reactions	**HEADACHE, FULLNESS IN HEAD**: Ask: "Does your head feel different? Does it feel like there is a band around your head?" Do not rate for dizziness or lightheadedness. Otherwise, rate severity. 0 not present 1 very mild 2 mild 3 moderate 4 moderately severe 5 severe 6 very severe 7 extremely severe

Table 16.1 (*Continued*)

AGITATION: Observation.	ORIENTATION & CLOUDING OF SENSORIUM: Ask: "What day is this? Where are you? Who am I?"
0 normal activity 1 somewhat more than normal activity 2 3 4 moderately fidgety and restless 5 6 7 paces back and forth during most of interview, or constantly thrashes about	0 oriented and can do serial additions 1 cannot do serial additions or is uncertain about date 2 disoriented for date by no more than 2 calendar days 3 disoriented for date by more than 2 calendar days 4 disoriented for place and/or person

Total Score:_____	Time:____	BP:____/____	HR:_____	Resp:___	Temp:____
Total Score:_____	Time:____	BP:____/____	HR:_____	Resp:___	Temp:____
Total Score:_____	Time:____	BP:____/____	HR:_____	Resp:___	Temp:____
Total Score:_____	Time:____	BP:____/____	HR:_____	Resp:___	Temp:____
Total Score:_____	Time:____	BP:____/____	HR:_____	Resp:___	Temp:____

CIWA–Ar is not copyrighted and may be used freely. Source: Sullivan JT, Sykora K, Schneiderman J, Naranjo CA, Sellers EM. Assessment of alcohol withdrawal: The revised Clinical Institute Withdrawal Assessment for Alcohol scale (CIWA–Ar). Br J Addict 1989;84:1353–7.

Physical and mental status exams
- Physical exam:
  - Vital signs.
  - Heavy alcohol consumption leading to liver failure or acute hepatotoxicity may manifest with jaundice, abdominal pain, decreased appetite and weight loss, ascites, caput medusa, and icteric sclerae.
  - **Opioid withdrawal** can present with mydriasis, yawning, rhinorrhea, lacrimation, gastrointestinal distress, joint and body pain, anxiety, insomnia, and restlessness.
  - **Methamphetamine and cocaine withdrawal** can present with severe psychomotor retardation, cognitive deficits, depression, and fatigue.
  - **Benzodiazepine, barbiturate, and alcohol withdrawal** can present with psychomotor agitation, hypertension, psychosis, seizures, and/or delirium.
  - **Cannabis withdrawal** can present with irritability, anger or aggression, nervousness or anxiety, sleep difficulties (insomnia), decreased appetite or weight loss, restlessness, depressed mood, and/or physical symptoms such as stomach pain, shakiness or tremors, sweating, fever, chills, and headache.
- Neurological exam should detail sensory abnormalities, nystagmus, motor weakness, abnormal reflexes, rigidity, bowel or bladder dysfunction, and any gait disturbance.
- Mental status exam:
  - Assessment for depression, psychosis, suicidality, homicidality, cognitive deficits, and altered sensorium is essential.

Useful clinical decision rules and calculators
- *Combining withdrawal rating scales with clinical and risk factor assessments can contribute to better patient care.*
  - High scores on the CIWA-Ar can predict development of more severe alcohol withdrawal, including seizures and delirium tremens. This scale facilitates clinical decisions regarding prescribing standing or PRN (e.g., symptom-triggered) medications for withdrawal.

Disease severity classification

- Severity of DSM-5 SUD is based on the number of criteria endorsed:
  - 2–3 criteria: mild;
  - 4–5 criteria: moderate;
  - ≥6: severe.

Laboratory diagnosis

List of diagnostic tests

- Currently, no laboratory test can confirm the presence/absence of SUD.
- Analysis of urine (most common), blood, sweat, and saliva via immunoassay screening or by confirmatory testing with gas chromatography/mass spectrometry (GC/MS) can detect recent drug use. Hair analysis can provide information on more protracted use. *These tests alone are not used, nor are they sufficient, to clinically diagnose SUD.*
- *Drug tests do not detect "dependence," intoxication, impairment, or addiction.* They detect drug use only within a designated time frame and at the minimal cut-off concentrations as set forth by each drug test.
- Certain medications or compounds, such as synthetic cannabinoids, methylphenidate, lorazepam, and some synthetic opioids (fentanyl, oxycodone) may not be detected on routine urine drug screens. Confirmatory testing should be pursued.

Lists of imaging techniques

- Currently, no imaging test or molecular marker is sufficiently specific to diagnose or predict vulnerability to SUD.
- However, neuroimaging to assess brain structure, function, and neurochemistry, in combination with advanced computational analytic methods, is a promising avenue for enhancing the study of the development, maintenance, and vulnerability to SUD.
  - For example, altered dopamine D2 receptor availability in the striatum is characteristic of numerous types of SUD (cocaine, alcohol, methamphetamine, heroin), and parallels functional changes in frontal cortical regions underlying self-control and value/salience attribution.

Diagnostic algorithm (Algorithm 16.1)

Potential pitfalls/common errors made regarding diagnosis of disease

- Differentiating between SUD, substance-induced psychiatric disorders, and other mental illness is a common and often challenging task for clinicians.
- *Drug tests do not detect "dependence," intoxication, impairment, or addiction.* Drug tests detect drug use, which may or may not present clinically and diagnostically as SUD.

Treatment

Treatment rationale

Treatments are usually multifaceted, with individual therapies (motivational, cognitive behavioral), self-help groups (Alcoholics Anonymous), and/or pharmacotherapy.

- Nicotine: use nicotine replacement therapy (NRT), varenicline, or bupropion.
- Alcohol:
  - Disulfiram interrupts the metabolism of alcohol, leading to an aversive physical reaction with alcohol intake.

Algorithm 16.1 Diagnostic algorithm for substance abuse. Reproduced with permission from AETC National Resource Center

Substance abuse or substance dependence:
- Correlates to increased incidence of psychiatric illness.
- Increases the difficulty in maintaining effective adherence to antiretroviral regimens.

Screening patients regularly using a non-judgmental, conversation style encourages patients to speak openly about their use of substances and assists the clinician in evaluating the patient's readiness to make a behavior change.

Occurrence of alcohol or drug use:
Self-report of problematic alcohol or drug use, family report of problematic use, clinical markers (e.g., positive toxicology screen), or physical symptomatology during exam

4 Question CAGE Screen
- Have you felt you ought to **cut** down on your drinking or drug use?
- Have people **annoyed** you by criticizing your drinking or drug use?
- Have you felt bad or **guilty** about your drinking or drug use?
- Have you ever had a drink or used drugs first thing in the morning to steady your nerves or to get rid of a hangover (**eye-opener**)?

0 "YES" responses → Probably not substance abuse/dependence. Continue periodic assessments.

1 "YES" response

Brief Intervention: FRAMES

Feedback	Address concerns about use: "I'm concerned about how alcohol is affecting your liver."(Your work, relationships, mood, behavior.)
Responsibility	Emphasize that change is up to patient: "Only you can decide to make your life better. There are programs that can help you."
Advice	Give your specific goals for the patient: "I want you to be evaluated at a treatment center."
Menu	Offer alternatives to advice: "You could go to an AA (or NA) meeting."
Empathy	Listen with empathy: "I imagine talking about this is difficult."
Self-efficacy	Encourage responses that support patient's confidence: "You deserve better – you can be better with help." or "Change can happen, but it takes time.

Assessment for withdrawal symptomatology
Alcohol, benzodiazepines, and opiates should be assessed for physiological withdrawal potential. All drugs will have psychological and social impact during withdrawal.

Drug/alcohol use escalates or consequences increase

Successful outcome resulting in abstinence or less chaotic use

≥2 "YES" responses

In-depth assessment of the following three dimensions:

Further screening:	Withdrawal potential:	Patient readiness:
■ AUDIT ■ DAST	Physiological for ETOH, opiates, and benzodiazepines	SOCRATES (available for both ETOH and other drugs)

Other options
- Family interview
- Intervention
- Watchful waiting
- Contingency agreement
- Pre-treatment programs

Patient refuses treatment

Relapse from treatment

Consider referral for specialized treatment

Successful intervention
Continue follow-up and relapse prevention

- Naltrexone, an opioid receptor antagonist, indirectly blocks the dopamine release associated with reinforcement and decreases drinking frequency and craving; it is relatively contraindicated in liver disease and requires careful monitoring of LFTs; also available in depot intramuscular form.
- Acamprosate reduces alcohol withdrawal by increasing GABAergic and inhibiting glutamatergic activity.
- Naloxone, a rapid opioid receptor blocker, is used in situations requiring immediate medical attention (e.g., slowed breathing, loss of consciousness) and to reverse opioid overdose.
- Opioids:
  - Substitution with either methadone or buprenorphine/naloxone; buprenorphine treatment is offered in the office-based setting. Patients with chronic pain and opioid addiction may benefit from either treatment, although tolerance must be taken into account for adequate analgesia.
  - Patients who fail substitution treatment, have a history of diverting buprenorphine, or abuse benzodiazepines or alcohol with opioids may do better with naltrexone treatment.
- There are as yet no FDA-approved pharmacological treatments for cocaine, methamphetamine, or cannabis use disorders.

When to hospitalize
- History of complicated alcohol, barbiturate, or benzodiazepine withdrawal (predisposing to seizures, delirium tremens).
- Acute medical crises (e.g., dehydration, sepsis, hemodynamic instability, seizures).
- Acute presentation of co-occurring psychiatric illness (e.g., agitated, psychotic, suicidal, homicidal, or delirious patients).
- Previously failed outpatient treatment for withdrawal.
- Pregnancy complicated by untreated SUD.

Managing the hospitalized patient
- Alcohol detoxification can be managed on a symptom-triggered or structured medication regimen, with benzodiazepines as first-line treatment.
- Opioid detoxification can be managed with methadone, buprenorphine, or clonidine (to reduce autonomic hyperactivity).
- With all patients, safety is of the utmost importance. The objective is to achieve hemodynamic, medical, and mental status stability.

Table of treatment

Pharmacotherapies	• *Nicotine addiction*
	    • Nicotine replacement therapy (NRT) (i.e., patch, gum, nasal spray)
	    • Varenicline
	    • Bupropion
	• *Alcohol addiction*
	    • Disulfiram
	    • Naltrexone
	    • Acamprosate
	• *Opioid addiction*
	    • Methadone maintenance
	    • Buprenorphine/naloxone
	    • Naltrexone

(Continued)

(Continued)

Psychotherapies	• Motivational enhancement therapy • Cognitive behavioral therapy • Twelve-step facilitation therapy • Network therapy • Group and family therapies • Contingency management • Voucher-based reinforcement therapy
Self-help fellowships	• Alcoholics Anonymous • Narcotics Anonymous • Cocaine Anonymous • Marijuana Anonymous • Crystal Meth Anonymous

Rehabilitation settings	• Inpatient treatment/detoxification
	• Therapeutic communities
	• Community-based treatments
	  ◦ Brief interventions in primary care
	  ◦ Employee assistance programs
	  ◦ Drug court programs
	  ◦ Day hospital/intensive outpatient treatment
	  ◦ Community residential facilities ("half-way houses")

Prevention/management of complications

- CNS depression precipitated by sedative hypnotics in patients on methadone or chronic opioids:
  - Obtain periodic drug testing to assess for drug misuse or compliance; consider reducing and/or discontinuing benzodiazepines, zolpidem, and other sedative hypnotics.
- Misuse of prescribed opioids in patients with SUD:
  - Assess for risk factors predicting misuse (see chapter case study on the companion website), obtain informed consent before prescribing, utilize a prescription monitoring program (if available in the state of practice) and use an opioid prescribing agreement.
- Peri- and post-operative pain in patients maintained on buprenorphine/naloxone:
  - Patients who undergo scheduled surgery and who require sufficient opioid analgesia will likely need to discontinue buprenorphine prior to surgery and reinstate treatment after completion of opioid pain management.
- Peri- and post-operative pain in patients maintained on methadone:
  - Patients may be able to continue their methadone dosing. Pain treatment will likely require additional opiates (beyond the methadone dosing).

Management/treatment algorithm (Algorithm 16.2 and Table 16.1)

- See http://buprenorphine.samhsa.gov/Bup_Guidelines.pdf, pages 53 and 55, for the Substance Abuse and Mental Health Services Association's algorithm for Suboxone (buprenorphine+naloxone) induction.

CLINICAL PEARLS
- Most people addicted to substances cannot quit on their own, making treatment essential for achieving abstinence.
- SUD treatment can be very specialized and often includes combining pharmacological, behavioral, community, and appropriate rehabilitation settings.

Algorithm 16.2 Pharmacological treatment algorithm for alcohol use disorder

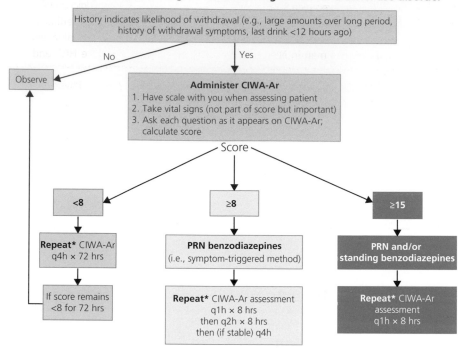

* Every time you repeat the CIWA-Ar for a given patient, use the algorithm to determine management based on the new score.
CIWA–Ar is not copyrighted and may be used freely. Source: Sullivan JT, et al., 1989.

Special populations
Pregnancy
- **Alcohol** use is associated with fetal alcohol spectrum disorders. Alcohol withdrawal during pregnancy should be managed in a high-risk maternity unit.
- **Cocaine** use is associated with preterm labor, placental abruption, and low birth weight newborns. Psychosocial interventions are most effective.
- Long-term maternal **smoking** is associated with reduction in birth weight and increased risk of sudden infant death syndrome.
- **Cannabis** use is associated with reduced birth weight.
- Untreated **opioid** addiction is associated with miscarriage, preterm labor, and intrauterine growth restriction. Methadone maintenance during pregnancy has been the gold standard treatment. *Neonatal abstinence syndrome* is common in infants born to mothers maintained on buprenorphine or methadone. The use of buprenorphine in pregnancy is still controversial but appears promising in newer studies, demonstrating good tolerability and less severe neonatal abstinence syndrome.

Others
- **In those with prescription drug abuse,** consider methadone or buprenorphine for opioid addiction and medications for ADHD with less liability for abuse.
- **LGBT, adolescent and young adults with SUD** may require more intensive treatment to address relapse triggers related to childhood trauma, internalized homophobia, and fragmented family dynamics.

- **Women with SUD** are more vulnerable to adverse medical consequences of addiction, often have comorbid mood disorders preceding SUD, and are less likely than men to enter addiction treatment.
- Treatment of **SUD with comorbid HIV/AIDS and/or hepatitis C** can be either primary prevention of HIV and HCV (e.g., attempts to target the methamphetamine epidemic among HIV-negative gay men in NYC) or secondary prevention to reduce HIV- and HCV-related morbidity.
- Treatment of **SUD among physicians** requires early intervention efforts. Physician Health Programs are widely available for support.

Prognosis

> **BOTTOM LINE/CLINICAL PEARLS**
> - Intoxication or withdrawal can present with psychosis, depression, or delirium, which can amplify the risk of suicide and violence.
> - SUD can co-occur with other psychiatric disorders, which should be treated concurrently.
> - SUD should be treated like any other chronic illness, with relapse serving as a trigger for renewed intervention.

Natural history of untreated disease
- Chronic alcohol use can lead to liver cirrhosis, hepatocellular carcinoma, and/or liver failure.

Prognosis for treated patients
- Relapse rates for drug addiction are similar to other chronic illnesses.
- SUD treatment can be helpful in achieving long-term abstinence.
- Extended abstinence can be predictive of sustainable recovery.

Follow-up tests and monitoring
- Monitor LFTs in patients on naltrexone or buprenorphine.
- Monitor QTc in patients on methadone. Obtain baseline EKG prior to initiation, 30 days after initiation, and annually thereafter. Be aware of any potential drug interactions that can also prolong QTc.
- Periodically monitor *urine drug toxicology* in patients with SUD who are prescribed controlled substances. Patients with SUD have an increased risk of medication misuse and also have the potential to relapse.

Reading list/references
Center for Substance Abuse Treatment. Treatment Improvement Protocol (TIP) Series. Rockville, MD: Substance Abuse and Mental Health Services Administration (US):
- TIP 34: Brief Interventions and Brief Therapies for Substance Abuse. 1999. http://www.ncbi.nlm.nih.gov/books/NBK64947/
- TIP 35: Enhancing Motivation for Change in Substance Abuse Treatment. 1999. http://www.ncbi.nlm.nih.gov/books/NBK64967/
- TIP 42: Substance Abuse Treatment for Persons With Co-Occurring Disorders. 2005. http://www.ncbi.nlm.nih.gov/books/NBK64197/
- TIP 45: Detoxification and Substance Abuse Treatment. 2006. http://www.ncbi.nlm.nih.gov/books/NBK64115/
- TIP 48: Managing Depressive Symptoms in Substance Abuse Clients During Early Recovery. 2008. http://www.ncbi.nlm.nih.gov/books/NBK64057/

- TIP 49: Incorporating Alcohol Pharmacotherapies Into Medical Practice. 2009. http://www. ncbi.nlm.nih.gov/books/NBK64041/
- TIP 54: Managing Chronic Pain in Adults With or in Recovery From Substance Use Disorders. 2012. http://www.ncbi.nlm.nih.gov/books/NBK92048/

Goldstein RZ, Volkow ND. Drug addiction and its underlying neurobiological basis: neuroimaging evidence for the involvement of the frontal cortex. Am J Psychiatry 2002;159(10):1642–52.

Humeniuk R, Ali R, Babor TF, et al. Validation of the Alcohol, Smoking And Substance Involvement Screening Test (ASSIST). Addiction 2008;103(6):1039–47.

Knight JR, Shrier LA, Bravender TD, Farrell M, Vander Bilt J, Shaffer HJ. A new brief screen for adolescent substance abuse. Arch Pediatr Adolesc Med 1999;153(6):591–6.

Saunders JB, Aasland OG, Babor TF, de la Fuente JR, Grant M. Development of the Alcohol Use Disorders Identification Test (AUDIT): WHO Collaborative Project on Early Detection of Persons with Harmful Alcohol Consumption – II. Addiction 1993;88(6):791–804.

Selzer ML. The Michigan alcoholism screening test: the quest for a new diagnostic instrument. Am J Psychiatry 1971;127(12):1653–8.

Substance Abuse and Mental Health Services Administration and National Institute on Alcohol Abuse and Alcoholism. Medication for the Treatment of Alcohol Use Disorder: A Brief Guide. HHS Publication No. (SMA) 15-4907. Rockville, MD: Substance Abuse and Mental Health Services Administration, 2015.

Sullivan JT, Sykora K, Schneiderman J, Naranjo CA, Sellers EM. Assessment of alcohol withdrawal: The revised Clinical Institute Withdrawal Assessment for Alcohol scale (CIWA–Ar). Br J Addict 1989;84:1353.

Volkow ND, Skolnick P. New medications for substance use disorders: challenges and opportunities. Neuropsychopharmacology 2012;37(1):290–2.

Suggested websites

American Academy of Addiction Psychiatry. http://www.aaap.org/

National Institute on Alcohol Abuse and Alcoholism. http://www.niaaa.nih.gov/

National Institute on Drug Abuse. http://www.drugabuse.gov/

Substance Abuse and Mental Health Services Association. http://www.samhsa.gov/

Guidelines
National society guidelines

- See the reading list for the Treatment Improvement Protocol (TIP) Series, which are best practice guidelines for the treatment of substance abuse published by the US Department of Health and Human Services, Substance Abuse and Mental Health Services Administration (SAMSA). The TIP Series is available free online at http://www.ncbi.nlm.nih.gov/books/NBK82999/.

Evidence

Type of evidence	Title and comment	Weblink
Federally funded RCT	The COMBINE Study: An Overview of the Largest Pharmacotherapy Study to Date for Treating Alcohol Dependence. **Comment:** This study included 1383 recently abstinent alcoholics from 11 US academic sites and evaluated the efficacy of naltrexone and acamprosate. Naltrexone plus medical management led to higher percentage of days abstinent, and naltrexone reduced the risk over time of heavy drinking days. An important implication of the COMBINE results is that naltrexone with medical management can be delivered in healthcare settings where traditional specialty treatment may be unavailable.	http://www.ncbi.nlm.nih.gov/pubmed/20877545

(Continued)

(Continued)

Type of evidence	Title and comment	Weblink
Multisite RCT	Project MATCH (Matching Alcoholism Treatments to Client Heterogeneity. **Comment:** Designed to investigate if matching patient with treatment modality improved treatment outcomes. 1726 subjects were randomly assigned to twelve-step facilitation (TSF), cognitive behavioral therapy (CBT), or motivational enhancement therapy (MET). *Only client anger* demonstrated the most consistent matching-related effects; those with high levels of anger fared better in MET than in CBT or TSF. The study demonstrates that once patients have reached a point at which they are willing to consider abstinence, their motivation and characteristics are likely to be better predictors of outcome than any specific aspect of the treatment program.	http://www.ncbi.nlm.nih.gov/pubmed/8979210 http://www.ncbi.nlm.nih.gov/pubmed/9756046 and http://www.ncbi.nlm.nih.gov/pubmed/10091964

Additional material for this chapter can be found online at: www.mountsinaiexpertguides.com/psychiatry

This includes advice for patients, a case study, ICD codes, and multiple choice questions.

CHAPTER 17

Personality Disorders: Assessment and Treatment

Antonia S. New[1], M. Mercedes Perez-Rodriguez[1], and Jake Rosenberg[2]

[1] Icahn School of Medicine at Mount Sinai, New York, NY, USA
[2] University of Pennsylvania School of Medicine, Philadelphia, PA, USA

OVERALL BOTTOM LINE

- DSM-5 retains the same diagnostic categories for personality disorders as DSM-IV (including all Cluster A, B, and C diagnoses).
- New to DSM-5 is that the personality disorders reside in Section 2 alongside other major psychiatric diagnostic categories and are no longer separated into a different "Axis."
- While advances have been made in the pharmacologic management of personality disorders, especially borderline personality disorder (BPD), the mainstay of treatment for these illnesses remains psychotherapy.
- Substantial improvements have been made in the development and validation of evidence-based psychotherapies for BPD.

Background

This chapter will focus on two personality disorders, BPD from Cluster B and avoidant personality disorder (AvPD) from Cluster C, as prototypes for their related disorders. Schizotypal personality disorder is covered in Chapter 15.

Borderline personality disorder

Definition of disease

BPD is defined in DSM-5 (as in DSM-IV) by meeting 5 of 9 criteria. The best instrument for the diagnosis of BPD is Zanarini's Diagnostic Interview for Borderline Personality Disorder (DIB-R). Scoring positively on 8/10 items is typically considered the appropriate score for a categorical diagnosis.

Disease classification

In the DSM-IV, BPD was placed on Axis II. In the new DSM-5, the personality disorders are placed in Section 2, alongside other major diagnostic categories such as mood disorders and anxiety disorders.

Incidence/prevalence

- The lifetime prevalence of BPD is estimated at 1.9–5.9%, with most authors agreeing on approximately 2% lifetime prevalence of BPD with sufficient severity to meet DIB-R criteria.

Mount Sinai Expert Guides: Psychiatry, First Edition. Edited by Asher B. Simon, Antonia S. New, and Wayne K. Goodman.
© 2017 John Wiley & Sons, Ltd. Published 2017 by John Wiley & Sons, Ltd.
Companion website: www.mountsinaiexpertguides.com/psychiatry

- The female:male ratio was over-estimated at 12:1 in the DSM-IV; more recent data using validated instruments suggest a ratio of approximately 1.5:1.

Economic impact

- Longitudinal studies show substantial impairment in interpersonal and vocational functioning in BPD. Even among "remitted" patients, almost 40% needed some government assistance (especially to maintain health insurance to cover the costs of their care).
- BPD patients are high consumers of medical care with high rates of pain syndromes (chronic fatigue, fibromyalgia, back pain, and headaches), obesity, diabetes, hypertension, smoking- and alcohol-related illnesses and lack of regular exercise.
- The financial burden to families with a BPD offspring in the year following diagnosis is high, with an average cost per year after diagnosis of approximately $14,000 out-of-pocket and $46,000 billed to insurance.

Etiology

- BPD is partially genetic, with calculated heritability scores (e.g., the degree to which the risk for BPD comes from genetic factors alone) of 51–71% from twin studies.
- Some forms of child abuse also contribute to the risk for BPD, especially "childhood neglect" and "childhood sexual abuse." However, meta-analyses suggest that these account for only a small part of the risk for BPD.

Pathophysiology

While the precise etiology of BPD is not known, one mechanism by which the genetic risk may predispose to the illness is an inherited difficulty in early attachment. Studies supporting this suggest that there may be delayed development of white matter tracts in the temporal lobe in BPD. In addition, BPD patients have smaller volumes of the anterior cingulate gyrus, a part of the brain involved in emotion regulation. Whether the poor early attachment leads to affective instability or affective instability leads to poor social attachment is unknown.

Predictive/risk factors

- Family history of BPD.
- Childhood sexual abuse or neglect.
- Low socioeconomic status.
- Poor social functioning with peers as early as elementary school.
- Unstable family environment.

Prevention

> **BOTTOM LINE/CLINICAL PEARLS**
> - Work from Australia showed that early intervention in teens with subsyndromal or syndromal BPD attenuates symptom severity in follow-up. This intervention involved case-management/ individual psychotherapy, brief family interventions, team-based care, group therapy, crisis management, and psychopharmacology as needed.
> - Screening: there are no good data on screening for BPD, but children and adolescents with poor emotion regulation and social skills, substance abuse, and turbulent peer relationships are at risk.

Diagnosis

> **BOTTOM LINE/CLINICAL PEARLS**
> - A history of disrupted interpersonal relationships is highly associated with BPD. While self-injury is a dramatic symptom of BPD, anxious and clinging attachments should raise a red flag.
> - People with BPD can appear very healthy on first evaluation, hiding their symptoms out of shame.
> - It is helpful to get collateral information from someone close to the patient; however, this must be done with the full collaboration of the patient.
> - The importance of transparency and honesty in interacting with someone with BPD cannot be overstressed. It is important to win the trust of patients with BPD to help them to overcome the emotional turmoil triggered by talking about feelings and establishing a therapeutic relationship. Educating patients about their diagnosis in a supportive way is helpful.
> - BPD is often diagnosed 6–10 years after first presentation. This is too long for patients to wait for evidence-based treatment.

Differential diagnosis

Differential diagnosis	Features
Complex posttraumatic stress disorder (PTSD)	Complex PTSD resembles BPD, with mood instability, self-injury, and dissociation. Complex PTSD, however, follows a specific traumatic experience. Chronic adversity in childhood is common in both disorders. Both respond to psychotherapy but only complex PTSD will respond to exposure-based therapy
Treatment-refractory depression	When a patient does not respond to usual antidepressant treatment, it is important to consider underlying BPD, which would guide recommendations for evidence-based psychotherapy
Substance abuse disorder	BPD is often comorbid with substance abuse. It is important to target both symptom domains for effective treatment. Substance abuse often masks BPD and the underlying diagnosis is often missed for years
Antisocial personality disorder (ASPD)	BPD in men is often misdiagnosed as ASPD. The impulsivity and interpersonal aggression in men with BPD is mistaken for the broad failure to behave in a law-abiding way seen in ASPD. Childhood conduct disorder also differentiates ASPD from BPD

Typical presentation
BPD patients typically present with anxiety and/or depression and often will have tried to self-medicate with cannabis or alcohol.

Clinical diagnosis
History
- The most important feature of assessing for BPD is not to be misled by comorbid diagnoses.

Physical and mental status exams
There are no diagnostic findings on clinical exam, although some patients will have scars from self-injury. The mental status exam of BPD patients is frequently normal unless they are emotionally activated.

Laboratory diagnosis
- There is no diagnostic lab test or imaging technique for BPD.

Potential pitfalls/common errors made regarding diagnosis of disease
- Missing the diagnosis of BPD since comorbid PTSD, substance abuse, depression, and anxiety can mask the underlying problem.
- Overlooking BPD in men.

Treatment
- Pharmacology: avoid over-medicating.
- Psychotherapy: greater efficacy than medication.

When to hospitalize
- Hospitalization is rarely helpful in BPD. When necessary for safety, hospitalizations should be brief and the patient should move to a setting of intensive outpatient treatment as soon as possible.
- However, the suicide completion rate in BPD is 10%. The fact that someone has BPD can be mistaken as a cause for less concern in the emergency department. BPD patients are at high risk for completed suicide and so should be protected in an acute episode as are patients with any other diagnosis.

Table of treatment

Medical **(Off-Label medications [there are no FDA-approved drugs targeting BPD specifically])**	
Second-generation antipsychotics • Aripiprazole 15 mg/day • Olanzapine 5–10 mg/day • Quetiapine 150–250 mg/day	• Olanzapine is less well tolerated due to weight gain • Second-generation antipsychotics are especially helpful for depression and anxiety in BPD • Raise dose slowly to enhance tolerability • Mood stabilizers are helpful with impulsivity and aggression
Mood stabilizers • Topiramate 50–250 mg/day • Lamotrigine 50–250 mg/day • Valproic acid (blood level 80–120 μg/mL) **Serotonin-selective reuptake inhibitors (SSRIs) if patient is in major depressive episode** • Fluoxetine 20–80 mg for depression	
Psychological	
There are a number of evidence-based psychotherapies for BPD with proven efficacy	• Dialectical behavior therapy (DBT) • Mentalization based therapy (MBT) • Transference focused psychotherapy (TFP) • STEPPS® • Cognitive analytic therapy (CAT) • Schema-focused therapy • General psychiatric management [Helping Young People Early (HYPE) for adolescents]
Complementary • Omega-3 fatty acids	

Prevention/management of complications
- Lamotrigine is associated with rashes and can cause Stevens–Johnson syndrome. If a rash appears, lamotrigine should be stopped and a dermatologist consulted.
- All pharmacologic interventions in BPD are of modest effect. Avoid polypharmacy and educate patients about the limits of psychopharmacology for this disorder, stressing the importance of evidence-based psychotherapy.
- Avoid benzodiazepines as they are rarely helpful and often increase impulsive behaviors.

CLINICAL PEARLS
- There are numerous evidence-based psychotherapies for BPD. Evidence of the superiority of one over another has not been proven.
- All the evidence-based psychotherapies focus on the development of a trusting treatment alliance and the need for transparency and authenticity in this alliance.
- All therapies also focus on present problems and tend to avoid a re-examination of early life experiences as a "cause" of the current symptoms.

Prognosis

BOTTOM LINE/CLINICAL PEARLS
- Studies suggest that, with treatment, more than 85% of patients go into remission over a 10-year period.
- BPD patients are at some lifetime risk of recurrence.
- A degree of functional impairment often persists, particularly in the area of professional/educational functioning.
- Notwithstanding the persistence of some symptoms, this disorder is treatable and patients should be educated about the opportunity for symptom relief.

Avoidant personality disorder
Definition of disease
AvPD is defined in DSM-5, as it was in DSM-IV, by meeting 4 of 7 criteria.

Disease classification
In the DSM-IV, AvPD was on Axis II, whereas in DSM-5 all the personality disorders are placed in Section 2.

Incidence/prevalence
Prevalence is up to 2.4% in the general population, and between 10 and 15.2% in the psychiatric population; AvPD is equally common in men and women.

Economic impact
In a nationally representative sample of US adults, AvPD was significantly associated with disability and with increased odds of receiving public assistance, especially Supplemental Security Income. This may be related to avoidance of occupational activities requiring interpersonal contact.

Etiology

While the etiology of AvPD is unknown and most evidence points to influence from both genetic and environmental factors, recent studies point to a common genetic vulnerability to AvPD and social phobia.

Pathophysiology

The genetic risk for AvPD may predispose to the illness through the presence of a highly sensitive fear network within the amygdaloid-hippocampal brain circuit.

Predictive/risk factors

- Family history of social anxiety and/or AvPD.
- Cormorbid anxiety disorders.
- Childhood temperament (high harm avoidance, shyness, anxiety, withdrawal, negative affectivity, low self-esteem).
- Parental neglect.

Prevention

> **BOTTOM LINE/CLINICAL PEARLS**
> - No intervention has been demonstrated to prevent the development of the disease.

Screening

There are no good data on screening for AvPD, but children and adolescents with high harm avoidance, shyness, anxiety, withdrawal, negative affectivity, and low self-esteem are at risk.

Diagnosis

> **BOTTOM LINE/CLINICAL PEARLS**
> - Those with childhood history of high harm avoidance, shyness, anxiety, withdrawal, negative affectivity, low self-esteem and parental neglect are at increased risk.
> - Those with family members with AvPD and/or social phobia are at increased risk.

Differential diagnosis

The high comorbidity and overlapping features of AvPD and social phobia may make them difficult to differentiate.

Differential diagnosis	Features
Social Phobia	High overlap between AvPD and social phobia; some hypothesize that they may be alternative conceptualizations of the same condition
Panic Disorder with Agoraphobia	In panic disorder with agoraphobia, avoidance typically starts after the onset of panic attacks and may vary based on their frequency and intensity. In AvPD, the avoidance tends to have an early onset, no clear precipitant, and a stable course
Dependent Personality Disorder	While the primary focus of concern in AvPD is avoidance of humiliation and rejection, in dependent personality disorder the focus is on being taken care of. However, they commonly co-occur

(Continued)

(Continued)

Differential diagnosis	Features
Schizoid and Schizotypal Personality Disorder	Individuals with AvPD want to have relationships with others and feel lonely, while those with schizoid or schizotypal personality disorder may prefer their social isolation
Paranoid Personality Disorder	In AvPD, the reluctance to confide in others is due more to a fear of embarrassment or being found inadequate than to a fear of others' malicious intent, as is the case in paranoid PD

Typical presentation
- AvPD patients typically present with feelings of inadequacy and sensitivity towards what others think, which leads to social inhibition and isolation.

Clinical diagnosis
History
- Screen for criteria as listed in DSM-5.
- Assess for commonly comorbid disorders such as social phobia, agoraphobia, and other personality disorders.

Physical and mental status exams
- There is no diagnostic finding on clinical exam. The mental status exam is frequently normal.

Laboratory diagnosis
There is no diagnostic lab test or imaging technique for AvPD.

Potential pitfalls/common errors made regarding diagnosis of disease
There is ongoing debate about whether AvPD and social phobia are separate diagnostic entities or reflect a spectrum of social anxiety.

Treatment
Due to the lack of evidence for treatment outcomes in AvPD, clinicians should apply treatment strategies that have primarily been developed for social anxiety/social phobia.

Treatment rationale
- Pharmacology: none.
- Psychotherapy: CBT including exposure and social skills training.

When to hospitalize
There is no good evidence about outcomes after hospitalization in AvPD specifically. Clinicians should make the decision to hospitalize a patient with AvPD as they would in a patient with any other psychiatric diagnosis

Table of treatment

Medical As in social phobia
Psychological CBT including exposure, and social skills training

Prognosis

> **BOTTOM LINE/CLINICAL PEARLS**
> Although no longitudinal study has assessed long-term outcomes, in clinical trials >50% of patients improve significantly after a brief psychotherapeutic intervention.

Reading list

Emmelkamp PM, Benner A, Kuipers A, Feiertag GA, Koster HC, van Apeldoorn FJ. Comparison of brief dynamic and cognitive-behavioural therapies in avoidant personality disorder. Br J Psychiatry 2006; 189:60–4.

Grant BF, Hasin DS, Stinson FS, et al. Prevalence, correlates, and disability of personality disorders in the United States: results from the national epidemiologic survey on alcohol and related conditions. J Clin Psychiatry 2004;65(7):948–58.

Herpertz SC, Zanarini M, Schultz CS, et al. World Federation of Societies of Biological Psychiatry (WFSBP) guidelines for biological treatment of personality disorders. World J Biol Psychiatry 2007;8(4):212–44.

Joyce PR, McKenzie JM, Luty SE, et al. Temperament, childhood environment and psychopathology as risk factors for avoidant and borderline personality disorders. Aust N Z J Psychiatry 2003;37(6):756–64.

Leichsenring F, Leibing E, Kruse J, New AS, Leweke F. Borderline personality disorder. Lancet 2011;377(9759):74–84.

Lieb K, Völlm B, Rücker G, Timmer A, Stoffers JM. Pharmacotherapy for borderline personality disorder: Cochrane systematic review of randomized trials. Br J Psychiatry 2010;196(1):4–12.

Livesley WJ. Moving beyond specialized therapies for borderline personality disorder: the importance of integrated domain-focused treatment. Psychodyn Psychiatry 2012;40(1):47–74.

McMain SF, Guimond T, Streiner DL, Cardish RJ, Links PS. Dialectical behavior therapy compared with general psychiatric management for borderline personality disorder: clinical outcomes and functioning over a 2-year follow-up. Am J Psychiatry 2012169(6):650–61.

Reichborn-Kjennerud, Czajkowski N, Torgersen S, et al. The relationship between avoidant personality disorder and social phobia: a population-based twin study. Am J Psychiatry 2007;164(11):1722–8.

Torgersen S, Myers J, Reichborn-Kjennerud T, Røysamb E, Kubarych TS, Kendler KS. The heritability of Cluster B personality disorders assessed both by personal interview and questionnaire. J Pers Disord 2012;26(6):848–66.

Suggested websites

Emotions Matter: http://emotionsmatterbpd.org/

http://BPD Resource Center

National Education Alliance for Borderline Personality Disorder. http://www.borderline personalitydisorder.com/

Treatment and Research Advocacy (TARA). http://www.tara4bpd.org

Guidelines
National society guidelines

Title	Source	Weblink
Guideline Watch: Practice Guideline for the Treatment of Patients With Borderline Personality Disorder	American Psychiatric Association (APA) sponsored PsychiatryOnline, 2001 and 2005	http://psychiatryonline.org/pb/assets/raw/ sitewide/practice_guidelines/guidelines/ bpd.pdf and http://psychiatryonline.org/pb/assets/raw/ sitewide/practice_guidelines/guidelines/ bpd-watch.pdf

International society guidelines

Title	Source	Weblink
Clinical Practice Guideline for the Management of Borderline Personality Disorder	Australian Government National Health and Medical Research Council (NHMRC), 2012	https://www.nhmrc.gov.au/guidelines-publications/mh25
Borderline personality disorder: recognition and management	United Kingdom NHS, 2009	https://www.nice.org.uk/guidance/cg78

Evidence (BPD)

Type of evidence	Title and comment	Weblink
Meta-analysis	Effectiveness of pharmacotherapy for severe personality disorders: meta-analyses of randomized controlled trials **Comment:** Utility or lack thereof for specific drugs for BPD.	http://www.ncbi.nlm.nih.gov/pubmed/19778496
Expert guidelines: Cochrane Database Systematic Review	Psychological therapies for people with borderline personality disorder. **Comment:** Evidence-based psychotherapies for BPD.	http://www.cochrane.org/CD005652/BEHAV_psychological-therapies-for-borderline-personality-disorder
Expert guidelines: Cochrane Database Systematic Review	Pharmacotherapy for borderline personality disorder: Cochrane systematic review of randomized trials. **Comment:** Evidence-based psychopharmacology for BPD.	http://www.ncbi.nlm.nih.gov/pubmed/20044651

There are no meta-analyses or systematic reviews on the treatment of AvPD.

Additional material for this chapter can be found online at:
www.mountsinaiexpertguides.com/psychiatry

This includes advice for patients, a case study, ICD codes, and multiple choice questions.

CHAPTER 18

Psychiatric Presentations of Primary Medical Illness

Adam Karz[1], Madeleine Fersh[2], Akhil Shenoy[3], and Kim Klipstein[3]
[1] Swedish Medical Group, Seattle, WA, USA
[2] Northwell Health, Glen Oaks, NY, USA
[3] Icahn School of Medicine at Mount Sinai, New York, NY, USA

OVERALL BOTTOM LINE
- Medically ill patients may present with psychiatric symptoms secondary to the illness itself.
- These symptoms are present in a wide variety of medical illnesses such as neurologic conditions, infectious diseases, endocrinopathies, oncologic illnesses, and metabolic disorders.
- It is important to differentiate primary psychiatric illnesses from psychiatric symptoms secondary to a non-psychiatric medical illness.
- Resolution of the medical illness may result in resolution of psychiatric symptoms.

Discussion of topic and guidelines

Many medical illnesses present with secondary psychiatric phenomena including depression, anxiety, mania, psychosis, personality changes, and cognitive dysfunction. These symptoms are present in a wide variety of medical illnesses such as neurologic conditions, infectious diseases, endocrinopathies, oncologic illnesses, and metabolic disorders. In many cases, treatment of the primary medical condition will improve the psychiatric symptoms. Common medical illnesses that result in significant psychiatric signs and symptoms are discussed further on.

Neurologic illness

- **Epilepsy** is a neurologic disorder that can lead to many psychiatric symptoms.
  - Psychosis is commonly seen and occurs most often post-ictally or inter-ictally. Psychotic episodes usually start 2–72 hours after a seizure and may take the form of delusions, hallucinations, or gross disorganization.
  - Depression and anxiety, including panic attacks, are seen in one-third of patients with epilepsy. Studies have shown a link between complex partial seizures and frontal lobe dysregulation resulting in depression.
  - Antiepileptics may contribute to the development of symptoms, particularly vigabatrin, which may precipitate psychotic and affective states in 3–10% of patients.
- **Multiple sclerosis (MS)** is a demyelinating disorder of the CNS with many psychiatric sequelae.
  - Symptoms initially seen include cognitive impairment, which often resembles a subcortical dementia.

Mount Sinai Expert Guides: Psychiatry, First Edition. Edited by Asher B. Simon, Antonia S. New, and Wayne K. Goodman.
© 2017 John Wiley & Sons, Ltd. Published 2017 by John Wiley & Sons, Ltd.
Companion website: www.mountsinaiexpertguides.com/psychiatry

- Mood symptoms including mania and emotional lability are frequent.
- Comorbid mood disorders are common with half of patients developing depressive symptoms over time.
- Patients have a greater risk of suicide than is seen in the general population.
- Substance-induced depression from interferon-beta treatment is seen in up to 40% of patients.
- Fatigue is one of the most common complaints, found in up to 80% of patients. Amantadine, pemoline, and modafinil may help to minimize this
- Pathological laughing and weeping is often present in advanced stages of the illness. Treatment options include tricyclic antidepressants, selective serotonin reuptake inhibitors (SSRIs) and dextromethorphan.
- **Cerebral vascular accidents** are acute CNS events that often result in significant psychiatric complications including cognitive impairment, mood symptoms, and psychosis.
  - 25% of patients will experience cognitive changes within 3 months of a stroke. Many will go on to have permanent changes consistent with amnestic syndromes or dementias.
  - Delirium is more typical following hemorrhagic strokes and is seen in 30–40% of patients within the first week. It is associated with a poorer prognosis and increased risk for dementia.
  - Depression is seen in one-third of stroke survivors and results in a higher morbidity and mortality. Early recognition and treatment help to maximize functional outcomes. Nortriptyline has been found to be more effective than fluoxetine for post-stroke depression, but SSRIs may be preferable due to better side effect profiles.
  - Anxiety is common in this population with a 4–28% prevalence. Post-stroke anxiety states may include posttraumatic stress disorder (PTSD), agoraphobia, and somatic preoccupation. Phobic states are more common in women.
  - Psychosis may be seen in approximately 1% of patients post stroke. It typically presents as a mania with associated delusions, hallucinations, and disorganization. Old age and a preexisting degenerative disease increase the risk.
  - Behavioral changes such as hypo- and hypersexuality, emotional lability, catastrophic reactions, disinhibition, and loss of empathy may also occur.
- **Systemic lupus erythematosus (SLE)** is an autoimmune vasculitis affecting the CNS with associated neuropsychiatric symptomatology in 75–90% of patients.
  - Psychiatric symptoms usually result from CNS injury, infection, systemic illness, or drug-induced side effects.
  - Autoimmune antibodies may play a direct role with antiribosomal-p and antineuronal antibodies being associated with psychosis and depression in some studies.
  - Most psychiatric symptoms with the exception of cognitive dysfunction often resolve within 2–3 weeks of corticosteroid treatment.
  - Cognitive dysfunction is the most common neuropsychiatric disorder, present in up to 80% of patients.
  - Depression is the second most common psychiatric finding, seen in up to 50% of patients. Chronic steroid use may precipitate depressive symptoms.
  - Anxiety is found in 13–24% of patients.
  - Mania is seen in 3–4% of patients and is most often the result of acute corticosteroid therapy.
  - Corticosteroid-induced psychosis may be difficult to differentiate from psychosis due to SLE and thus an empirical trial of corticosteroids to treat psychosis may be warranted.

- **Creutzfeldt–Jakob disease**, a prion disease, is a rare, degenerative neurologic disorder with predominant psychiatric manifestations. Etiology can be familial, sporadic, or acquired (variant).
  - Symptoms include memory loss, personality changes, hallucinations, paranoia, and obsessive-compulsive symptoms.
  - Sporadic forms of the illness present with a rapid, progressive dementia and early behavioral changes. Death occurs within 4 months after onset.
  - Variant forms of the illness may first present with anxiety or depression and progress more slowly, taking 14 months from time of onset to death.

Neoplastic Illness

- Brain tumors, both primary and secondary, are the most likely neoplasms to present with psychiatric symptoms including depression, anxiety, psychosis, confusion, cognitive dysfunction, and personality changes.
- Psychiatric phenomena often correlate with location of the tumor. Frontal pole tumors tend to be "neurologically silent," not manifesting psychiatrically until they are fairly large and have dramatically affected personality and neurocognitive function.
- Right-sided lesions have classically been associated with manic symptoms while left-sided lesions have been linked more often to depression.
- Temporal lobe lesions are the most likely to cause psychosis, including auditory and olfactory hallucinations.
- Occipital tumors may produce visual hallucinations and illusions.
- **Paraneoplastic syndromes (PNS)** illustrate how non-CNS neoplasms can influence the nervous system unique from direct invasion or metastasis.
  - Patients may present with irritability, depression, hallucinations, personality changes, and short-term memory deficits. Sleep disturbance, confusion, and seizures may also be found.
  - Neurologic and psychiatric symptoms are thought to be due to cross-reactivity of autoantibodies to CNS structures.
  - The most common cancers associated with PNS are those of breast, ovarian, and lung.
  - The most common PNS is limbic encephalitis, characterized by the subacute development of short-term memory dysfunction and the subsequent onset of irritability, sleep disturbance, delusions, hallucinations, agitation, seizures, and psychosis. This syndrome is most commonly associated with small cell lung cancer and the presence of anti-Hu antibodies.
  - Anti-Ma2 antibodies tend to be associated with testicular germ cell tumors and can manifest as obsessive-compulsive disorder.
  - Anti-NMDA receptor encephalitis, most often seen in conjunction with ovarian teratomas, may present with mania, personality changes, cognitive dysfunction, paranoia, and catatonia.
  - Once thought to be rare, the paraneoplastic syndromes are now considered under-reported and under-estimated.

Vitamin deficiencies

- Deficiencies in the B-complex vitamins can present with neuropsychiatric complications including subacute dementia, delirium, psychosis, anxiety, and mood disorders.
- Thiamine (B_1) deficiency can lead to the life-threatening Wernicke–Korsakoff syndrome.
  - The classic triad of confusion, ataxia, and eye findings (nystagmus or intranuclear ophthalmoplegia) may be seen in a minority of patients with Wernicke's encephalopathy.
  - Alcoholism, chronic gastrointestinal disease, and eating disorders may lead to this deficiency.

- 80% of alcoholics who develop Wernicke's will progress to Korsakoff's psychosis.
- Korsakoff's psychosis is an amnestic syndrome characterized by memory impairment, confabulation, confusion, and personality changes.
- Half of Korsakoff patients will recover, although recovery can take years.
- Treatment includes immediate IV or IM thiamine (a minimum of 200 mg) followed by 100 mg IV/IM for 3 days and then oral thiamine (50–100 mg) 2–3 times daily for several weeks.
- B_{12} deficiency can lead to depression and reversible dementia as well as associated neuropathies and blood dyscrasias.
  - Mania, psychosis, fatigue, irritability, cognitive deficits, and personality changes have also been reported.
  - If deficiency is suspected, checking levels of homocysteine and methylmalonic acid is warranted as serum B_{12} levels do not always correlate with symptoms.
  - Both oral and parenteral forms of supplementation have been found to be helpful in treating symptoms.
  - It is important to be aware that folate supplementation may mask B_{12} deficiency.

Endocrinopathies

- Endocrinopathies are some of the most frequent causes of secondary psychiatric symptomatology.
- Thyroid dysfunction is the most common endocrinopathy to cause psychiatric symptoms. Both hyperthyroidism and hypothyroidism are associated with a variety of cognitive and psychiatric changes:
  - The most common form of hyperthyroidism is Graves' disease, an autoimmune disorder that can present with depression, hypomania, anxiety, and cognitive dysfunction. Psychiatric symptoms correlate poorly with hormone levels.
  - Hyperthyroidism may present differently, depending on the age of the patient, with hyperactivity or an anxious dysphoria seen in younger patients, and apathy or depression seen in the elderly.
  - Hypothyroidism may be commonly mistaken for a primary depression with symptoms such as somnolence, fatigue, and depressed mood.
  - Untreated hypothyroidism can present as an acute psychotic state, termed "myxedema madness." Once thyroid stimulating hormone (TSH) levels return to normal, the psychosis remits.
  - Hashimoto's encephalopathy is a rare potential complication of hypothyroidism that may present as delirium with psychosis. Anti-thyroid antibodies are often detected in the serum.
- Cushing's syndrome is a result of abnormally elevated levels of cortisol and other corticosteroids.
  - Depression is the most common psychiatric symptom seen in this illness.
  - A full depressive syndrome has been reported in 50–70% of cases.
  - Anxiety, hypomania, and psychosis including erotomanic delusions, paranoia, and hallucinations have also been reported.
  - The syndrome may be misdiagnosed as bipolar disorder.

Infections

- Psychiatric symptoms are a part of the clinical presentation of many systemic and CNS infections:
  - HIV-infected individuals may commonly exhibit depression, anxiety, mania, delirium, and dementia.

- Rates of depression in HIV are as high as 60% in some studies. Risk factors include a personal or family history of depression, female gender, not telling others of HIV-positive status, and poor social support.
- Delirium may be a presenting symptom of HIV with increased risk seen in patients with underlying dementia. Common etiologies include CNS infections such as toxoplasmosis, Cryptococcus, and progressive multifocal leukoencephalopathy.
- Direct HIV infection of the CNS may also produce acute encephalopathy.
- HIV-associated mania has been reported and is thought to be due to infection of the brain by the virus itself. It is most common in patients with low CD4 count and has declined in incidence since the widespread use of highly active antiretroviral therapy.
- Treatment with antiretrovirals may also produce psychiatric symptoms. Efavirenz is associated with insomnia, nightmares, confusion, memory disturbance, depression, and rarely psychosis.
- **Syphilis** is a chronic systemic disease caused by the spirochetal bacterium *Treponema pallidum*.
  - Tertiary syphilis leads to a host of neuropsychiatric symptoms.
  - A century ago, syphilis was the leading diagnosis seen in psychiatric hospitals due to it causing a frank psychosis resembling schizophrenia. Incidence has declined, however, with the advent of antibiotics.
  - Today, psychiatric presentations of this illness are more subtle with dementia, depression, and grandiosity seen most often.
  - Treatment with neuroleptics may be helpful, but caution is advised as patients may be more susceptible to extrapyramidal side effects.
- **Herpes simplex encephalitis** is the most common of the viral encephalitides to present with psychiatric phenomenology.
  - Due to its predilection for the temporoparietal areas of the brain, HSV encephalitis can present with focal seizures, olfactory hallucinations, and personality changes.
  - Other presenting symptoms can include dysphasia, ataxia, delirium, psychosis, and focal neurological symptoms.
  - Klüver–Bucy syndrome is a rare potential sequela of the infection due to bilateral damage of the temporal lobes. It is characterized by hyperorality, irritability, hypersexuality, and placidity.

Reading list

Bialer PA, Wallack JJ, McDaniel S. Human immunodeficiency virus and AIDS. In: Stoudemire A, Fogel B, Greenberg D (eds). Psychiatric Care of the Medical Patient, 2nd edn. New York: Oxford University Press, 2000, pp. 871–87.

Caroff SN, Mann SC, Glittoo MF, et al. Psychiatric manifestations of acute viral encephalitis. Psychiatr Ann 2001;31:193–204.

Filley CM, Kleinschmidt-DeMasters BK. Neurobehavioral presentations of brain neoplasms. West J Med 1995;163(1):19–25.

Hall R, Popkin M, Devaul R, Faillace L, Stickney S. Physical illness presenting as psychiatric disease. Arch Gen Psychiatry 1978;35:1315–20.

Kayser MS, Kohler CG, Dalmau J. Psychiatric manifestations of paraneoplastic disorders. Am J Psychiatry 2010;167(9):1039–50.

Kudrjavcev T. Neurologic complications of thyroid dysfunction. Adv Neurol 1978;19:619–36.

Kumar N. Acute and subacute encephalopathies: deficiency states (nutritional). Semin Neurol 2011;31(2):169–83.

Levenson JL. The American Psychiatric Publishing Textbook of Psychosomatic Medicine, 2nd edn. VA: APA, 2010.

Sonino N, Fava GA. Psychosomatic aspects of Cushing's disease. Psychother Psychosom 1998;67:140–6.

Testa A, Giannuzzi R, Daini S, Bernardini L, Petrongolo L, Gentiloni Silveri N. Psychiatric emergencies (part III): psychiatric symptoms resulting from organic diseases. Eur Rev Med Pharmacol Sci 2013;17 Suppl 1:86–99.

Additional material for this chapter can be found online at: www.mountsinaiexpertguides.com/psychiatry

This includes advice for patients, a case study, and multiple choice questions.

CHAPTER 19

Neuropsychiatric Illnesses

Silvana Riggio[1], Zorica Filipovic-Jewell[1], and Devendra S. Thakur[2]

[1] Icahn School of Medicine at Mount Sinai, New York, NY, USA
[2] Geisel School of Medicine at Dartmouth College, Hanover, NH, USA

OVERALL BOTTOM LINE
- Neuropsychiatry addresses behavioral and/or psychiatric manifestations of neurologic diseases; symptoms often result from alterations in neurotransmitters, hormones, neuropathological changes, epileptogenic discharges, and/or medications.
- Many neurologic diseases present with psychiatric manifestations, and systematic and comprehensive evaluations are essential, including incorporating psychosocial aspects into the total management strategy.
- Post-concussive syndrome (PCS) and nonconvulsive status epilepticus (NCSE) are model neuropsychiatric diseases and will be the focus of this chapter.

Background
Definition of disease
- **Post-concussive syndrome (PCS)**: somatic, neurologic, and psychiatric symptoms which occur after mild traumatic brain injury (TBI); mild TBI is commonly known as a concussion.
- **Nonconvulsive status epilepticus (NCSE)**: continuous seizure activity for ≥30 minutes, with change in mental status or behavior, minimal or no motor findings, and diagnostic electroencephalogram (EEG) changes.

Incidence/prevalence
PCS
- 1.7 million TBI presentations per year to US emergency departments.
  - 1.4 million are treated/released (most are categorized as concussion); 275,000 require hospitalization; 52,000 die.
- Millions never seek medical care.
- >300,000 soldiers from Iraq and Afghanistan wars have reported concussion.

NCSE
- Incidence: 1.5 per 100,000/year
- May account for up to 20% of all cases of status epilepticus and up to 8% of all cases of patients with impaired consciousness.

Mount Sinai Expert Guides: Psychiatry, First Edition. Edited by Asher B. Simon, Antonia S. New, and Wayne K. Goodman.
© 2017 John Wiley & Sons, Ltd. Published 2017 by John Wiley & Sons, Ltd.
Companion website: www.mountsinaiexpertguides.com/psychiatry

Economic impact

PCS

- Acute medical care, rehabilitation, and other care for TBI costs $60 billion yearly in the US.

NCSE

- Not clearly established, although delay in diagnosis increases costs due to associated morbidity and prolonged hospitalization.

Etiology

PCS

- Among US civilians, the leading cause is TBI from falls, motor vehicle-related injuries, and blows to the head (including occupational injuries, sports-related injuries, and assault); pressure forces (e.g., blast injury) have also been implicated.
- The ApoE4 allele may increase risk for dementia in context of a brain injury.

NCSE

- Medication non-compliance in patients with known seizure disorders is the most common etiology, although a significant percentage of patients found to be in NCSE have no previous history of seizures.
- Underlying etiologies include structural lesions or processes causing neuronal excitability (e.g., metabolic abnormality, drug/ethyl alcohol toxicity or withdrawal, pregnancy, infection).
- No good data on genetic predisposition.

Pathophysiology

PCS

- Trauma to brain tissue at the site of impact (coup) and from the brain rebounding off the skull opposite the impact (contre-coup) causes focal injury.
  - Glutamate is released through depolarization of compressed neurons and damaged cell membranes; resulting Ca^{2+} release results in excitotoxicity.
- Diffuse axonal injury (DAI; white matter damage) results from rapid acceleration–deceleration or rotational forces to the brain.
  - Brain structures are differentially anchored to the skull base and to each other, and sudden forces lead to differential shearing, stretching, and compression; dysfunction can also be due to diffuse vascular injury and/or edema.

NCSE

- Not completely understood.
- The excessive neuronal activity may itself be injurious, and brain injury and epileptogenesis can result from status epilepticus.

Predictive/risk factors

PCS

- Male.
- Age: highest in children <5, followed by adolescents (15–19), then adults ≥75.
- Military personnel (blast exposure).
- Loss of consciousness (LOC).
- Posttraumatic amnesia (PTA).

NCSE

- Medication non-compliance.
- Sleep deprivation.
- Intoxication/withdrawal.
- Metabolic abnormalities (e.g., hyponatremia, hypoglycemia, hypocalcemia, hypoxia).

Prevention

> **BOTTOM LINE/CLINICAL PEARLS**
> **PCS**
> - Limit primary causes of concussion.
> - To minimize sequelae, limit risk of re-injury by physical and mental rest.
> **NCSE**
> - Early identification/treatment of reversible underlying etiologies.
> - Adherence with antiepileptic drug (AED) therapy.

Screening

PCS
- Neurological or psychiatric changes after injury should prompt complete neurological/neuropsychiatric exams.
- No universally agreed upon screening tool to evaluate concussion and sequelae.
  - Screens in acute setting include symptom checklists, neurologic exam including balance and coordination, and assessment of attention including reaction time and memory; SCAT3 is the most commonly used screen in sports.

NCSE
- Consider screening patients who manifest new or prolonged change in mental status.
  - 14% of those who appear to be in a "prolonged postictal state" after convulsive status epilepticus may be in NCSE.
- Routine EEG and/or sleep-deprived EEG; 24-hour video EEG when needed.

Secondary (and primary) prevention

PCS
- Education to prevent concussion and re-injury:
  - Use car seats and seat belts; never drive intoxicated; use appropriate headgear during sports.
  - In households with children: use window guards; safety gates at top/bottom of stairs.
  - In households with elderly persons: remove fall hazards (e.g., clutter, throw rugs); use non-slip mats and handrails; improve lighting.
  - Social policy should address violence and substance use.
- Education at time of discharge decreases intensity and duration of PCS:
  - Avoid athletics until full return to baseline, including balance and reaction time.

NCSE
- Adherence to anti-epileptic drug (AED) therapy.
  - Ensure that patient is on appropriate AED for seizure type.
- Minimize physiologic and mental stress.

Diagnosis

> **BOTTOM LINE/CLINICAL PEARLS**
> **PCS**
> - Mild neurological and psychiatric symptoms may be nonspecific and resolve within days to weeks.
> - Diagnosis is important to facilitate recovery.
> - Imaging will not make the diagnosis.

> **NCSE**
> - Frequently forgotten in differential diagnosis of altered mental status.
> - Symptoms are often misdiagnosed as a primary psychiatric disorder.
> - EEG is essential.

Differential diagnosis

PCS

Differential diagnosis	Features
Primary mood or anxiety disorder	Mood/anxiety symptoms prior to injury
Personality disorder	Established pattern of behavior pre-dating injury
Substance use disorder	Correlation between symptoms and substance use
Seizure	Brief stereotypic episodes, confirmed by video EEG, with intervening periods of normalcy
Other brain lesion	Neurological exam consistent with focal lesion or lesion seen on imaging
Other medical illness	Confirmatory history and laboratory values (e.g., in a patient with depressive symptoms and history of insult to the head, presence of abnormally low TSH would suggest depression due to hypothyroidism)

NCSE

Differential diagnosis	Features
Psychiatric disorders (psychosis, anxiety, etc.)	See individual disorders
Metabolic encephalopathy	Clinical and EEG disturbance improve following correction of metabolic disturbances
Toxic encephalopathy	Clinical and EEG disturbance improve after toxin is eliminated
Structural lesion	Focal slowing on EEG

Typical presentation

PCS

Most commonly, patients present after a concussion with mild neurobehavioral and somatic symptoms which resolve within days to weeks. Some cases have persisting neurobehavioral symptoms after mild TBI.

NCSE

Can appear *de novo* or atop a history of seizure disorder; there is usually no prior history of psychiatric illness. Patients typically present with an acute change in mental status with minimal or no motor involvement. Duration ranges from minutes to months. Misdiagnosis and delayed diagnosis are common due to physician unfamiliarity with NCSE; patients may be on psychiatric units for weeks before the diagnosis is made. Key to diagnosis is abrupt onset, fluctuating symptoms, and possible presence of automatisms, associated with EEG changes.

Clinical diagnosis

History
PCS
- Establish circumstances of event, nature and severity of injury, neuropsychiatric symptoms, and comorbidities.
  - Neurological/somatic symptoms may be nonspecific: headache, dizziness, nausea/vomiting, blurred vision, difficulty concentrating, memory loss, sleep disturbances, etc.
  - Psychiatric symptoms may include depression, anxiety, irritability, or behavioral changes.
  - LOC and PTA not required for diagnosis.
- Rule out other causes or complications (e.g., preexisting psychiatric/neurological illness, substance use, other medical comorbidities).
- A psychiatrist or neuropsychiatrist should be involved in the care of patients whose symptoms persist for months.

NCSE
- Evaluate for new-onset altered mental status and/or changes in behavior.
- Determine the history of seizure disorder and adherence to meds.
- Mental status changes may fluctuate and vary in degree:
  - subtle changes in level of consciousness all the way to coma;
  - mild to severe cognitive impairment;
  - affective or psychotic symptoms; confabulation;
  - speech disturbance, mutism, echolalia, aphasia, reduced fluency;
  - bizarre behavior: repetitive motor activity, laughing, singing, dancing, autonomic disturbances (e.g., borborygmi, flatulence, belching), sensory and/or psychic phenomena.
- Abnormal motor activity is absent or minimal: automatisms (eye fluttering, lip smacking, yawning, chewing, picking, eyelid/facial twitching), apraxia, clumsiness, positioning, raising, flexion/extension of extremities, head deviation.

Physical and mental status exams
PCS
- Physical exam: focus on neurologic deficits, particularly balance and cranial nerves.
- Mental status exam: formally evaluate cognition, particularly orientation, attention, memory.

NCSE
- Physical exam: begin with vital signs, O_2 saturation, and blood glucose to determine stability; assess for trauma and infection.
  - Focus on neurologic deficits, including automatisms.
- Mental status exam: assess for acute affective or psychotic phenomena; formally evaluate cognition, particularly orientation, attention, immediate and delayed recall.

Disease severity classification
PCS
- TBI is categorized based on level of consciousness: severe (coma), moderate (lethargy), mild (alertness).
  - Glasgow Coma Scale (GCS), PTA, and LOC have been used for classification but have little diagnostic/prognostic value in mild TBI (concussion).

NCSE
- Varies in severity, but duration must be >30 minutes.

- Subcategorized by change in level of consciousness and/or behavior.
  - Complex partial status epilepticus (CPSE) is focal in origin.
  - Absence status epilepticus (ASE) is primarily generalized.

Laboratory diagnosis
List of diagnostic tests
PCS

- None.
- While the biomarker S100B is sensitive for damage to brain and traumatic lesions on head CT, it is not correlated with development of PCS.

NCSE

- EEG: consider if new change in mental status with normal labs and CT scan.
  - Benzodiazepine challenge during EEG with improvement in both EEG and clinical picture are confirmatory.
  - If the event has clinically resolved, a single EEG might not identify NCSE.
- Metabolic/electrolyte profile; pregnancy test in women.
  - Hyponatremia is the most common metabolic abnormality in NCS.
- Usually no lactic acidosis or hyperprolactinemia (as in convulsive status).
- If on AED, check drug level.
- Urine toxicology.
- CSF if suspicion for infectious etiology.

Lists of imaging techniques
PCS

- Non-contrast CT in acute evaluation to assess for hematoma and/or hemorrhage, particularly if alteration in consciousness, severe headache, vomiting, intoxication, or if patient is on antithrombotic medication.
- MRI not indicated in acute evaluation; used to assess DAI when symptoms persist.

NCSE

- Neuroimaging in all cases of suspected new NCSE.
  - First: non-contrast CT to assess for space-occupying lesion or intracerebral hemorrhage.
  - Second: MRI±gadolinium in patients with negative CT and undetermined etiology for symptoms.

Potential pitfalls/common errors made regarding diagnosis of disease
PCS

- Ascribing neuropsychiatric symptoms to TBI before evaluating for other confounding factors (e.g., mood/anxiety/personality/substance disorders, etc.).
- Clinical symptoms can be due to other physical injuries in head, neck, and body (e.g., cervical strain, ocular nerve palsy, musculoskeletal pain, etc.).
- Relying on imaging to diagnose TBI (no abnormality is found in most cases of concussion/PCS).

NCSE

- Failing to consider NCSE in patients with acute mental status change.
- Failing to recognize that NCSE can present broadly, from psychosis, to subtle behavior changes, to coma, and does not require abnormal motor activity.
- Discounting diagnosis based on a single negative EEG, especially if symptoms have resolved.
- Treating a patient in NCSE with benzodiazepine prior to EEG.

Treatment
Treatment rationale
PCS
- Prevention remains essential; no accepted treatment addresses the underlying pathology of TBI.
- Symptomatic treatment for somatic/psychiatric symptoms; treat concomitant psychopathology.
- In recovery, no therapy has demonstrated superiority to abstinence from activity.
NCSE
- First-line treatment is benzodiazepine.
  - Lorazepam: favored due to long duration of anticonvulsant effects (up to 12 hours); best in patients in alcohol withdrawal due to reduced liver metabolism.
  - Diazepam: enters CNS quickly but redistributes out within 15 minutes, thus losing the anti-convulsant benefit.
- Long-term therapy depends on underlying etiology, EEG, and neuroimaging.

When to hospitalize
PCS
- Rarely needed.
NCSE
- Almost always.

Managing the hospitalized patient
NCSE
- Requires admission to a monitoring area with strict seizure precautions; patients are at risk for evolving into a convulsive event.

Table of treatment
PCS

Medical • Rest from activities • Physical rehabilitation	• No intervention proven superior to rest
Psychological • Cognitive rehabilitation • Education about illness	• Education decreases incidence and can facilitate recovery

NCSE

Medical • NCSE due to seizure disorder requires AED therapy and referral to neurologist • Metabolic, structural, infectious, or toxic etiologies require treatment	• If etiology is due to reversible cause, treatment does not necessarily include an AED

Prevention/management of complications
PCS
- Rest facilitates recovery.
- Education about PCS helps normalize the clinical course for the patient.
- Refer to a provider experienced in concussion management.
NCSE
- Benzodiazepines may rarely cause transient respiratory depression, requiring a brief period of bag mask ventilation.

CLINICAL PEARLS

PCS

- Prevention is the primary focus in at-risk populations.
- When a patient with history of TBI and neurobehavioral disturbances presents for clinical attention, the psychiatrist must systematically assess for all possible contributing factors besides TBI.

NCSE

- Benzodiazepines are first-line treatment.
- NCSE can continue after convulsive status is terminated, and a convulsive seizure can evolve in patients in NCSE.
- Although morbidity related to duration of NCSE is unclear, management should focus on rapid termination of seizure.

Special populations

Pregnancy

Pregnancy is a risk factor for NCSE.

Prognosis

BOTTOM LINE/CLINICAL PEARLS

PCS

- Symptoms usually resolve within days or weeks.
- Can be complicated by contributing factors, and a subset of patients have persisting neurobehavioral sequelae.
- Repeated insults can lead to a progressing neurodegenerative dementia (i.e., dementia pugilistica or chronic traumatic encephalopathy).

NCSE

- Overall prognosis is good.
- Unclear morbidity, although biomarker studies document the release of neuronal peptides associated with cellular injury.
- Unknown whether the neuronal damage that occurs in convulsive status epilepticus also occurs in NCSE.
- Underlying etiology and comorbidities affect prognosis.

Reading list

PCS

Kashluba S, Paniak C, Blake T, Reynolds S, Toller-Lobe G, Nagy J. A longitudinal, controlled study of patient complaints following treated mild traumatic brain injury. Arch Clin Neuropsychol 2004;19(6):805–16.

Marshall S, Bayley M, McCullagh S, Velikonja D, Berrigan L. Clinical practice guidelines for mild traumatic brain injury and persistent symptoms. Can Fam Physician 2012;58(3):257–67, e128–40.

McCrea M, Kelly JP, Randolph C, Cisler R, Berger L. Immediate neurocognitive effects of concussion. Neurosurgery 2002;50(5):1032–40.

McCrory P. Sports concussion and the risk of chronic neurological impairment. Clin J Sport Med 2011;21(1):6–12.

Meares S, Shores EA, Taylor AJ, et al. The prospective course of postconcussion syndrome: the role of mild traumatic brain injury. Neuropsychology 2011;25(4):454–65.

Riggio S. Traumatic brain injury and its neurobehavioral sequelae. Neurol Clin 2011;29(1):35–47.

Ruff RM, Iverson GL, Barth JT, Bush SS, Broshek DK; NAN Policy and Planning Committee. Recommendations for diagnosing a mild traumatic brain injury: A National Academy of Neuropsychology education paper. Arch Clin Neuropsychol 2009;24(1):3–10.

NCSE

Kaplan P. The clinical features, diagnosis, and prognosis of nonconvulsive status epilepticus. Neurologist 2005;11(6):348–61.

Riggio S. Psychiatric manifestations of nonconvulsive status epilepticus. Mt Sinai J Med 2006;73(7):960–6.

Sutter R, Kaplan P. Electroencephalographic criteria for nonconvulsive status epilepticus: Synopsis and comprehensive survey. Epilepsia 2012;53 Suppl 3:1–51.

van Rijckevorsel K, Boon P, Hauman H, et al. Standards of care for non-convulsive status epilepticus: Belgian consensus recommendations. Acta Neurol Belg 2006;106(3):117–24.

Walker MC. Treatment of nonconvulsive status epilepticus. Int Rev Neurobiol 2007;81:287–97.

Suggested websites

PCS

Brain Injury.com. http://www.braininjury.com

Centers for Disease Control and Prevention. http://www.cdc.gov/TraumaticBrainInjury/index.html and http://www.cdc.gov/headsup/youthsports/index.html

NCSE

Epilepsy Foundation. http://www.epilepsyfoundation.org

National Institute of Neurological Disorders and Stroke. http://www.ninds.nih.gov/disorders/epilepsy/detail_epilepsy.htm

Guidelines

PCS

Title	Source	Weblink
Clinical Report – Sport-Related Concussion in Children and Adolescents	American Academy of Pediatrics (AAP), 2010	http://pediatrics.aappublications.org/content/126/3/597
Summary of evidence based guideline update: evaluation and management of concussion in sports	American Academy of Neurology, 2013	http://www.ncbi.nlm.nih.gov/pubmed/23508730

NCSE

Title	Source	Weblink
Standards of care for non-convulsive status epilepticus: Belgian consensus recommendations	Group of Belgian Neurologists, 2006	http://www.ncbi.nlm.nih.gov/pubmed/17091614

Additional material for this chapter can be found online at:
www.mountsinaiexpertguides.com/psychiatry

This includes advice for patients, a case study, ICD codes, and multiple choice questions.

CHAPTER 20

Somatic Symptom and Related Disorders, Including Illness Anxiety, Factitious, Malingering, and Conversion Disorders

Hansel Arroyo, Kim Klipstein, Carrie L. Ernst, and Jennifer Finkel
Icahn School of Medicine at Mount Sinai, New York, NY, USA

OVERALL BOTTOM LINE
- Somatic symptom and related disorders are unique psychiatric illnesses characterized by disproportionate thoughts, feelings, or behaviors related to bodily symptoms.
- Presentation involves the manifestation of physical symptoms or anxiety about physical symptoms or illnesses, with resultant distress and impairment in functioning.
- DSM-5 contains major changes in the categorization of these illnesses.

Background
Definition of disease
For diagnosis, each entity below requires clinically significant distress or functional impairment:
- **Somatic symptom disorder**: ≥1 physical complaint over ≥6 months, accompanied by abnormal feelings, thoughts, and behaviors about the symptoms.
- **Illness anxiety disorder**: preoccupation over ≥6 months with having/acquiring a serious illness. Physical symptoms are either not present or are mild.
- **Factitious disorder**: falsification of physical/psychological signs and symptoms (in oneself or others) in the absence of external gain; patients exaggerate, misrepresent, or induce symptoms for the primary motivation of assuming the sick role.
- **Malingering**: intentional production of physical/psychological symptoms, motivated by external incentives. Not considered a psychiatric disorder. Classified as "Other Conditions That May Be a Focus of Clinical Attention."
- **Conversion disorder (functional neurological symptom)**: psychological factors or "psychic conflicts" affecting voluntary motor or sensory functions suggestive of a neurological or general medical condition. Symptoms are not intentionally produced or feigned. Production of and motivation for the symptoms are unconsciously mediated.

Disease classification
- Significant classification changes in DSM-5 attempt to reduce redundancies and clarify diagnoses for non-psychiatric providers.

Mount Sinai Expert Guides: Psychiatry, First Edition. Edited by Asher B. Simon, Antonia S. New, and Wayne K. Goodman.
© 2017 John Wiley & Sons, Ltd. Published 2017 by John Wiley & Sons, Ltd.
Companion website: www.mountsinaiexpertguides.com/psychiatry

- Creation of new category: Somatic Symptom and Related Disorders.
  - DSM-IV Somatoform Disorders (somatization disorder, hypochondriasis, pain disorder, undifferentiated somatoform disorder) is now either DSM-5 Somatic Symptom Disorder (if somatic symptoms predominate) or Illness Anxiety Disorder (if somatic symptoms are not present but the patient is preoccupied with having an illness).
  - Factitious disorder is now included in this category.
  - Conversion disorder is kept relatively intact.

Incidence/prevalence
Somatic symptom
- ~5–7%; female predominance.

Illness anxiety
- 1.3–10% in general population.
- 3–9% in ambulatory medical clinics.
- Male:female = 1:1.
- Onset at any age but most common at 20–30 years.

Factitious
- ~1% in hospital settings.

Conversion
- 1–3% in general hospitals.

Economic impact
- ~$256 billion/year.

Etiology
Somatic symptom and Illness anxiety: multifactorial.
- Genetics: first-degree female relatives have higher rates. Male relatives are more likely to have antisocial personality and substance use disorders.
- Physiological somatosensory amplification:
  - Misinterpretation of bodily sensations and somatosensory inputs; inability to habituate to repetitive stimuli.
- Development and learning theory:
  - Physical symptoms are a form of interpersonal communication and attachment.
  - Being sick may offer escape from noxious obligations.
- Psychological:
  - Alexithymia: impaired ability to identify and describe one's emotions and distinguish between them and bodily sensations.
  - Introspectiveness: the tendency to think about oneself is associated with an increase in the reporting of physical symptoms.
  - Negative affectivity: tendency to experience and report negative emotions.
  - Psychodynamic theory: aggressive wishes are disavowed into physical complaints; attachment to caregiver is preserved.

Factitious disorder
- Primary gain: unconsciously motivated symptoms allow one to assume the sick role.
  - May be connected to childhood abuse and emotional deprivation.
- Most often presents in early adulthood and after hospitalization for a medical condition or a mental disorder.
- Symptoms can be reinforced by medical providers.

Conversion

- Psychodynamic theory: internal conflict is converted to neurological sensory or motor symptoms, keeping the conflict out of conscious awareness.
- Learning theory: learned maladaptive response to stress leads to support or attention.

Pathophysiology

See Etiology section.

Predictive/risk factors

Somatic symptom and Illness anxiety

- Family history
- Sexual/physical abuse or neglect
- Childhood experience of illness or models of illness
- Low socioeconomic status; less education; older age
- History of depression, anxiety, or personality disorder
- Medical/psychiatric illness

Factitious

- Female
- Health-related job or training
- Childhood experience of illness or models of illness

Conversion

- Extreme stress; recent trauma
- Rural upbringing; low socioeconomic status; adolescence or early adulthood
- Female gender
- Family history
- Physical or sexual abuse
- Personality disorder

Prevention

> **BOTTOM LINE/CLINICAL PEARLS**
> - No intervention has been demonstrated to prevent the development of these illnesses.

Screening

Somatic symptom and Illness anxiety

- Brief, well-validated measures for detecting and monitoring depression, anxiety, and somatization: Patient Health Questionnaire (PHQ)-9, Generalized Anxiety Disorder Assessment (GAD)-7.

Conversion

- Minnesota Multiphasic Personality Inventory-2 (MMPI-2): conversion V pattern reflects elevated scores on hypochondriasis and hysteria and lower on depression scales; this pattern suggests that the patient uses somatic symptoms to avoid dealing with psychological issues.

Secondary (and primary) prevention

- Outpatient psychological treatment as a conduit for emotional expressivity, affect tolerance, and coping skills.

Diagnosis

> **BOTTOM LINE/CLINICAL PEARLS**
>
> **Somatic symptom**
> - Somatic symptoms predominate and lead to distorted thoughts, feelings, and behaviors for ≥6 months.
>
> **Illness anxiety**
> - Preoccupation with, or fear of, illness is central. Somatic symptoms are minimal or absent.
>
> **Factitious**
> - Recurrent presentations and atypical courses or treatment responses.
> - Discrepancies between stated history and objective findings on exam.
> - Diagnosis is confirmed only by objective evidence of symptom falsification or self-induced injury or disease, in the absence of obvious external rewards.
>
> **Conversion**
> - Voluntary motor or sensory dysfunction, not consciously produced.
> - Associated with recent stressors/conflicts.
> - Symptoms typically do not conform to known anatomical pathways or physiological mechanisms.

Differential diagnosis

Differential diagnosis	Features
Medical/neurological disorders (e.g., multiple sclerosis, systemic lupus erythematosus, Lyme disease)	- Lab/imaging findings - Physical abnormalities on exam consistent with known anatomic pathways - No evidence/suspicion that symptoms are deliberately fabricated
Mood and anxiety disorders	- Somatic symptoms tend to be temporally limited and resolve with treatment
Substance use disorders	- Urine toxicology
Psychotic disorders	- Delusions, hallucinations, formal thought disorder
Borderline personality disorder	- Deliberate self-harm does not occur in the context of deception
Malingering	- Conscious production of symptoms for secondary gain (medicolegal context, antisocial personality, external incentives)

Typical presentation

In all illnesses below, typical presentation is first and often to non-psychiatric physicians, and patients tend to be resistant to psychiatric evaluation.

Somatic symptom
- Poor historians with vague and circumstantial descriptions of medical history.
- Frequent inability to distinguish between current and past symptoms.
- Physical complaints can be dramatic and exaggerated.

Illness anxiety
- Frequent use of medical services and extensive medical tests.
- Reassurance is often ineffective.
- Increased vigilance toward bodily sensations.
  - Somatic symptoms are minimal or absent and may involve normal bodily functions or incidental abnormal physical states, but the patient is preoccupied with having illness.
  - Fear of illness becomes the central feature of life.

Factitious
- Repeatedly present as ill, impaired, or injured.
- Deceptive behaviors include feigning or exaggerating symptoms, manipulating laboratory tests, falsifying medical records, ingesting substances, or self-injurious behaviors to precipitate illness.

Conversion
- Sudden onset of neurologic deficit after a significant life stressor.
- Patients do not consciously produce or feign symptoms.

Clinical diagnosis

History

Somatic symptom and Illness anxiety
- Diagnosis is based on exam, review of medical records, and collateral information.
- Focus on chronology and chronicity of symptoms, preoccupations, or illness anxieties.
- Explore symptoms in the context of current life stressors as well as past life events.
- Assess social, functional, and occupational impairment.
- Of those previously diagnosed with Hypochondriasis, 75% fit Somatic Symptom Disorder and 25% fit Illness Anxiety Disorder.

Factitious and Malingering
- History-taking is challenging as many patients are resistant to psychiatric intervention.
- Obtain additional information from collateral sources and thoroughly review the medical record.
- Look for evidence of falsification of symptoms, inconsistencies between reported history and objective findings, atypical illness course, failure to respond to usual therapies, unusual acquiescence to invasive tests, recurrent presentations to healthcare providers, and resistance to releasing medical records.
- Explore the patient's perception of being a patient and inquire about possible external gain (e.g., legal, financial, housing, substance use).

Conversion
- The most frequent complaints are weakness, paralysis, non-epileptic seizures, involuntary movements, and sensory disturbances.
- Assess level of distress and level of functioning.
- Inquire about current stressors.

Physical and mental status exams
- *Physical evaluation is essential for all.*

Somatic symptom
- Focus on the patient's quality of descriptions, emotional responses, symptom amplifications, and meaning attributed to illness.

Illness anxiety
- Explore the level of flexibility or fixation with the disease to differentiate from delusional disorder.

Factitious
- Long, complicated, refractory, and chronic medical histories; inconsistencies between objective findings and subjective reports.

Conversion
- Physical exam
  - Motor/sensory deficits do not conform to anatomic distribution.
  - Inconsistent findings.
  - Hoover's sign (involuntary extension of the affected leg when the unaffected leg is flexing against resistance).
  - Pseudoclonus.
  - Distractible symptoms.
  - Generalized seizures without accompanying change in level of consciousness.
  - Bizarre movements.
- Mental status exam: "la belle indifference," a classic feature in which patient demonstrates a paradoxical lack of emotional distress in relation to symptoms.

Disease severity classification

Somatic symptom
- Mild, moderate, or severe: severe tends to be associated with multiple somatic complaints.
- With predominant pain: pain symptoms predominate (Pain Disorder in DSM-IV).

Illness anxiety
- Care-seeking type: multiple visits/tests.
- Care-avoidant type: medical care is rarely used.

Factitious
- Imposed on one's self or on another (e.g., falsifying illness in another person, such as a child; previously called "by proxy").
- Single or recurrent episodes can be specified.

Laboratory diagnosis

List of diagnostic tests
- Dependent on presenting physical symptoms; the goal is to rule out medical illness.
- Psychological testing may help rule out malingering or other underlying psychiatric illness.

Potential pitfalls/common errors made regarding diagnosis of disease

Somatic symptom and Illness anxiety
- Avoid implying that symptoms are "imaginary"; patients experience symptoms as real and this implication can sever the therapeutic alliance.
- Diagnosis no longer requires that symptoms be medically unexplained.

Factitious and Malingering
- Failing to thoroughly review medical records.
- Failing to rule out other psychiatric or medical disorders that may explain symptoms
- Failing to recognize that the patient may have a combination of feigned and actual illness.
- Overuse of unnecessary diagnostic tests and procedures.

Conversion

- Failing to rule out other psychiatric or medical disorders that may explain symptoms.
- Failing to recognize that the patient may have a combination of feigned and actual illness.
- Overuse of unnecessary diagnostic tests and procedures.
- Patients may exhibit minimal distress but they suffer functional impairment.

Treatment

Treatment rationale

Somatic symptom and Illness anxiety

- Schedule short but regular medical follow-up visits; set limits while providing reassurance.
- Pharmacotherapy to treat comorbid mood and anxiety symptoms.
  - Antidepressants may help modulate changes in somatic experiences in non-depressed, non-anxious patients.
- Psychotherapeutic goals: draw connections between physical states and emotional states in a non-judgmental manner.

Factitious and Malingering

- Delicate, indirect confrontation allows the patient to save face and quietly relinquish factitious signs or symptoms.
  - Techniques such as inexact interpretations or therapeutic double binds may minimize confrontation.
  - If confronting a malingerer, prepare for an angry or defensive reaction and ensure adequate security measures.
- Behavioral and other psychotherapies may be useful over the long term.
- Treatment should be collaborative and involve close communication among all providers.
- Invasive procedures should be minimized.
- In cases where the factitious disorder is imposed on another individual, first ensure the safety of the suspected victim.
- Treat comorbid medical and psychiatric disorders.

Conversion

- Provide a thorough, clear, and non-judgmental explanation to the patient, along with reassurance that the disorder is "a real illness" and usually reversible.
- Often spontaneously remits.
- Psychotherapy can address underlying psychic stressors.

Table of treatment

Somatic symptom and Illness anxiety

Medical 1. SSRIs 2. SNRIs	• Treats comorbid mood and anxiety • May modulate somatic experiences • Treats pain
Psychological 1. Cognitive behavioral therapy (CBT) 2. Insight-oriented psychotherapy 3. Supportive psychotherapy 4. Biofeedback, relaxation techniques, meditation	• Connect physical symptoms and emotions • Set limits • CBT has been proven to reduce somatization, healthcare visits, health preoccupation, and misinterpretations of non-pathological body sensations

Conversion

Medical 1. Benzodiazepines 2. Amytal interview	• Although not evidence-based, some clinicians use benzodiazepines to initiate treatment • Historically, patients were sedated with amytal and questioned about the psychological precipitants of the symptoms to allow unconscious conflicts to come into conscious awareness
Psychological interventions 1. CBT 2. Supportive therapy 3. Hypnosis	• Reduce and manage stress

Prevention/management of complications

• Non-compliance with psychiatric treatment is common.
• Minimal medical work-ups help minimize iatrogenic complications.

CLINICAL PEARLS
• *For all, use minimal/judicious medical interventions to avoid iatrogenic complications and treat comorbid medical and psychiatric disorders.*
Somatic symptom and Illness anxiety
• Develop a therapeutic alliance and set regular office visits.
• Validate the patient's somatic complaints and provide reassurance.
Factitious
• Begin with delicate confrontation.
• Collaborate with all members of the treatment team.
• There is great resistance to psychiatric treatment.
• Insight-oriented psychotherapy may be useful in understanding the unconsciously-motivated behavior.
Conversion
• Explain the mind–body connection that leads to the disorder.
• Encourage psychiatric treatment.

Prognosis

BOTTOM LINE/CLINICAL PEARLS
Somatic symptom and Illness anxiety
• Tend to be chronic, fluctuating, and relapsing.
• Health-related anxiety and somatization increases with age.
• Favorable prognosis if there is early acute onset, mild symptoms, high socioeconomic status, comorbid medical condition, and absence of secondary gain.
Factitious and Malingering: unknown
Conversion
• In most hospitalized cases, symptoms fully resolve within 2 weeks.
• 20–25% will recur within a year.
• Favorable prognosis if there is acute onset, a clearly identifiable stressor, and a short time between onset and treatment.

Natural history of untreated disease
- Untreated patients are at higher risk of iatrogenic complications due to unnecessary diagnostic investigations, polypharmacy, and polysurgery.

Prognosis for treated patients
- Treatment reduces healthcare visits, physical complaints, bodily preoccupation, and medication use.

Reading list

Abramowitz JS, Schwartz SA, Whiteside SP. A contemporary model of hypochondriasis. Mayo Clin Proc 2002;77(12):1323–30.

Allen LA, Escobar JI, Lehrer PM, Gara MA, Woolfolk RL. Psychosocial treatment for multiple unexplained physical symptoms: a review of the literature. Psychosom Med 2002;64:939–50.

American Psychiatric Association. Diagnostic and Statistical Manual of Mental Disorders, 5th edn. Washington, DC: American Psychiatric Publishing, 2013.

Blumenfield M, Strain J (eds). Textbook of Psychosomatic Medicine. Philadelphia, PA: Lippincott Williams & Wilkins, 2006.

Kroenke K, Swindle R. Cognitive-behavioral therapy for somatization and symptom syndromes: a critical review of controlled clinic trials. Psychother Psychosom 2000;69:205–15.

Levenson JL (ed.). The American Psychiatric Publishing Textbook of Psychosomatic Medicine, 2nd edn. Washington, DC: American Psychiatric Publishing, 2005.

Noyes R Jr, Happel RL, Muller BA, et al. Fluvoxamine for somatoform disorders: an open trial. Gen Hosp Psychiatry 1998;20:339–44.

Evidence

Type of evidence	Title and comment	Weblink
Systematic review	Cognitive-behavioral therapy for somatization and symptom syndromes: a critical review of controlled clinical trials. **Comment:** Treatment reduces healthcare visits, physical complaints, bodily preoccupation, and medication use.	http://www.ncbi.nlm.nih.gov/pubmed/10867588
Systematic review	A contemporary conceptual model of hypochondriasis. **Comment:** CBT is effective treatment.	http://www.ncbi.nlm.nih.gov/pubmed/12479520

Additional material for this chapter can be found online at: www.mountsinaiexpertguides.com/psychiatry

This includes advice for patients, a case study, ICD codes, and multiple choice questions.

CHAPTER 21

Sexual Dysfunctions, Gender Dysphoria, and Paraphilic Disorders

Stephen Snyder[1], William Byne[1], and Sara Lozyniak[2]
[1] Icahn School of Medicine at Mount Sinai, New York, NY, USA
[2] Cambridge Health Alliance/Harvard Medical School, Cambridge, MA, USA

OVERALL BOTTOM LINE

- **Sexual Dysfunctions:** multiple causal factors involved (e.g., psychiatric, medical, sociocultural, medication); the best treatments combine medical and psychological approaches.
- **Gender Dysphoria:** the goal of modern treatment is to promote authentic gender expression, which may involve gender transition.
- **Paraphilic Disorders:** paraphilias are no longer automatically considered mental disorders; they are only diagnosed if the patient acts on urges with a non-consenting person, or if urges cause distress or impairment.

Background
Definition of disease
Sexual Dysfunctions
Male:

- **Erectile Disorder (ED):** marked difficulty obtaining/maintaining erection or decrease in rigidity.
- **Premature Ejaculation (PE):** ≤1 minute after vaginal penetration and before the man wishes it.
- **Delayed Ejaculation (DE):** marked delay, infrequency, or absence of ejaculation during partnered sexual activity.
- **Male Hypoactive Sexual Desire Disorder (MHSDD):** deficiency/absence of sexual thoughts/ desire.

Female:

- **Female Sexual Interest/Arousal Disorder (FSIAD):** criteria new to DSM-5; ≥3 of the following are absent or reduced: (1) sexual interest, (2) thoughts/fantasies, (3) initiation or receptivity to initiation, (4) excitement/pleasure during sex, (5) response to erotic cues, (6) genital/non-genital sensations during sex.
- **Female Orgasmic Disorder (FOD):** marked delay, infrequency, absence, or reduced intensity of orgasms.
- **Genito-Pelvic Pain-Penetration Disorder (GPPPD):** criteria new to DSM-5; ≥1 of the following: difficult vaginal penetration, marked pain during intercourse or attempted penetration, marked fear/anxiety about penetration-related pain, marked pelvic floor muscle tensing during attempted penetration.

Mount Sinai Expert Guides: Psychiatry, First Edition. Edited by Asher B. Simon, Antonia S. New, and Wayne K. Goodman.
© 2017 John Wiley & Sons, Ltd. Published 2017 by John Wiley & Sons, Ltd.
Companion website: www.mountsinaiexpertguides.com/psychiatry

Gender Dysphoria

- Disparity between experienced/expressed and assigned gender associated with clinically significant distress or impairment; Gender Dysphoria in Children is a separate diagnosis from Gender Dysphoria in Adolescents and Adults, and has different diagnostic criteria.

Paraphilic Disorders

- A paraphilia is any persistent and intense sexual interest other than from genital stimulation or preparatory fondling with phenotypically normal, physically mature, consenting adults.
- A Paraphilic Disorder is only diagnosed if the individual has acted on paraphilic urges with a non-consenting person or has distress or impairment.
  - Paraphilic Disorders include Voyeuristic Disorder, Exhibitionistic Disorder, Frotteuristic Disorder, Sexual Masochism Disorder, Sexual Sadism Disorder, Pedophilic Disorder, Fetishistic Disorder, Transvestic Disorder.

Incidence/prevalence

Disorder	Prevalence
ED	Increases with age: ≤10% below 40 to ≥50% above 70
MHSDD	Generalized form uncommon in younger men, but increases with age; situational form common at all ages
PE/DE	15–25% for PE; unknown for DE
FSIAD	Unknown; low interest without clinically significant distress is extremely common and often conceptualized as normal
FOD	Orgasmic problems in 10–42%; unclear how many are sufficiently distressed to meet criteria
GPPPD	Unknown; provoked vestibulodynia (PVD) may be the most common premenopausal pattern

- Prevalence of Gender Dysphoria is unknown; Paraphilic Disorder varies with disorder.

Etiology

Note that pathophysiology is also included in this section.

Disorder	Etiology, pathophysiology
ED	Neuropsychiatric, psychological, endocrine, vascular, smooth muscle, endothelial; impairment in cavernosal blood flow and veno-occlusion
MHSDD	Endocrine, neuropsychiatric, psychological
PE	Most common form involves low ejaculatory threshold
DE	High ejaculatory threshold and/or history of forceful masturbation technique; decreased penile erotic sensitivity due to age, medical condition, or medications
FSIAD	Unknown in most cases; endocrine, neuropsychiatric, psychological, sociocultural
FOD	Unknown; wide variation in orgasmic capability/experience as well as degree of importance an individual attaches to it
GPPPD	Conditions involving vulva, vagina, vestibule, pelvic floor, pudendal nerve, etc., as well as psychological

- Gender Dysphoria and Paraphilic Disorders: unknown.

Predictive/risk factors

Sexual Dysfunction	Risk factor
ED	• Age • Medical (e.g., diabetes mellitus, atherosclerosis, hypertension, obesity, hypogonadism, prostatectomy, Peyronie's disease) • Medications (e.g. finasteride, SSRIs, diuretics) • Psychiatric (e.g., mood/anxiety disorders) • Psychological conditions not conducive to sexual arousal
MHSDD	• Generalized form: age, diminished health status, ED • Specific form: relationship problems, compulsive masturbation, frequent pornography use • Medical (hypogonadism, hyperprolactinemia, endocrinopathies) • Medication/substance (e.g., alcohol) • Psychiatric
PE	• Younger age (mild PE only; severe lifelong form rarely resolves with age) • ED
DE	• Forceful masturbation • Medication (PDE5I, SSRI, others) • Decreased penile erotic sensitivity due to age, condom use, medical illness
FSIAD	• Age and overall health status • Endocrine (e.g., androgen deficiency, post bilateral oophorectomy) • Chemotherapy • Psychiatric • Other sexual dysfunctions, including in partner • Medications (e.g., SSRI, oral contraceptive) • Adverse psychological, sexual, relational, cultural, or economic conditions • History of childhood sexual abuse • Negative body image • Unsatisfying sexual experiences
FOD	• Medical (e.g., multiple sclerosis, vulvovaginal atrophy) • Medications (e.g., SSRI) • Sexual inexperience ("pre-orgasmic")
GPPPD	• Vaginal infections and dermatoses • Pelvic floor muscle dysfunction • Disease of adjacent structures (e.g., hip, spine)

Prevention

> **BOTTOM LINE/CLINICAL PEARLS**
> • Minimize/treat risk factors.
> • Actively assess for sexual dysfunction and include sexual health/education in psychiatric and medical care.

Screening
• ED: Sexual Health Inventory for Men (SHIM; Rosen et al., 1999) for men over age 40 in general medical settings.
• The authors are unaware of any validated screening tools for female DSM-5 Sexual Dysfunctions brief enough for routine clinical use.

Secondary (and primary) prevention

• Treat ongoing and episodic conditions.

Diagnosis

BOTTOM LINE/CLINICAL PEARLS

• Do not expect patients to describe sexual dysfunction without prompting. Diagnosis requires active inquiry and minimization of stigma.

ED	• Physical exam may indicate risk factors; refer all but the most obviously psychogenic to a urologist
MHSDD	• Determine generalized vs specific • Ask about frequency of masturbation and pornography use
PE	• Most common sexual dysfunction in younger men; ~33% have comorbid ED
DE	• Determine lifelong vs acquired • Determine generalized vs situational • Assess masturbation frequency and technique
FSIAD	• Only diagnose if patient is distressed by the condition • Screen for other sexual dysfunctions
FOD	• Patient may be unsure whether she has had orgasms • Patients often only experience orgasms alone • Some patients do not discover necessary requirements for achieving orgasm until early adulthood or mid-life
GPPPD	• Varied presentations of pain (e.g., independent of sex; only with penetration) • May have history of pain with tampon insertion or pelvic exams • Patients previously categorized as dyspareunia or vaginismus

---

• Individuals with Gender Dysphoria retain that diagnosis even post gender transition.
• Paraphilic Disorders: presence of a paraphilia is not automatically a disorder.

Differential diagnosis

	Differential diagnosis	Features
ED	MHSDD, PE, DE (often comorbid)	Erections preserved (unless comorbid)
MHSDD	Medical/psychiatric illness; substance/medication use; psychological conditions not conducive to sexual desire	History, exam, drug screen
PE	ED (often comorbid)	Loss of erection before ejaculation
	Normal ejaculatory control	Able to control ejaculation for several minutes, but patient or partner desires better control
DE	Retrograde ejaculation	Intact sensation of orgasm
	Other impediments to intravaginal ejaculation	Inability to penetrate (e.g., due to partner's GPPPD)

(Continued)

(Continued)

FSIAD	Desire discrepancy with partner	Desire is intact but discrepant
	Medical/psychiatric illness; substance/medication use; response to adverse psychological, sexual, relational, cultural, or economic conditions	History, exam
	Normal variant	Individual's usual pattern
FOD	Medical illness; substance/medication use; response to adverse psychological, sexual, relational, cultural, or economic conditions	History, exam
GPPPD	Persistent Genital Arousal Disorder (PGAD)	Complaints of pain usually not prominent
	GPPPD in setting of vulvar infections and dermatoses; pelvic floor muscle dysfunction; neurological disorders (e.g., pudendal nerve entrapment); urological disorders (e.g., interstitial cystitis); orthopedic disorders (e.g., femoro-acetabular impingement)	Specialized assessments as indicated by gynecology, physical therapy, neurology, urology, orthopedics
Gender Dysphoria	Transvestic Disorder	Cross-dressing associated with sexual excitement and clinically significant distress or impairment
	Non-conformity to gender roles	Atypical gender expression without strong desire to be the other gender
Paraphilic Disorders	Paraphilia (i.e., not a disorder)	Individual does not act on urges with non-consenting persons, and does not experience distress or impairment

Typical presentation

ED	Patient or partner is worried/discouraged/avoids sex
MHSDD	Partner complains that patient rarely initiates sex; patient reports that sexual cues are no longer of interest
PE	Minimal stimulation required for ejaculation
DE	Subjective feeling that sex has become laborious; infertility due to absence of intravaginal ejaculation
FSIAD	Avoidance of sexual, non-sexual physical contact; relationship difficulties
FOD	Pressure from partner for woman to reach orgasm; comorbid desire/arousal complaints are common
GPPPD	Provoked pain during penetration; or if pain is generalized, distress and interference with activities of daily life
Gender Dysphoria	Patient reports discrepancy between experienced gender and sex assigned at birth; may be in various stages of social, hormonal, or surgical transition
Paraphilic Disorders	Most often seen in forensic settings; legal involvement

Clinical diagnosis

History

- Diagnosis of a Sexual Dysfunction:
  - generally requires ≥6 months and clinically significant distress;
  - excluded if symptoms are better explained by non-sexual mental disorder, severe relationship distress or other significant stressors, effects of substance/medication, or medical condition.
- General assessment guidelines:
  - determine (1) generalized vs situational, and (2) lifelong vs acquired;
  - medical/psychiatric history; medication/substance use; partner/relationship issues; cultural/religious factors; sexual impulsivity/compulsivity, including pornography use; body image concerns; history of sexual/physical/emotional abuse; presence of other sexual dysfunctions in patient and/or partner.

Specific assessment of key features	
ED	• Rigidity with partner, with masturbation, on awakening • SHIM rating scale (Rosen et al., 1999)
MHSDD	• Level of subjective arousal in solitary vs partnered sexual activity
PE	• Subjective lack of ejaculatory control • Ejaculation with minimal stimulation, before patient or partner wishes it, and/or before or shortly after penetration
DE	• Ability to ejaculate alone vs with partner • Masturbation frequency/technique • Specific conflicts (e.g., fear of pregnancy; strict cultural/religious beliefs; shame re sexuality)
FSIAD	• Presence/absence of erotic thoughts/fantasies/subjective arousal, either spontaneously or in response to erotic cues • Degree of lubrication (often does not correlate with subjective arousal) • Masturbation techniques • Sexual practices with partner
FOD	• Presence/absence of orgasm with masturbation • Details of masturbation and sex techniques
GPPPD	• Onset, course, character, triggers • Pain superficial or deep • Experiences with attempted penetration, tampon insertion, pelvic exams • Impact of problem on mood and relationships
Gender Dysphoria	• History/duration of cross-gender identification • Distress or impairment • Medical/surgical treatments planned/performed
Paraphilic Disorders	• Acting on paraphilic urges with non-consenting persons or has distress/impairment

Physical and mental status exams

- Assess for psychiatric comorbidity and medical risk factors.
- Refer for genitourinary and pelvic exams if there is no clear psychiatric etiology.
- Patients may be anxious/timid about areas of discussion and may feel particularly vulnerable during the physical exam.

Laboratory diagnosis
List of diagnostic tests

ED and MHSDD	General health screening labs; HbA1c; fasting glucose; TSH; morning total and free testosterone (if testosterone is low, repeat and obtain LH, prolactin)
FSIAD	General health screening labs; HbA1c; fasting glucose; TSH; reproductive hormone profile if indicated (e.g., perimenopause, post bilateral oophorectomy); note that only certain labs can accurately and reliably measure testosterone at the low levels typically seen in women, and serum testosterone levels are not well correlated with desire in otherwise healthy women
PE, DE, FOD, and GPPPD	As indicated by physical findings

Lists of imaging techniques
- As indicated by clinical findings (e.g., brain MRI to rule out pituitary abnormality if high prolactin).
- For ED, consider color duplex Doppler ultrasonography or Nocturnal Penile Tumescence (NPT) measurement.

Potential pitfalls/common errors made regarding diagnosis of disease

ED	Failing to assess for ED; assuming psychological cause in younger men
MHSDD	Failing to screen for comorbid ED
PE	Failing to screen for comorbid ED
DE	Misdiagnosis as ED, since prolonged sexual activity without ejaculation often leads to erectile failure
FSIAD	Failing to inquire about all relevant factors; failure to assess for other sexual dysfunctions in patient/partner
FOD	Failing to assess for other sexual dysfunctions in patient/partner; failing to get details of masturbation and partner sex practices
GPPPD	Attributing pain solely to psychological factors; failing to conduct a thorough medical assessment
Gender Dysphoria	Failing to appreciate the reality of the patient's experienced gender
Paraphilic Disorders	Diagnosing in individuals who only engage in paraphilic activity (e.g., transvestism) alone or with other consenting adults, and in whom paraphilic urges do not cause distress or impaired function

Treatment
Treatment rationale

ED	• If predominant psychological factors, first-line therapy is psychotherapy and/or PDE5 inhibitor • If predominant medical factors, first-line therapy is PDE5 inhibitor and medical treatment
MHSDD	• As indicated by clinical findings
PE	• If acquired, treat underlying medical, psychiatric, or relational problem • If lifelong, psychotherapy for mild cases; medical ± psychotherapy for more severe cases

(Continued)

(Continued)

DE	• If acquired, treat underlying medical, psychiatric, or relational problem • If lifelong, refer to sex therapist for masturbation retraining, enhancing arousal during sexual activity with partner, and attending to individual and relational issues
FSIAD	• As indicated by clinical findings
FOD	• If acquired, address situational and/or medical factors • If lifelong, help patient discover what conditions she requires for orgasm
GPPPD	• As indicated by clinical findings
Gender Dysphoria	• Explore patient's gender transition goals • May include medical/surgical treatment • Gender transition usually follows a stepwise course starting with reversible (e.g., name change, cross-gender dressing), then partially-reversible (e.g., hormonal treatments), then irreversible measures (e.g., sex reassignment surgeries) • Coexisting psychiatric disorders should be diagnosed and treated
Paraphilic Disorders	• Goal is to reduce paraphilic urges and promote adaptive behavior

When to hospitalize

• Most do not require hospitalization, with the exception of paraphilic behavior not controllable in the outpatient setting.

Table of treatment

ED

Medical PDE5 inhibitor: • Sildenafil 25–100 mg prn • Vardenafil 5–20 mg prn, or 10 mg oral disintegrating tab prn • Tadalafil 5–20 mg prn or 2.5–5 mg daily • Avanafil 50–200 mg prn	• PDE5 inhibitor is usually first line • Refer non-responders to a urologist for other and combination treatments • Avoid all with nitrates
Device-based • Vacuum device	• Available without prescription
Psychological • Various individual and couples therapies	• As indicated by clinical findings

MHSDD

Medical • Testosterone replacement • Treatment of medical disorders **Psychological** • Various individual and couples therapies	• As indicated by clinical findings

PE

Medical • SSRI (off-label) daily or prn • Dapoxetine (short-acting on-demand SSRI, not yet approved in US) • Lidocaine or lidocaine/prilocaine spray • PDE5 inhibitor for mixed ED/PE	• Often combined with psychotherapy

Device-based • Condom	• Minimizes risk of medication transfer to partner when used with anesthetizing spray
Psychological • Stop/start in response to premonitory sensations • Breathing/relaxation techniques • Various individual and couples therapies	• First line in mild PE • Combine with medical approaches for more severe PE

DE

• As indicated by clinical findings.

FSIAD

Medical • Flibanserin 100 mg qHS is FDA-approved for premenopausal women with acquired, generalized DSM-IV-TR Hypoactive Sexual Desire Disorder (HSDD)	• No studies yet on women with DSM-5 FSIAD
Device-based • Clitoral vacuum device	• Rarely used
Psychological • Psychotherapy, couples therapy, sex therapy, erotica	• Wide variety of techniques. Diversity of clinical situations makes outcomes research difficult

FOD

Psychological • Genital self-exploration; masturbation practice; challenging sex-negative attitudes, promoting sex-positive ones	• Books/videos are often helpful

GPPPD

Medical • General supportive (e.g., avoid soap on vulva; protective ointment) • Pelvic floor physical therapy • Topical (e.g., corticosteroids, lidocaine) • Injected (botulinum toxin) • Psychopharmacology for pain (e.g., tricyclic antidepressants, gabapentin)	• Care providers should have experience with GPPPD
Psychological • Cognitive behavioral therapy, pain management techniques, sex therapy	• Care providers should have experience with GPPPD
Surgical • Vestibulectomy for PVD	• Most impressive outcome data of any treatment for PVD, but long-term results of CBT may be equivalent

Gender Dysphoria

Medical • Medical and surgical gender affirming treatments	Stepwise (reversible and partially-reversible before irreversible) to the extent desired by patient
Psychological • Various individual therapies	As needed or desired, to explore modes of authentic gender expression, desire and commitment to cross-gender transition, or for related distress

Paraphilic Disorders

Medical • Hormonal (e.g., antiandrogen, GnRH agonists) • Psychotropic (e.g., SSRIs) **Psychological** • Various individual and group interventions

Prevention/management of complications
• Avoid using SSRIs for PE in men with ED.
• Adverse effects on erections and semen quality have been reported with longer-term SSRI use.
• Patients with asphyxiophilia who practice near-suffocation are at risk of accidental death from suffocation.

CLINICAL PEARLS
• **ED:** a ban on intercourse is often helpful at first to minimize performance pressure; with a PDE5 inhibitor, insure adequate sexual stimulation, take on an empty stomach, try on several occasions in order to maximize success.
• **MHSDD:** brief office evaluation is rarely adequate; consider referral to a sex specialist.
• **PE:** consider SSRI+PDE5 inhibitor in refractory cases.
• **DE:** options in refractory cases include self-stimulation to orgasm after intercourse, and acceptance of non-ejaculation during partner sex.
• **FSIAD:** it is sometimes best to accept, understand, and accommodate low desire, rather than trying to "fix" it.
• **FOD:** treatment needs vary widely depending on clinical situation.
• **GPPPD:** can have a devastating effect on quality of life; multi-modal assessment and treatment are generally required.
• **Gender Dysphoria:** show respect by using the patient's preferred name and pronouns consistent with gender identity.
• **Paraphilic Disorders:** most present in a forensic setting; many do not seek treatment because of legal/social concerns.

Special populations
Others
• If a patient with FSIAD has undergone natural or surgical menopause, refer to an endocrinologist to assess risks/benefits of off-label transdermal testosterone, with or without estrogen.

Prognosis

BOTTOM LINE/CLINICAL PEARLS

- **ED:** often worsens if untreated; the goal is to restore full rigidity and erectile confidence.
- **MHSDD:** varies with clinical situation.
- **PE:** social impact can be substantial; severe lifelong PE rarely resolves with increasing age; if on long-term SSRI treatment, periodically screen for ED; consider semen analysis if planning to conceive.
- **DE:** newer psychological techniques (masturbation retraining and enhancing arousal) have improved prognosis.
- **FSIAD:** varies with clinical situation.
- **FOD:** prognosis is more favorable than most other sexual dysfunctions; reported success rate with masturbation practice is 80–90% for women with lifelong anorgasmia.
- **GPPPD:** many cases become chronic.
- **Gender Dysphoria:** most individuals who choose gender transition report subjective improvement; correlates of regret following hormonal and surgical gender transition treatment include inadequately treated psychiatric disorders, poor cosmetic results, and poor social support.
- **Paraphilic Disorders:** tend to be chronic; fantasies/urges tend to be recurrent but with significant variation in frequency/intensity in response to psychosocial stressors and psychiatric disorders; advancing age tends to reduce both paraphilic and normophilic sexual behavior; response to treatment depends on patient motivation and adherence.

Reading list

American Psychiatric Association. Diagnostic and Statistical Manual of Mental Disorders, 5th edn. Washington, DC: American Psychiatric Publishing, 2013.

Byne W, Bradley S, Green R, et al. Report of the American Psychiatric Association Task Force on Treatment of Gender Identity Disorder. Arch Sex Behav 2012;41:759–96.

Brotto L, Atallah S, Johnson-Agbakwu C, et al. Psychological and Interpersonal Dimensions of Sexual Function and Dysfunction. J Sex Med 2016;13:538–571.

Laws DR, O'Donohue WT. Sexual Deviance – Theory, Assessment, and Treatment. New York: Guilford Press, 2008.

Meana M. Sexual Dysfunction in Women (Advances in Psychotherapy – Evidence-Based Practice). Cambridge: Hogrefe Publishing, 2012.

Rosen RC, Cappelleri JC, Smith MD, Lipsky J, Pena BM. Development and evaluation of an abridged, 5-item version of the international index of erectile dysfunction (IIEF-5) as a diagnostic tool for erectile dysfunction. Int J Impot Res 1999;14:226–44.

Rowland DL. Sexual Dysfunction in Men (Advances in Psychotherapy – Evidence-Based Practice). Cambridge: Hogrefe Publishing, 2012.

Rowland DL, Incrocci L (eds). Handbook of Sexual and Gender Identity Disorders. Hoboken: John Wiley and Sons, 2008.

Segraves RT, Balon R. Sexual Pharmacology Fast Facts. New York: W. W. Norton & Co., 2003.

Thibaut F, De La Barra F, Gordon H, Cosyns P, Bradford JM. The World Federation of Societies of Biological Psychiatry (WFSBP) guidelines for the biological treatment of paraphilias. World J Biol Psychiatry 2010;11(4):604–55.

Suggested websites

American Association of Sexuality Educators, Counselors and Therapists (AASECT). https://www.aasect.org

The Society for Sex Therapy and Research (SSTAR). http://www.sstarnet.org

Association of Peyronie's Disease Advocates. http://www.peyroniesassociation.org

Multidisciplinary Vulvodynia Program of the Gordon and Leslie Diamond Health Care Centre at Vancouver General Hospital – Vancouver, British Columbia. http://www.mvprogram.org

World Professional Association for Transgender Health. http://www.wpath.org

Guidelines
National society guidelines

Title	Source	Weblink
AUA Guideline on the Pharmacologic Management of Premature Ejaculation	American Urological Association (AUA), 2004	https://www.auanet.org/ education/guidelines/ premature-ejaculation.cfm

International society guidelines

Title	Source	Weblink
Guidelines on Male Sexual Dysfunction: Erectile Dysfunction and Premature Ejaculation	European Association of Urology (EAU), 2016	https://uroweb.org/guideline/ male-sexual-dysfunction/
Sexual desire and hypoactive sexual desire disorder in women. Introduction and overview. Standard operating procedure (SOP Part 1)	International Society for Sexual Medicine, 2012	http://www.ncbi.nlm.nih.gov/ pubmed/22974089
Treatment Algorithm for Premature Ejaculation (2013) Guidelines on the Management of Sexual Problems in Men and Women — the Role of Androgens (2010) Guidelines for the Management of Erectile Dysfunction (2013)	British Society for Sexual Medicine	All available at: http://www. bssm.org.uk/downloads/
Hormone Therapy Position Statement	The North American Menopause Society, 2012	http://www.ncbi.nlm.nih.gov/ pubmed/22367731
Women's Sexual Pain and Its Management	Journal of Sexual Medicine, 2005	http://www.ncbi.nlm.nih.gov/ pubmed/16422861
Standard operating procedures for female genital sexual pain	Journal of Sexual Medicine, 2013	http://www.ncbi.nlm.nih.gov/ pubmed/22970822
Standards of Care for the Health of Transsexual, Transgender and Gender-Nonconforming People, Version 7	World Professional Association for Transgender Health (WPATH), 2011	http://www.wpath.org/site_ page.cfm?pk_association_ webpage_menu=1351&pk_ association_webpage=3926
Guidelines for the Biological Treatment of Paraphilias	World Federation of Societies of Biological Psychiatry (WFSBP), 2010	http://www.ncbi.nlm.nih.gov/ pubmed/20459370

Evidence

Type of evidence	Title and comment	Weblink
RCT	A randomized comparison of group cognitive-behavioral therapy, surface EMG biofeedback, and vestibulectomy in the treatment of dyspareunia from vulvar vestibulitis. **Comment:** In women with provoked vestibulodynia disorder (PVD) group cognitive behavioral therapy, surface EMG biofeedback, and vestibulectomy all produced significant pain reduction at 6-month follow-up. Vestibulectomy appeared to be the most advantageous treatment, although there was some doubt about this finding.	http://www.ncbi.nlm.nih.gov/pubmed/11275387

Additional material for this chapter can be found online at:
www.mountsinaiexpertguides.com/psychiatry

This includes advice for patients, a case study, ICD codes,
and multiple choice questions.

CHAPTER 22

Eating Disorders

Thomas B. Hildebrandt[1], Sharon M. Batista[1], Matthew Shear[2], and Yadira Alonso[3]

[1] Icahn School of Medicine at Mount Sinai, New York, NY, USA
[2] Weil Cornell Medical College, White Plains, NY, USA
[3] Harvard Medical School, Boston, MA, USA

OVERALL BOTTOM LINE

- The eating disorders are psychiatric conditions with two primary features: disturbances in eating behaviors and body image disturbance.
- This summary contains data about incidence, prevalence, and treatment; the data are based on DSM-IV diagnostic criteria. While the overall diagnostic and treatment approach to eating disorders is largely unchanged, we refer to the specific changes in diagnostic criteria in DSM-5. Please also refer to the DSM-5 for full descriptions of the adult eating disorders.
- The feeding and eating disorders are:
  - Pica;
  - Rumination Disorder;
  - Avoidant/Restrictive Food Intake Disorder;
  - Anorexia Nervosa;
  - Bulimia Nervosa;
  - Binge-Eating Disorder;
  - Other Specified Feeding or Eating Disorder;
  - Unspecified Feeding or Eating Disorder.

The chapter focuses on anorexia nervosa (AN), bulimia nervosa (BN), and binge-eating disorder (BED), the diagnoses retained in DSM-5. These eating disorders are chronic conditions, with frequent relapse.

Predictive/risk factors

- Etiology of any eating disorder is multifactorial: genetic, biological, and environmental.
  - Relatives of patients with AN are 11.3 times as likely to have AN as controls with an estimated heritability of 58%.
  - Relatives of patients with BN are 4.4 times as likely to have BN as controls with an estimated heritability of 62%.
- All eating disorders are more common in women than men (ranging from 3:1 to 1.7:1), typically develop in adolescence, and have chronic courses.

Prevention
Screening

- Common screening tools for eating disorders are: (1) the Eating Disorder Examination (EDE), focusing on eating, shape, weight concern, and dietary habits; (2) the Eating Disorders Inventory (EDI), focusing on psychological features associated with eating disorders.

Mount Sinai Expert Guides: Psychiatry, First Edition. Edited by Asher B. Simon, Antonia S. New, and Wayne K. Goodman.
© 2017 John Wiley & Sons, Ltd. Published 2017 by John Wiley & Sons, Ltd.
Companion website: www.mountsinaiexpertguides.com/psychiatry

Primary prevention

- Multiple prevention programs exist; most use cognitive dissonance to challenge belief systems about thinness that leave individuals vulnerable to unhealthy attempts to change shape/weight.

Secondary prevention

- For AN, longer hospitalization stays associated with a higher body mass index (BMI) at discharge are associated with a lower likelihood of relapse.
- Partial hospital or residential treatment programs are commonly used to manage chronicity but have little empirical support.

Approaches to the complex patient with comorbidities and associated symptoms

- Medical and psychiatric comorbidity are often present with eating disorders. Multidisciplinary treatment is often necessary for these cases acutely, and harm reduction methods for management of chronic and severe cases in the community.

Clinical diagnosis
Anorexia nervosa

AN is characterized by:
1. restriction of energy intake relative to requirements, leading to a significantly low body weight in the context of age, sex, developmental trajectory, and physical health;
2. intense fear of gaining weight or of becoming fat, or persistent behavior that interferes with weight gain, even though at a significantly low weight;
3. disturbance in the way in which one's body weight or shape is experienced, undue influence of body weight or shape on self-evaluation, or persistent lack of recognition of the seriousness of the current low body weight.

Subtypes include:
- **Restricting type:** this subtype describes presentations in which weight loss is accomplished primarily through dieting, fasting, and/or excessive exercise.
- **Binge-eating/purging type:** during the last 3 months, the individual has engaged in recurrent episodes of binge eating or purging behavior (i.e., self-induced vomiting or the misuse of laxatives, diuretics, or enemas).

The minimum level of severity is based, for adults, on current BMI or, for children and adolescents, on BMI percentile. The level of severity may be increased to reflect clinical symptoms, the degree of functional disability, and the need for supervision.

Etiology

- The etiology of AN is unknown, but certain personality disorders may be risk factors.

Bulimia nervosa

Bulima nervosa is characterized by:
1. Recurrent episodes of binge eating. An episode of binge eating is characterized by both of the following:
   - eating, in a discrete period of time (e.g., within any 2-hour period), an amount of food that is definitely larger than what most individuals would eat in a similar period of time under similar circumstances;

- a sense of lack of control over eating during the episode (e.g., a feeling that one cannot stop eating or control what or how much one is eating).
2. Recurrent inappropriate compensatory behaviors in order to prevent weight gain, such as self-induced vomiting; misuse of laxatives, diuretics, or other medications; fasting; or excessive exercise.
3. The binge eating and inappropriate compensatory behaviors both occur, on average, at least once a week for 3 months.
4. Self-evaluation is unduly influenced by body shape and weight.
5. The disturbance does not occur exclusively during episodes of AN.

The minimum level of severity is based on the frequency of inappropriate compensatory behaviors (see below). The level of severity may be increased to reflect other symptoms and the degree of functional disability.

Etiology
- Unknown.

Binge-eating disorder
Binge-eating disorder is characterized by:
1. Recurrent episodes of binge eating. An episode of binge eating is characterized by both of the following:
   - eating, in a discrete period of time (e.g., within any 2-hour period), an amount of food that is definitely larger than what most people would eat in a similar period of time under similar circumstances;
   - a sense of lack of control over eating during the episode.
2. The binge-eating episodes are associated with three (or more) of the following:
   - eating much more rapidly than normal;
   - eating until feeling uncomfortably full;
   - eating large amounts of food when not feeling physically hungry;
   - eating alone because of feeling embarrassed by how much one is eating;
   - feeling disgusted with oneself, depressed, or very guilty afterward.
3. Marked distress regarding binge eating is present.
4. The binge eating occurs, on average, at least once a week for 3 months.
5. The binge eating is not associated with the recurrent use of inappropriate compensatory behavior as in BN and does not occur exclusively during the course of BN or AN.

Diagnosis

BOTTOM LINE/CLINICAL PEARLS
- Eating disorders present with a variety of symptoms.
- AN may be associated with a history of low body weight, menstrual irregularities, unexplained gastrointestinal problems, and unexplained food allergies.
- BN may be associated with electrolyte abnormalities, bloating, abdominal pain, and dental problems.
- Patients are often successful at disguising symptoms so secondary sources of information are important.
- While the physical complications of eating disorders can be wide-ranging, affecting multiple organ systems, patients often have a normal physical exam due to physiologic adapatation to the illness.

- When treating children and adolescents, one must obtain accurate height and weight measurements and, if possible, to compare to patients' own growth curves.
- Important items to assess for include: overexercise (including compulsive exercise), use of laxatives or emetic agents, and use of diet pills or supplements.

Differential diagnosis
- Malignancy, immunodeficiency, hyperthyroidism, gastrointestinal disease, polycystic ovarian syndrome (PCOS).
- Depressive disorder.
- Psychotic or delusional disorder.
- Obsessive-compulsive disorder.

Typical physical examination and mental status exam findings
- AN: cachexia, hair loss, bradycardia, orthostatic hypotension, lanugo.
- BN: salivary gland enlargement (sialadenosis), knuckle calluses, erosion of tooth enamel.
- BED: may not have physical manifestations other than obesity, PCOS.
- Patients with eating disorders often wear clothing that masks symptoms, draws attention away from their shape or bodies, and masks their weight loss.
- Anxiety, particularly related to food and weight gain, or depressed mood.
- Obsessions related to weight loss, dieting, or ritualized eating habits.
- Distorted body image and misperception of weight and/or appearance.
Beware: the physical examination may be normal!

Common emotional complaints and useful items to assess on interview
- Preoccupation with weight, food and nutrition, body image.
- Feeling out of control around food and/or eating more than intended.
- Specific foods may be avoided or feared.
- Eating may be different when with others vs alone.
- May avoid eating in social settings.
- Calorie counting.
- Strict diets including fad diets, veganism as means of calorie restriction.
- Food behaviors may correlate to specific settings, e.g., binges may occur while watching TV or in kitchen but not in other places.
- Guilty feelings after eating.
- Drive to "undo" effects of eating, i.e., compensate for eating through use of substances, medications, restriction of future food intake, exercise.
- Compulsion to exercise.
- Forcefully regurgitating.
- Mood and anxiety may dramatically change when finding out weight.
- Excessively prolonged meals and food rituals.

Common physical complaints in AN and/or BN
- Weakness and low energy.
- Weight loss.
- Apathy, poor concentration.
- Bone pain with exercise.

- Muscle aches.
- Limited sexual maturation or interest, loss of libido.
- Cold intolerance.
- Abdominal pain.
- Vomiting, bloating, constipation, obstipation.
- Edema.
- Excessive facial hair (lanugo).
- Painless swelling of cheeks (parotid glands) and neck to produce appearance of facial swelling.
- Irritability.
- Fertility problems.
- Amenorrhea.
- Dental decay.
- Palpitations.
- Headaches.
- Persistent heartburn.
- Dry, dull skin and hair.
- Disturbed sleep, frequent urination overnight.
  Urgent referral for medical assessment and/or hospitalization are indicated when any of following is present:
- using emetics: ipecac is cardiotoxic;
- signs of cardiovascular instability: rapid weight loss, chest pain when exercising, irregular heartbeat or skipped heartbeats, bradycardia, hypertension or hypotension, palpitations;
- hematemesis or persistent heartburn;
- symptoms of hypo- or hyperglycemia.

Laboratory diagnosis and other diagnostic tests

- AN and BN:
  - Screening laboratory tests for AN include complete blood count (for leukopenia), metabolic panel (for electrolye abnormalities – hypochloremia, hypokalemia, and metabolic alkalosis caused by purging), liver function tests, and thyroid function.
  - EKG may show bradycardia, a prolonged QT interval, and, for patients who have been underweight for >6 months, dual energy x-ray absorptiometry (DEXA scan) can be useful to assess for osteoporosis or osteopenia.
- Limited clinical utility:
  - Fasting serum glucose (low) and salivary amylase (high) concentrations if patients are vomiting; thiamine and leptin levels (markers of malnutrition).

Treatment

Overall treatment goals for all eating disorders:

- Medical stability.
- Normalized eating including variety, nutritional balance, comfort with food.
- Absence of compensatory behaviors associated with eating.
- Improved mental health.
- Relapse prevention.
- For adult AN, medically stabilize and increase weight, preferably to BMI >19.0.

- For children and adolescents, symptom focused family therapy is an effective treatment for refeeding AN patients and preventing relapse. For BN, family or individual cognitive behavioral therapy (CBT) is an effective treatment.
- Relapse prevention for adult AN should include CBT and may need step-down (partial hospital or day program) care for those with significant comorbidity.
- For BN, first-line treatment is CBT and second-line treatments are interpersonal therapy (IPT) or antidepressant medication.
- For BED, first-line treatments are CBT and IPT; second-line treatments involve antidepressant medications.

Management of medical emergencies and hospitalization

- Hospitalization is appropriate either for medical necessity (usually cardiovascular instability) or inability to maintain weight (below 20% expected weight) as an outpatient.
- Patients may be hospitalized for unstable vital signs, orthostatic hypotension, hypothermia, seizures, severe laboratory abnormalities, or EKG changes.
- The goal of hospitalization and of treatment of AN is to restore the patient's nutritional status.
- Patients with BN and BED are less likely to be hospitalized than patients with AN, because these patients have reduced frequency of life-threatening complications of illness in comparison with AN.
- Oral refeeding is optimal, but nasogastric and parenteral feeds may be used when patients refuse to eat.
- Inpatient hospitalization involves a meal plan, establishing weight gain expectations, constant monitoring of vital signs, monitoring for signs of refeeding syndrome (see further on), and consultation with other psychiatric and/or medical services when necessary.

Prevention/management of treatment complications

- Refeeding syndrome is a rare but potentially fatal complication that can occur during the refeeding of malnourished patients. It is the result of large fluid and electrolyte shifts that occur as the body moves from using carbohydrates to using fats and proteins as primary energy sources.

Psychopharmacology in eating disorders

- Medication is generally considered an adjunctive intervention, and often reserved for comorbid psychiatric conditions. There is no FDA-approved medication for the treatment of AN. For BN, fluoxetine is the only FDA-approved medication.
- In malnutrition states, care must be taken particularly in the effect of electrolyte abnormalities on drug function and metabolism, and liver and renal function; care must be taken to monitor the QTc.

Table of treatment

Evidence-based (meta-analyses, clinical trials)	Comments
Fluoxetine 60 mg/day	- No evidence for use in the treatment of AN - FDA-approved for bulimia - Decreases binging and purging behavior in BN, with better results at higher dose of 60 mg/day - Carries risk for hyponatremia

(Continued)

(Continued)

Olanzapine 1.25 mg/day	• Reduces ruminative thinking in AN • Mixed results in terms of significant weight gain in AN • Carries high risk for metabolic syndrome
Topiramate 100 mg/day (range 25–400 mg/day)	• Decreases binging and purging behaviors, and weight in BN and BED • Can increase lactic acid and cause acidosis, kidney stones • Can cause sedation and slowed thought process
IGF-1 and estrogen • estrogen 100 mcg patch/ 2x week • oral ethinyl estradiol (3.75 mcg daily for the first 6 months, 7.5 mcg daily for the second 6 months, and 11.25 mcg daily for the last 6 months) for immature • rhIGF-1: 30 microg/kg s.c. twice daily	• The combination of IGF-1 and oral contraception has been shown to improve bone density in patients with AN
No evidence base	
Cannabinoids	• No published studies to support use
Mirtazapine	• Very little evidence in the form of case reports that show weight gain via 5HT2C and H1 antagonism
Often clinically used but no evidence base • Lorazapem • Clonazepam • Paroxetine	
Use with caution	
Lithium • MAOIs • Stimulants	• Causes increased thirst, decreased appetite • Risk for hyponatremia, renal and thyroid toxicity
Contraindicated overall	
Bupropion	• Contraindicated in AN and BN, it lowers the seizure threshold; especially problematic in BN
Tricyclic antidepressants	• Side effect profile and toxicity concerns outweigh the benefits of weight gain shown in some studies

- *Medication side effects to be aware of overall:*
  - Zolpidem can cause binge eating and/or night eating and possible amnesia in persons with or without formal diagnosis of eating disorder.
  - Most psychotropic medications (especially antidepressants, mood stabilizers, and antipsychotics) carry risk of weight gain.
  - Stimulants may be abused for weight loss.

Special populations
Pregnancy
- Women with AN have lower fertility rates because of the effects of starvation on the hypothalamic-pituitary-ovarian axis.
- Women with eating disorders who do become pregnant are at a higher risk for spontaneous abortion, and are more likely than healthy women to give birth to children of low birth weight.
- While eating disorder symptoms often improve during pregnancy, relapse post partum is common.

Men
- Men are less likely than women to seek treatment.
- Men with eating disorders may not strive for thinness, but rather for a muscular build. As a result, assessments and diagnostic criteria that focus on thinness may lead to an underestimation of disordered eating behavior in men. This problem often emerges in adolescence.

Middle age/late-onset eating disorders
- Menopause presents as a potential risk for onset of eating pathology.
- There are very few data on course or outcome in this population.

Prognosis

BOTTOM LINE/CLINICAL PEARLS
- For AN, about 30–50% will have chronic course with 5–10% dying from the disorder.
- For BN, about 30–40% will have a chronic course with about 5% dying from the disorder.
- For BED, little is known about the course of illness. It is associated with obesity and resistance to weight intervention strategies.

Natural history of untreated disease
Morbidity and mortality
- The crude mortality rate for AN is 5.0%, and among surviving patients the majority do not obtain a full and sustained recovery. While medical complications can be the cause of mortality, individuals with AN are at especially heightened risk for suicide, with suicide rates reported as high as 7.3%. Mortality rates are lower and remission rates are higher for patients who develop AN during adolescence, as compared to other age groups.
- Crude mortality rates for BN are estimated at 0–2%.
- Crude mortality rates for BED are estimated at 2.9%.

Reading list
American Psychiatric Association. Diagnostic and Statistical Manual of Mental Disorders, 5th edn. San Francisco, CA: American Psychiatric Association, 2013.

Bulik CM, Berkman ND, Brownley KA, Sedway JA, Lohr KN. Anorexia nervosa treatment: A systematic review of randomized controlled trials. Int J Eat Disord 2007;40:310–20.

Fairburn CG. Cognitive Behavior Therapy and Eating Disorders. New York: Guilford Press, 2008.

Garner D, Olmsted M. Development and validation of a multidimensional eating disorder inventory for anorexia nervosa and bulimia. Int J Eat Disorder 1983;2:15–34.

Greetfeld M, Cuntz U, Voderholzer U. [Pharmacotherapy of anorexia nervosa and bulimia nervosa: state of the art.] Fortschr Neurol 2012;80(1):9–16.

Keel P, Brown T. Update on course and outcome in eating disorders. Int J Eat Disord 2010;43:195–204.

Lock J, Le Grande D. Treatment Manual for Anorexia Nervosa. A Family-Based Approach. New York: Guilford Press, 2001.

Setnick J. Eating disorders. Clinical Pocket Guide: Quick Reference for Healthcare Professionals. Snack Time Press. Dallas, Tx, 2005.

Shapiro J, Berkman N. Bulimia nervosa treatment. A systemic review of randomized controlled trials. Int J Eat Disord 2007;40:321–36.

Wilson GT. Treatment of binge eating disorder. PsychiatrClin North Am 2011;34(4):773–83.

Suggested websites

Academy for Eating Disorders. http://www.aedweb.org

https://www.nationaleatingdisorders.org/

Additional material for this chapter can be found online at:
www.mountsinaiexpertguides.com/psychiatry

This includes advice for patients, a case study, and multiple choice questions.

CHAPTER 23

Sleep-Wake Disorders

Akhil Shenoy[1], Rachel Fischer[1], and Amir Garakani[1,2]
[1] Icahn School of Medicine at Mount Sinai, New York, NY, USA
[2] Yale School of Medicine, New Haven, CT, USA

OVERALL BOTTOM LINE
- Sleep debt leads to fatigue, daytime sleepiness, and cognitive dysfunction.
- DSM-5 can help clinicians more easily identify individual sleep-wake disorders and minimizes the diagnosis of nonspecific categories.
- Some sleep-wake disorders have become defined by their etiology, while insomnia disorder, the most common disorder, continues to be characterized by symptom criteria.
- For insomnia disorder, the primary focus of this chapter, first-line approaches should be non-pharmacologic.

Background
Definition of disease and disease classification
The sleep-wake disorders are a heterogeneous group:
- Insomnia Disorder;
- Hypersomnia Disorder;
- Narcolepsy;
- Breathing-Related Sleep Disorders;
- Restless Legs Syndrome;
- NREM Sleep Arousal Disorders;
- Nightmare Disorder;
- REM Sleep Behavior Disorder;
- Circadian Rhythm Disorders;
- Substance or Medication Induced Sleep Disorder.

DSM-5 has removed the prior classification system of dyssomnias and parasomnias to highlight the known etiological differences between individual disorders:
- A subtype of narcolepsy with hypocretin deficiency has been identified.
- Breathing-related sleep disorders can be diagnosed effectively by polysomnography.
- Parasomnias have been re-categorized by their respective sleep stage and recognized as disorders of arousal.
- No specific etiology has been found for *primary* insomnia, which continues to be described by its symptom profile.

Insomnia, being one of the most common patient complaints in clinical medicine, will be the focus of this chapter. As both a symptom and a sign, insomnia demands clinical attention for its own sake and also points the clinician toward broader psychiatric and medical disorders.

Mount Sinai Expert Guides: Psychiatry, First Edition. Edited by Asher B. Simon, Antonia S. New, and Wayne K. Goodman.
© 2017 John Wiley & Sons, Ltd. Published 2017 by John Wiley & Sons, Ltd.
Companion website: www.mountsinaiexpertguides.com/psychiatry

While DSM-5 lists new diagnoses to highlight present knowledge of sleep-wake disorders, it has simplified the diagnosis of insomnia disorder, lumping all insomnia disorders without regard for intrinsic or extrinsic etiology.

Incidence/prevalence
- Prevalence of insomnia disorder = 6–10%.
- Prevalence of insomnia symptoms over one year in adults = 30–45%.

Economic impact
Sleep debt may lead to a loss of $150 billion/year from accidents and lost productivity.

Etiology and pathophysiology
Genetics are unknown at present. Normal sleep is regulated by the interaction between the homeostatic sleep drive and the circadian rhythm (involving melatonin). While no specific etiology has been found for insomnia disorder, it is often precipitated by a triggering event or rapid change in sleep schedule, and it is often characterized by a higher metabolic rate, less heart-rate variability, and higher cortisol secretion, all of which may be responsible for maintaining the disorder.

Risk factors
- Anxious or worry-prone temperament.
- Female gender.
- Increasing age.
- Some familial disposition.

Prevention
Screening
Screening for sleep disturbance should be part of every medical evaluation.

Secondary (and primary) prevention
- Maintaining good sleep hygiene.
- Environmental changes.
- Treating anxiety and mood disorders.

Diagnosis
- Most sleep-wake disorders, including insomnia disorder, are clinical diagnoses and rely on patient reports of disturbed sleep or daytime sleepiness.
- Polysomnography (sleep study) is useful in ruling out breathing-related sleep disorders.
- New to DSM-5, Insomnia Disorder can be diagnosed alongside other mental or medical disorders.

Differential diagnosis

Differential diagnosis	Features
Normal sleep variations	Sleep state misperception may lead to misdiagnosis
Substance or medication induced sleep disorder	Tobacco, caffeine, and other stimulants should be reviewed
Primary psychiatric condition (e.g., mood/anxiety disorders)	Predominance of mood/anxiety symptoms meeting diagnostic criteria

Typical presentation

Patients often complain of sleep difficulty. Coexisting clinical conditions are the rule, not the exception. Patients with sleep-wake disorders go undiagnosed 75% of the time.

Clinical diagnosis

History

- Insomnia Disorder requires patient's report of difficulty initiating or maintaining sleep ≥3 times per week for ≥3 months, with resultant daytime impairment or distress and continuing despite efforts to effect change.
- Take a detailed history of the patient's sleep habits, substance use, and new medications (see Box 23.1).
- Explore sleep hygiene practices and environment (noise, light, and temperature of bedroom).
- Modern sleep bands or actigraphs may overestimate total sleep as compared to the gold standard polysomnograph, but are more accurate than a sleep log.

BOX 23.1 MEDICATIONS THAT COULD CONTRIUTE TO INSOMNIA

Over-the-counter (OTC) and commonly prescribed medications may contribute to insomnia by affecting REM sleep, by inducing nightmares, by side effects of restlessness/agitation/anxiety, or by physical side effects that disturb sleep, such as frequent urination or arthralgias/myalgias.

- α blockers
- β blockers
- Statins
- Diuretics
- Angiotensin converting enzyme (ACE) inhibitors/ angiotensin receptor blockers (ARBs)
- Interferon
- Levodopa
- Anticonvulsants
- Selective serotonin reuptake inhibitors (SSRIs)
- Methylphenidate

- Dextroamphetamine
- Corticosteroids
- Thyroid hormone
- Cholinesterase inhibitors
- Second-generation H1 antagonists
- OTC cold medications
- OTC headache medications with caffeine
- Stimulant laxatives
- Oral contraceptives

Physical and mental status exams

The patient can appear haggard or "wired." Worry-prone patients often ruminate about bedtime or the fear of not being able to sleep, which perpetuates their condition. Those with sleep debt may present with cognitive dysfunction, particularly in executive tasks and working memory.

Disease severity classification

Insomnia disorder has been further qualified as episodic, persistent, and/or recurrent.

Laboratory diagnosis

CSF hypocretin to rule out a variant of narcolepsy.

List of diagnostic tests

Although polysomnography remains the sole diagnostic study designed to evaluate the biophysical changes that occur during sleep, it is seldom used in clinical practice. Indications for polysomnography include diagnosing a sleep-related breathing disorder, sleep-related movement disorder, or evaluation of sleep-related behaviors that may be potentially violent or harmful to the patient or others.

Diagnostic algorithm (Algorithm 23.1)

Algorithm 23.1 Diagnostic algorithm for insomnia. Differential diagnosis for nine major insomnia-related sleep-wake disorders in DSM-5

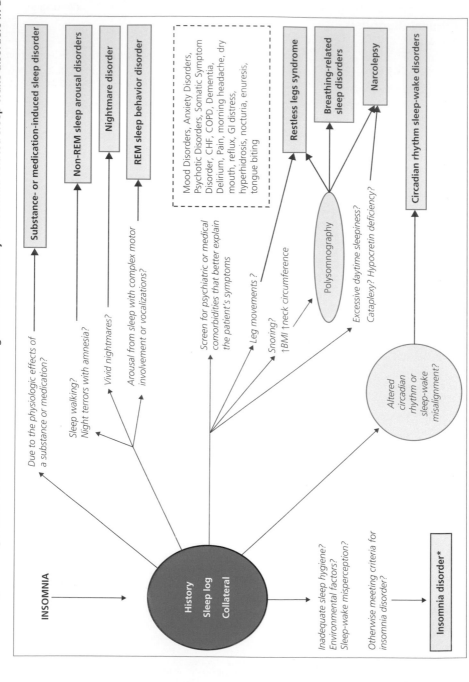

* Insomnia disorder may be co-diagnosed with specifiers of "with non-sleep disorder mental comorbidity" or "with other medical comorbidity"

Potential pitfalls/common errors made regarding diagnosis of disease

Patients complaining of insomnia tend to underestimate their sleep. Collateral from a bed partner is not always available. Polysomnography to help diagnose insomnia is not currently covered by major insurance. Sleep-wake disorders tend to be under-recognized by physicians and under-diagnosed.

Treatment
Treatment rationale

For primary insomnias, non-pharmacologic approaches are first line. Patients should be educated on stimulus control, sleep restriction, and sleep hygiene.

- Stimulus control involves maintaining the same sleep schedule, avoiding "clock-watching" in bed, and instructing patients to get out of bed and engage in a relaxing activity if they are not asleep after 20 minutes.
- Sleep restriction involves avoiding daytime naps and advising patients to reduce time in bed to only when they are sleeping.
- Sleep hygiene techniques:
  - Ensure adequate natural light during the day.
  - Avoid daytime naps.
  - Avoid television, electronic screens, and bright lights before bedtime.
  - Avoid alcohol, caffeine, or other stimulating substances in the hours before bedtime.
  - Avoid heavy meals before bedtime, but also avoid going to bed hungry.
  - Avoid heavy exercise at least 3 hours before bedtime.
  - Maintain the same bedtime and awake time.
  - Keep the bedroom dark, quiet, and at a comfortable temperature.
  - Use the bed and bedroom only for sleeping and intimate contact.
  - CBT for managing anxiety around bedtime.

Treating patients with comorbid medical or psychiatric conditions may require adjusting doses or selecting different medications.

- Cognitive disorders, the elderly, and/or lower body weight.
  - Use half the regular healthy adult dose.
- Breathing disorders (e.g. COPD).
  - Monitor the patient closely, as hypnotic medications may increase the risk of respiratory depression.
- Comorbid anxiety.
  - May benefit from anxiolytic agents that aid sleep (e.g., mirtazapine, antihistamines).
  - Avoiding benzodiazepines may be prudent given their side effect of decreasing REM sleep.
- Posttraumatic stress disorder (PTSD).
  - Screen for nightmares, which may cause insomnia by autonomic hyperactivity and fear of sleep; consider treatment with prazosin.
- Bipolar disorder and/or psychosis.
  - Medicate as indicated but dose sedating medications at bedtime to help increase sleep time. Use of antipsychotics for primary insomnia is not recommended given the high risk of severe adverse effects, even at low doses.

When to hospitalize

- Patients with *primary insomnia* would rarely, if ever, require psychiatric hospitalization for their sleep disturbance.
- Patients with nonspecific insomnia may require hospitalization due to one of several under-lying psychiatric conditions: (1) mania in the context of bipolar disorder; (2) disorganization

and psychosis in a schizophrenia spectrum disorder; (3) insomnia with suicidal thoughts in a depressive disorder.

Managing the hospitalized patient

The diagnosis of a sleep-wake disorder in a medically hospitalized patient warrants care in the consideration of the emergent medical condition and/or new medications that the patient is taking.

Table of treatment

Medication class	Medication	Half-life (hours)	Dose range (mg)	FDA indication(s)	Effect on REM sleep
Benzodiazepines (GABA-A agonists)	Flurazepam (Dalmane)	2–3 40–100 (metabolite)	15–30	Sleep maintenance (short term, 7–10 days)	↓
	Quazepam (Doral)	25–40 28–115 (metabolite)	7.5–15	Sleep maintenance (short term, 7–10 days)	↓
	Estazolam (Prosom)	8–24	0.5–2	Sleep maintenance (short term, 7–10 days)	↓
	Temazepam (Restoril)	6–16	7.5–30	Sleep maintenance (short term, 7–10 days)	↓
	Triazolam (Halcion)	2–5 40–50 (metabolite)	0.125–0.5	Sleep onset (short term, 7–10 days)	↓
	Clonazepam (Klonopin)	24–56	0.5–2	REM Sleep Behavior Disorder	↓
Benzodiazepine receptor agonists (α1 selective to GABA-A receptor)	Zolpidem (Ambien)	2.5–3.1	5–10	Sleep onset (short term, 7–14 days)	↓
	Zolpidem CR (Ambien CR)	2.5–3.1	6.25–12.5	Sleep onset and maintenance (chronic use)	↓
	Zolpidem sublingual (Intermezzo)	2.5–3.1	1.75–3.5	Middle of the night awakening (short term, 7–10 days)	↓

(Continued)

Medication class	Medication	Half-life (hours)	Dose range (mg)	FDA indication(s)	Effect on REM sleep
	Zaleplon (Sonata)	1	5–10	Sleep onset and middle-of-the-night awakening (short term, 7–10 days)	←→
	Eszopiclone (Lunesta)	6	1–3	Sleep maintenance (chronic use)	←→
GABA-B agonist	Sodium oxybate (Xyrem)	0.5–1	4.5–9.0 g	Narcolepsy and cataplexy	↓
Orexin receptor (OXR1–OXR2) antagonist	Suvorexant (Belsomra)	12	5–20	Sleep onset and/or maintenance	↑
Melatonin receptor (MT1–MT2) agonist	Ramelteon (Rozerem)	1–2.6 2–5 (metabolite)	8	Sleep onset (chronic)	←→
Melatonin agonist	Melatonin	0.5–1	1–5	Not approved	←→
GABA enhancer	Gabapentin (Neurontin)	5–7	100–600	Neuralgia, partial seizures	↑ (?)
	Valerian	1.1±0.6	400–600	Not approved	←→
Antihistamines (H1-antagonists)	Diphen-hydramine (Benadryl, Unisom)	2–10	12.5–50	Sleep onset (short term)	↓
	Doxylamine (Unisom SleepTab)	10	12.5–50	Sleep onset (short term)	↓
	Hydroxyzine (Vistaril, Atarax)	20–25	25–100	Anxiety, pruritus, anesthesia, sedation	↓
Antidepressants (mostly H1-antagonists)	Trazodone (Desyrel)	4–9	25–200	Major depressive disorder	←→
Mirtazapine with also 5-HT2 inhibition	Mirtazapine (Remeron)	20–40	7.5–15	Major depressive disorder	←→
	Doxepin (Silenor)	15.3 31 (metabolite)	3–6	Sleep maintenance (chronic use)	↓
Wakefulness promoting agent	Modafinil (Provigil)	10–12	100–400 Morning dose	Narcolepsy, obstructive sleep apnea, shift-work sleep disorder	NA
	Armodafinil (Nuvigil)	15	150–250 Morning dose	Narcolepsy, obstructive sleep apnea, shift-work sleep disorder	NA

Prevention/management of complications

- Benzodiazepines and benzodiazepine receptor agonists carry the risk of tolerance and dependence and should be used with caution in high-risk populations such as persons with past or current substance use disorders.
- Reports of nocturnal activity with zolpidem include sleep-walking, sleep-eating, and sleep-driving.
- Trazodone may rarely cause priapism.
- Certain sedative antidepressants (trazodone, doxepin) can lead to serotonin syndrome if combined with other serotonergic medications (e.g., triptans for migraines, or tramadol for pain).

CLINICAL PEARLS

- First-line treatment for primary insomnia should be stimulus control and sleep hygiene, followed by referral for cognitive therapy.
- Antihistamines have short-term efficacy for insomnia, but tolerance can develop quickly.
- Non-habit-forming agents (e.g., trazodone, mirtazapine, doxepin) may be used for longer-term treatment, especially in patients with comorbid anxiety and depression, but some agents do carry the risk of cardiac side effects and drug–drug interactions.
- Benzodiazepine receptor agonists are preferred to benzodiazepines as they target the hypnotic receptors of GABA; patients should be advised about the risks of tolerance and dependence with both classes of these medications. Some agents may be used for longer, chronic treatment (e.g., eszopiclone and zolpidem CR) but all medications in these classes should not be stopped abruptly due to the risk of withdrawal.
- Suvorexant, an orexin receptor antagonist, was approved by the FDA in 2014. It represents a novel mechanism for treating insomnia. It is contraindicated in narcolepsy. It may also increase suicidal thinking. Suvorexant became available in US pharmacies as of spring 2015.

Special populations
Pregnancy
- Maternal use of benzodiazepine receptor agonists does not appear to carry a teratogenic risk, although it is recommended to consider alternative treatments.

Prognosis

BOTTOM LINE/CLINICAL PEARLS

- While 30–50% of adults report insomnia over the course of a year, only 10% become chronic.
- Poor sleep habits, excessive use of coffee, irregular schedules, and fear of not sleeping perpetuate the cycle of insomnia.
- Long-term use of sedatives may not improve quality of sleep.

Natural history of untreated disease
Chronic insomnia can lead to daytime irritability, poor concentration, and occupational problems. Decreased attention and concentration are related to higher rates of accidents. Persistent insomnia is a risk factor for major depressive disorder.

Reading list

Buysse DJ. Insomnia. JAMA 2013;309(7):706–16.

Gulyani S, Salas RE, Gamaldo CE. Sleep medicine pharmacotherapeutics overview: today, tomorrow, and the future (Part 1: insomnia and circadian rhythm disorders). Chest 2012;142(6):1659–68.

Morgenthaler T, Kramer M, Alessi C, et al.; American Academy of Sleep Medicine. Practice parameters for the psychological and behavioral treatment of insomnia: an update. An American Academy of Sleep Medicine report. Sleep 2006;29(11):1415–9.

Morin AK, Jarvis CI, Lynch AM. Therapeutic options for sleep-maintenance and sleep-onset insomnia. Pharmacotherapy 2007;27(1):89–110.

Winkelman JW. Insomnia disorder. NEJM 2015;373:1437–44.

Guidelines
National society guidelines

Title	Source	Weblink
Clinical Guideline for the Evaluation and Management of Chronic Insomnia in Adults	American Academy of Sleep Medicine (AASM), 2008	http://www.aasmnet. org/Resources/clinical guidelines/040515.pdf

International society guidelines

Title	Source	Weblink
Insomnia – Clinical Knowledge Summaries	National Institute for Health and Clinical Excellence (NICE), 2009	http://cks.nice.org.uk/ insomnia

Evidence

Type of evidence	Title and comment	Weblink
Meta-analysis	Drug treatment of primary insomnia: a meta-analysis of polysomnographic randomized controlled trials. **Comment:** Benzodiazepine receptor agonists and classical benzodiazepines are significantly more effective than antidepressants in reducing the sleep onset latency. Benzodiazepine receptor agonists produced greater objective total sleep time compared to other medications.	http://www.ncbi. nlm.nih.gov/ pubmed/25168785
Meta-analysis	Effectiveness of non-benzodiazepine hypnotics in treatment of adult insomnia: meta-analysis of data submitted to the Food and Drug Administration, BMJ, Dec 2012. **Comment:** Benzodiazepine receptor agonists produced a large clinical response in both subjective and polysomnographic sleep latency but only a slight improvement over placebo.	http://www.ncbi. nlm.nih.gov/ pubmed/23248080
Review	Chronic insomnia. **Comment:** CBT is an effective alternative to medications for chronic insomnia. Although more time consuming than drug management, CBT produces sleep improvements that are sustained over time.	http://www.ncbi. nlm.nih.gov/ pubmed/22265700

Additional material for this chapter can be found online at:
www.mountsinaiexpertguides.com/psychiatry

This includes advice for patients, a case study, ICD codes,
and multiple choice questions.

PART 3

Child/Adolescent Disorders

CHAPTER 24

Assessment of Child Development

Suzanne Garfinkle[1], Mary M. LaLonde[2], and John O'Brien[1]
[1] Icahn School of Medicine at Mount Sinai, New York, NY, USA
[2] Private Practice, Scarsdale, NY, USA

OVERALL BOTTOM LINE
- Developmental assessment takes into account four main areas of functioning: motor, language, cognitive, and social-emotional.
- Early intervention for developmental delays improves IQ, raises academic achievement, increases adult employment, decreases criminality, and may be more effective than interventions later in life.
- Providers should have a low threshold for immediate referral to a specialist if any red flags are identified.
- As it is difficult for young children to talk about their feelings directly to a physician, play may be the best method to assess psychological development.

Discussion of topic and guidelines
- Development refers to the progression of function, skill, thought, and behavior, resulting from interactions between the child and his/her environment.
  - There are four main areas of assessment: motor, language, cognitive, social-emotional.
- Approximately 17% of children in the US have ≥1 developmental delay.
  - This leads to significant morbidity/cost.
  - Even subtle disabilities are associated with poorer health status and higher rates of school failure, in-grade retention, and special education.
  - Early intervention improves IQ, raises academic achievement, increases adult employment, and decreases criminality. Later interventions may be less effective.
  - Centers for Disease Control and Prevention recommends brief assessment to identify children who should receive intensive evaluation.

Caregiver interview
Obtain:
- Careful description of the presenting problem.
- Reason for seeking help now.
- Previous attempts to obtain help; prior assessments/interventions.
- Prenatal, perinatal, postnatal problems: maternal health during pregnancy; delivery mode; birth condition; Apgar scores; birth weight; head circumference; newborn hearing screen.
- History of previous illnesses and accidents.
- Acquisition of developmental milestones.

Mount Sinai Expert Guides: Psychiatry, First Edition. Edited by Asher B. Simon, Antonia S. New, and Wayne K. Goodman.
© 2017 John Wiley & Sons, Ltd. Published 2017 by John Wiley & Sons, Ltd.
Companion website: www.mountsinaiexpertguides.com/psychiatry

- Environmental, social, and family history including:
  - family history of developmental problems, learning difficulties, psychiatric illness, substance use, domestic violence, trauma, consanguinity;
  - education history;
  - history of biological functions: appetite, sleep, bladder and bowel control, puberty;
  - child's relationships within the nuclear and extended family and with peers;
  - significant events, such as separations, losses, illnesses, accidents, abuse, and deaths.
- Current psychosocial aspects including:
  - childcare and extended family arrangements;
  - child's psychological role in family;
  - caregiver perceptions and expectations of child;
  - stability of home/family environment;
  - family functioning, stress, and coping mechanisms.

Evaluation and observation of the child

- Physical health, appearance, growth parameters, sensory, gross motor, fine motor, communication, cognition, and language assessment.
- See Table 24.1 for normal and problematic development.
- Very low threshold for immediate referral to specialist:
  - If there are moderate to severe delays.
  - If there are any red flags (Table 24.1).

Table 24.1 Normal developmental milestones in social, emotional, and behavioral domains, and red flags in all domains.

Age	Social, emotional, and behavioral domains	Red flags (including motor, language, etc.)
6 weeks	Smiles	Unresponsive to sound or visual stimuli
3 months	Regards hand, laughs, and squeals	Lack of social response or vocalization
6 months	May finger feed self	Poor head control, low tone, not reaching
9 months	Waves bye-bye, plays pat-a-cake, indicates wants, stranger anxiety begins	Cannot sit unsupported, no babble
12 months	Imitates activities, indicates wants, object permanence, stranger anxiety	Not communicating with gestures such as pointing, not weight-bearing through legs
18 months	Uses spoon, symbolic play ("talking" on telephone), mimics domestic chores	Not walking, no symbolic play, no words
2 years	Can remove some clothes	Not joining 2 words, not running, no symbolic play, perseveration in play
3 years	Eats with fork and spoon, puts on clothes, may be toilet trained	Not communicating with words, cannot climb stairs
4 years	Makes up stories, plays in a group, goes to toilet independently	
5 years	Names several friends, interactional play with rules, imitative play	
7 years	Capable of empathy, able to contemplate mental states of others, conservation, reversibility	
12+ years	Likely will have best friend and close circle of friends, increased self-reliance and independence, has empathy	

- If any of the following: loss of developmental skills at any age; concern about vision, fixing, or following an object at any age; hearing loss at any age; persistently low muscle tone; no speech by 18 months, especially if the child does not attempt to communicate by other means; loss of previously acquired speech; asymmetry of movements; persistent toe walking; complex disabilities; height curve (HC) >99.6th percentile or if HC has crossed two centiles (up or down) on growth chart.
  - Delay in referral can impede possible improvement.
  - Concurrent referral to early intervention/early childhood services.
- Observe the child's developing sense of self, social relatedness, interest in environment, coping skills, capacity for affect regulation and for symbolic representation and play.
  - Observe the child entering and moving about the office, interacting with age-appropriate toys, and relating with interviewer and caregiver.
  - Videos may identify problems not manifested in the office.
  - Obtain reports from other caregivers and teachers.
  - Observe how the child uses the caregiver for support and reassurance, and the caregiver's responsiveness to the child's affective state and efforts.
- No universally accepted screening tool is appropriate for all ages and populations (Table 24.2).
  - Common causes of deviated development can be elicited through history and physical exam (e.g., late talking and walking may be familial; language development may seem delayed in bilingual families; undernutrition; social isolation of family; maternal depression).

Table 24.2 Tools for developmental assessment.

Tool	Ages (months)	Format	Weblink
Ages and Stages Questionnaire (ASQ)	6–60	Parent report 30 items 10–15 min	http://agesandstages.com
Parents' Evaluation of Developmental Status	0–96	Parent report 10 items 2–5 min	http://www.pedstest.com
Child Development Inventory	5–72	Parent report 300 items 30–50 min	http://www.childdevrev.com/page15/page17/cdi.html
Infant Development Inventory	0–18	Parent report 60 items 5–10 min	http://www.childdevrev.com/page15/page28/idi.html
Bayley Infant Neurodevelopmental Screener	3–24	Clinician-administered 66–78 items 15–20 min	http://www.pearsonassessments.com
Denver Developmental Screening Test	0–72	Clinician-administered 125 items 20–30 min	http://www.denverii.com
Modified checklist for autism in toddlers (M-CHAT)	16–48	Parent/teacher report 23 items 5–10 min	http://www.firstsigns.org/downloads/m-chat.pdf
Child Behavior Checklist (CBCL) 1½ –5 and 6–18	18-18 years	Parent/teacher report 99 items 15–20 min	http://www.aseba.org/

Assessment of social-emotional development
- The first 5 years are crucial for social-emotional development.
- Approximately 10–15% of children age 0–5 experience social-emotional problems that negatively impact functioning, development, and school readiness.
- A substantial number of children with social-emotional difficulties are not being identified in primary care.

Infancy and preschool
- It is nearly impossible for young children to talk about their feelings directly to a physician until 4–5 years of age.
- Use play to assess psychological development.
  - Dolls and dollhouses, blocks, crayons and paper, animal figures; use age- and gender-appropriate activities.
- Assessments may be made by playing with a child and observing the child's interaction with toys.
  - Motor dexterity.
  - Aspects of temperament (e.g., activity level; ability to sustain attention).
  - Ask the child to explain her/his "rules" for the game. (While young children are not expected to play rule-driven games, they often have their own ideas about how games ought to be played.)
  - Observe for repetitive play; assess flexibility by trying to change course.
  - Observe for frustration and response to reassurance, redirection, or other interventions.
  - Observe intensity/quality of affect; is it fun to play with this child?
  - A child >2 can begin to venture past the repetitive games of infancy into more symbolic play (e.g., pretending to go to sleep and wake up, pretending to feed a doll, pretending to be a doggie).
  - Observe perseverance and level of curiosity about new games or new forms of play.
  - In preschoolers and beyond, observe competitiveness and response to winning and losing.
  - Ask all children to help tidy up after play; observe ability to participate.
- Drawing is a useful assessment activity for children of almost all ages.
  - Drawings of people reflect a great deal about development: motor dexterity, maturity level (based on anatomical accuracy and complexity of the drawing), self-esteem (Is the child big and bold or small and insignificant?), mood (Is the child smiling? Is there vibrant color?), and relationships (Are the family members connected but nicely spaced apart? Crowding each other? Are some engulfing others? Are they detached and floating in their own worlds? Are members of the family omitted?).

School age
- Children ≥7 can be assessed through play, talk, and observation.
- Toys and games can display motor, cognitive, and language skills, and can be a distraction that frees children to speak openly about emotional issues.
- School-related activities are the primary focus of development.
  - Goal for this period (Erikson): solidify self-esteem grounded in a sense of one's unique talents and interests, and acquiring a place in society beyond one's immediate family.
- Myelination of the brain is almost complete by age 7, and cognition switches from pre-operational (language without logic; magical thinking) to logical thinking (Piaget). New logical concepts emerge for the child:
  - Conservation (maintaining inherent properties when shapes of objects change).
  - Seriation (putting things in order according to specific properties).

- Reversibility (matter can shift between two forms).
- Classification (organizing objects by characteristic).
- Decreased egocentrism (although empathy begins at 2–3, school-age children are better able to sustain empathy).
- Children become able to judge actions more in accordance with intentions. Children typically develop "conventional" morality, measuring actions against the rules of society and the views of significant adults.
- Role models are required for self-esteem. Children identify with characteristics of parents and teachers. A healthy-school age child should be able to describe one or more key adult figures.
- Assess older children and adolescents primarily through conversation.
- Typically begin by asking children some basics about their lives:
  - *How old are you?*
  - *Who do you live with?*
  - *Where do you go to school; what grade are you in?*
- Move into the realm of feelings:
  - *Do you like school?*
  - *What are your favorite activities?*
  - *What do you want to be when you get older?*
  - *Would you say you are mostly a happy kid? An angry kid? A sad kid? A scared kid?*
  - *If you could have three wishes, what would they be?*
  - *If you could change one thing about your life, what would it be?*
- Finally, ask about their relationships:
  - *Do you have friends?*
  - *Do you have a best friend? What do you like most about that person?*
  - *Is your mom nice? Is your dad nice? Is your teacher nice?*
  - *If you were lost in a forest, who would come and find you?*
  - *If you could take one person on a trip with you to the moon, who would it be and why?*

Adolescence

- A culturally-determined period of time beginning with puberty and ending when a person becomes an "adult."
  - Biological changes include hormonal status, metabolic rate, appetite, and sleep pattern phase shifted later in the day.
  - Neurological changes allow greater cognitive and emotional complexity and self-regulation.
- Capacity for abstraction begins.
  - Ability to see a situation from another's point of view.
  - Ability to think of multiple possibilities when solving a problem.
  - Ability to develop and test hypotheses, test reality, reason deductively, and think in terms of probabilities.
  - Further decrease in egocentrism and growth in social perspective.
- Core conflict: "identity versus role confusion" (Erikson).
  - Struggle to cultivate a self-image that feels authentic and culturally sanctioned.
  - Focus shifts away from nuclear family and toward peer groups.
  - A successful adolescent is able to envision the future with optimism about the realistic role s/he might play in society.
- Observe parents' reactions to the separation process.
  - Common areas of difficulty for parents include being de-idealized and helping their teenager acquire autonomy despite lack of proficiency in many adult tasks.

- Most adolescents regard relationships with parents as stable, trusting, and sustaining.
  - Assess for psychosocial disturbances in families with a great deal of conflict; do not explain this away as part of normal adolescence.
- The adolescent's body is both rapidly changing and over-emphasized in importance, and there is often a high level of physical dissatisfaction.
  - These concerns should be balanced by other interests, and not interfere with most activities.
- Assessment must include drug and alcohol use, sex, and risk-taking behaviors.
  - Experimenting with illicit substances is common, but any sign of substance abuse or dependence, or repeated risk-taking, warrants psychiatric consultation.
  - Teens at greatest risk typically lack stabilizing forces in their lives, such as stable family situations and authority figures.

Reading list

Brauner CB, Stephens BC. Estimating the Prevalence of Early Childhood Serious Emotional/Behavioral Disorder: Challenges and Recommendations. Public Health Rep 2006;121(3):303–10.

Crain WC. Theories of Development: Concepts and Applications, 5th edn. Upper Saddle River, NJ: Pearson, 2005.

Dulcan MK. Dulcan's Textbook of Child and Adolescent Psychiatry, 1st edn. Washington, DC: American Psychiatric Publishing, 2010.

Ebert MH, Loosen PT, Nurcombe B, Leckman JF. Current Diagnosis and Treatment: Psychiatry, 2nd edn. New York: McGraw Hill, 2000.

Karoly LA, Kilburn R, Cannon J. Early Childhood Interventions: Proven Results, Future Promises. Santa Monica, CA: RAND Corporation, 2005.

Suggested websites

Centers for Disease Control and Prevention. Child development: Developmental Monitoring and Screening for Health Professionals. http://www.cdc.gov/ncbddd/childdevelopment/screening.html

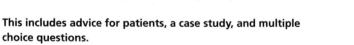

Additional material for this chapter can be found online at:
www.mountsinaiexpertguides.com/psychiatry

This includes advice for patients, a case study, and multiple choice questions.

CHAPTER 25

Autism Spectrum Disorder

Benjamin N. Angarita and Alexander Kolevzon

Icahn School of Medicine at Mount Sinai, New York, NY, USA

OVERALL BOTTOM LINE
- Autism spectrum disorder (ASD) is characterized by deficits in social communication and restricted and repetitive behaviors and interests.
- The etiology is considered primarily genetic.
- Applied behavior analysis (ABA) is the first-line treatment for ASD.
- Risperidone and aripiprazole are approved by the FDA for the treatment of irritability associated with ASD in children and adolescents.

Background
Definition of disease
- ASD is a chronic neurodevelopmental disorder with early childhood onset of impaired social communication (affecting social-emotional reciprocity, non-verbal communication, and peer relationships) and restricted and repetitive behaviors and interests (e.g., stereotyped or repetitive speech, excessive adherence to routines, highly restricted or fixed interests, hyper- or hypo-reactivity to sensory input).
- It may co-occur as a feature of various genetic syndromes.

Incidence/prevalence
- Prevalence = 1/88 children.
- Male predominance: 1/54 boys; 1/252 girls.
- Occurs across all ethnic, racial, and socioeconomic groups.

Economic impact
- Average annual medical costs for children with ASD are ~6 times higher than for unaffected children.
- In addition to medical costs, intensive behavioral interventions may cost ~ $50,000/child/year.

Mount Sinai Expert Guides: Psychiatry, First Edition. Edited by Asher B. Simon, Antonia S. New, and Wayne K. Goodman.
© 2017 John Wiley & Sons, Ltd. Published 2017 by John Wiley & Sons, Ltd.
Companion website: www.mountsinaiexpertguides.com/psychiatry

Etiology
- Primarily genetic; twin studies estimate heritability at ~90%.
- Toxic, metabolic, and perinatal risk factors may influence the development of ASD.

Pathophysiology
- 10–15% of ASD is caused by rare genetic variants.
- Certain genes which have been shown to cause ASD disrupt pathways that regulate synaptic neurotransmission; as a result, ASD is sometimes referred to as a "synaptopathy."
  - Phelan–McDermid syndrome (PMS; characterized by global developmental delay, severe intellectual disability, hypotonia, delayed or absent speech, and ASD) is a single-gene cause of ASD that results from deletions/mutations in the *SHANK3* gene located at terminal end of chromosome 22. *SHANK3* codes for a master scaffolding protein in the postsynaptic density of glutamatergic synapses; deficiency of *SHANK3* disrupts the integrity of nerve cell connections.

Predictive/risk factors
- Male.
- Family history.
- Advanced paternal age (>40).
- Advanced maternal age (>35).
- Preterm birth.
- Low birth weight.
- Intrauterine exposure to divalproex sodium.

Prevention

> **BOTTOM LINE/CLINICAL PEARLS**
> - Vaccines do not cause autism. Large epidemiological studies in the US, UK, and Japan using gold standard population-based case control and birth cohort studies have found no evidence supporting a link.

Screening
- Chromosomal microarray analysis is recommended for all children with suspected ASD, regardless of age.
  - Genetic testing (chromosomal microarray analysis; whole exome sequencing) can identify causes of ASD in 10–15% of cases.
- Screen all children aged 16–24 months with the Modified Checklist for Autism in Toddlers, Revised (M-CHAT-R).
- Screen with Grodberg's Autism Mental Status Exam:
  - poor eye contact;
  - lack of interest in others;
  - lack of pointing to show or share interest;
  - impaired language, including pragmatics of language (reciprocal conversation);
  - repetitive behaviors and motor stereotypies;
  - unusual or encompassing preoccupations;
  - unusual sensitivities.

Diagnosis

BOTTOM LINE/CLINICAL PEARLS
- Persistent deficits in social communication across multiple contexts manifested by deficits in:
  - social-emotional reciprocity;
  - non-verbal communicative behavior;
  - developing and maintaining relationships.
- Restricted, repetitive patterns of behavior, interests, or activities, shown by ≥2 of:
  - stereotyped or repetitive use of speech, objects, or motor movements;
  - excessive adherence to routines, ritualized patterns of non-verbal or verbal behavior, or excessive resistance to change;
  - highly restricted, fixated interest that is abnormal in focus or intensity;
  - hyper-or hypo-reactivity to sensory input.
- Symptoms must present in early childhood and must impair everyday functioning.

Differential diagnosis

Diagnosis	Features
Speech Delay	ASD includes deficits in non-verbal communication and social interaction
Schizophrenia	ASD is not characterized by psychosis
Social Phobia	In ASD, social withdrawal is pervasive and not situation-dependent. ASD includes other developmental delays
Attention-Deficit/Hyperactivity Disorder (ADHD)	Significant deficits in emotion-recognition and perspective-taking are evident in ASD and less common in ADHD

Typical presentation

A 3-year-old boy is referred to a child and adolescent psychiatrist for an evaluation for ASD because his pediatrician is concerned about language delay. The child is using single words but is not speaking in phrases and is not interested in other children. The patient's mother reports that he does not respond to his name when called and that he does not make consistent eye contact when others speak to him. His diet is very restricted: he prefers to eat only crunchy foods and tends to eat the same things repetitively.

Clinical diagnosis

History

- Inquire about developmental history and relationships with peers.
- Assess the patient's ability to demonstrate perspective-taking and empathy toward others (e.g., if the caregiver appears upset during interview, observe how the child reacts and whether s/he pays attention).
- Caregivers often report that children with ASD have difficulty with transitions or when routines are disrupted.
- Major changes have been made in the criteria for Pervasive Developmental Disorders (PDDs) from DSM-IV-TR to DSM-5.
  - Autistic Disorder, Asperger's Disorder, and Pervasive Developmental Disorder Not Otherwise Specified (PDD NOS) are collapsed into a single diagnostic entity called Autism Spectrum Disorder.

- Criteria for "deficits in social interaction" and "delays in communication" are collapsed into one category titled "social communication."
- Hyper- or hypo-reactivity to sensory input or unusual sensory-seeking behavior is added to the "repetitive behavior" domain.
- Age of onset is no longer strictly defined as 3 years; instead delays must begin in the "early developmental period."

Physical and mental status exams

- No specific findings on physical exam, except in some single-gene causes of ASD (e.g., fragile X or Phelan–McDermid syndromes) in which dysmorphic physical features are common and other organ systems may be affected.
- Mental status exam often includes poor eye contact, lack of response to name, and deficits in joint attention and pragmatic language.
  - The child may insist on speaking only about a specific topic of interest and show little interest in interacting with the examiner.
  - See Grodberg's Autism Mental Status Exam (above, in "Screening" section).

Laboratory diagnosis

List of diagnostic tests

- Chromosomal microarray analysis for all children with suspected ASD.

Lists of imaging techniques

- Not routinely recommended for clinical diagnosis or management.
  - For known genetic syndromes associated with ASD, consider magnetic resonance imaging (MRI) to rule out structural brain abnormalities.
- Given the high prevalence of comorbid seizure disorders (~25%), consider electroencephalography (EEG) if there is clinical concern.

Diagnostic algorithm (Algorithm 25.1)

Algorithm 25.1 Diagnosis of ASD

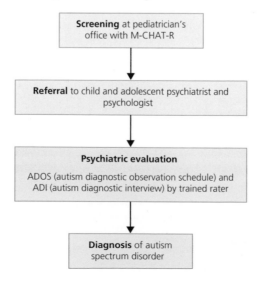

Screening at pediatrician's office with M-CHAT-R

Referral to child and adolescent psychiatrist and psychologist

Psychiatric evaluation

ADOS (autism diagnostic observation schedule) and ADI (autism diagnostic interview) by trained rater

Diagnosis of autism spectrum disorder

Potential pitfalls/common errors made regarding diagnosis of disease
- Failure to spend enough time observing the child.
- Failure to collect developmental history to assess extent of delays and confirm childhood onset of symptoms.
- Failure to get corroborative information to confirm that symptoms are pervasive across situations.

Treatment
Treatment rationale
- Intensive ABA is first-line treatment and is provided by a specialized therapist who works individually with the patient and family.
- A specialized school setting may be necessary and should include a highly structured environment with a low student-to-teacher ratio.
- No medication is currently available to treat core symptoms.
  - Medications target associated symptoms, such as irritability, anxiety, and hyperactivity.
  - Risperidone and aripiprazole are FDA approved to treat irritability in children and adolescents with ASD; however, significant side effect profiles warrant cautious use, typically only after more benign treatment has failed.
- Although many small pilot trials have shown promise for psychopharmacological treatment of ASD, most large-scale, randomized, placebo-controlled studies have not demonstrated statistical separation from placebo, except in the cases of risperidone and aripiprazole.
  - One notable exception is a large randomized controlled trial with methylphenidate that showed significant improvement of hyperactivity in ASD. Approximately 50% of individuals with ASD also have symptoms of ADHD that interfere with learning and require treatment.

When to hospitalize
- Self-injurious behaviors and/or aggression toward others that cannot be managed with outpatient interventions.

Managing the hospitalized patient
- Medication targets associated features, including aggression and self-injury.
- A structured behavioral reinforcement system on the inpatient unit with careful planning of transitions between activities and visual schedules provides predictability and may ease anxiety.
- Careful discharge planning facilitates a more structured home environment and a higher level of outpatient care.

Table of treatment

FDA-approved medications • Risperidone: 1–2.5 mg/day • Aripiprazole: 5–15 mg/day	Start at a low dose and titrate slowly
Psychosocial interventions • ABA • Speech therapy • Social skills groups • Occupational therapy • Physical therapy	ABA is first-line treatment Speech therapy is often an integral part of treatment
Parental and sibling support • Support groups	www.autismspeaks.org has a list of resources for children, siblings, and parents

Prevention/management of complications
- If using antipsychotics, monitor weight every month and blood chemistries, lipid panel, and hemoglobin A1c every 6 months.
- If using stimulants, monitor height, weight, and vital signs with each dose increase and regularly during follow-up.

Management/treatment algorithm (Algorithm 25.2)

Algorithm 25.2 Management of ASD

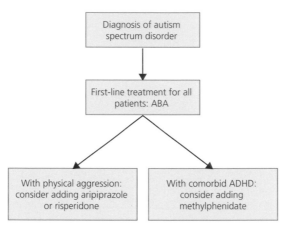

CLINICAL PEARLS
- Intensive ABA is first-line treatment.
- Risperidone and aripiprazole are effective treatments for aggression and self-injurious behavior.
- Children are especially sensitive to side effects from medications, and doses should be started very low and titrated slowly over time, depending on tolerability and evidence of benefit.

Prognosis
- ASD is a lifelong disability, but evidence from early intervention studies using intensive ABA suggests that treatment produces significant improvements in cognition, adaptive behavior, and severity of symptoms.
- Level of language and cognitive abilities are the best predictors of outcome.
- Older children and adolescents with ASD may present with or develop depressive symptoms as they become more aware of their social and communication impairments.

Reading list
Buxbaum J, Hof PR (eds). The Neuroscience of Autism Spectrum Disorders. New York: Elsevier, 2013.
Hollander E, Kolevzon A, Coyle JT (eds). Textbook of Autism Spectrum Disorders. Washington, DC: American Psychiatric Publishing, 2011.

Lounds Taylor J, Dove D, Veenstra-VanderWeele J, et al. Interventions for Adolescents and Young Adults With Autism Spectrum Disorders. Comparative Effectiveness Review No. 65. AHRQ Publication No. 12-EHC063-EF. Rockville, MD: Agency for Healthcare Research and Quality, 2012. www.effectivehealthcare.ahrq.gov/reports/final.cfm

Rogers SJ, Estes A, Lord C, et al. Effects of a brief Early Start Denver model (ESDM)-based parent intervention on toddlers at risk for autism spectrum disorders: a randomized controlled trial. JAACAP 2012;51(10):1052–65.

Volkmar F (ed.). Autism and Pervasive Developmental Disorders. New York: Cambridge University Press, 2007.

Suggested websites

http://autismmentalstatusexam.com.

Free access to the Autism Mental Status Exam as well as training modules that teach a clinician how to use the instrument. http://www.autismspeaks.org/

Access to news, research updates, and family services for individuals with ASD. http://www.autismsciencefoundation.org/

Funding for investigators and information and support for individuals with ASD. http://www.cdc.gov/ncbddd/autism/index.html

CDC website on ASD that includes information for providers and patients.

Guidelines
National society guidelines

Title	Source	Weblink
Caring for Children with Autism Spectrum Disorder: A Resource Toolkit for Clinicians	American Academy of Pediatrics (AAP), 2012, 2nd edn	https://www.aap.org/en-us/advocacy-and-policy/aap-health-initiatives/pages/Caring-for-Children-with-Autism-Spectrum-Disorders-A-Resource-Toolkit-for-Clinicians.aspx

Evidence

Type of evidence	Title and comment	Weblink
Randomized, controlled trial (RCT)	Randomized, controlled trial of an intervention for toddlers with autism: the Early Start Denver Model. **Comment:** ABA improves IQ and adaptive behavior and reduces severity of ASD symptoms.	http://www.ncbi.nlm.nih.gov/pubmed/19948568
Multisite, randomized, double-blind, placebo controlled trial (RDBPCT)	Risperidone in children with autism and serious behavioral problems. **Comment:** Risperidone improves irritability, including symptoms of aggression and self-injurious behaviors.	http://www.ncbi.nlm.nih.gov/pubmed/12151468
Multisite RDBPCT	A placebo-controlled, fixed-dose study of aripiprazole in children and adolescents with irritability associated with autistic disorder. **Comment:** Aripiprazole improves irritability, including symptoms of aggression and self-injurious behaviors.	http://www.ncbi.nlm.nih.gov/pubmed/19797985

(Continued)

(Continued)

Type of evidence	Title and comment	Weblink
RDBPCT	Divalproex sodium vs placebo for the treatment of irritability in children and adolescents with autism spectrum disorders. **Comment:** Divalproex sodium improves irritability, including symptoms of aggression and self-injurious behaviors.	http://www.ncbi.nlm.nih.gov/pubmed/20010551
RDBPC cross-over trial	Randomized, controlled, crossover trial of methylphenidate in pervasive developmental disorders with hyperactivity. **Comment:** Methylphenidate improves hyperactivity in ASD.	http://www.ncbi.nlm.nih.gov/pubmed/16275814

Additional material for this chapter can be found online at:
www.mountsinaiexpertguides.com/psychiatry

This includes advice for patients, a case study, ICD codes, and multiple choice questions.

CHAPTER 26

Intellectual Developmental Disorders in Children and into Adulthood

Jesse L. Costales[1], Asher B. Simon[1], and Katharine A. Stratigos[2]

[1] Icahn School of Medicine at Mount Sinai, New York, NY, USA
[2] Columbia University/New York State Psychiatric Institute, New York, NY, USA

OVERALL BOTTOM LINE
- Intellectual disability (ID) is a multifaceted disease that affects approximately 1% of the US population.
- Rates of psychopathology among those with ID are 4–6× the general population.
- Psychiatric treatment focuses on management of both behavioral symptoms and comorbid psychiatric disorders.
- Assessment must explore:
  1. The nature of the intellectual disability
  2. Related developmental, cognitive, or language issues
  3. Presence of DSM-5 diagnoses
  4. Nonspecific problematic behaviors.
- Treatment includes:
  1. Environmental modification
  2. Behavioral techniques
  3. Parent/caregiver strategies
  4. Psychopharmacology.

Background
Definition of disease
- Based upon DSM-5, ID is a disorder with onset during the developmental period with deficits in adaptive and intellectual functioning.

Disease classification
- Mild, moderate, severe, or profound based upon adaptive and intellectual functioning and level of need for supports.

Incidence/prevalence
- Approximately 1% of US population.
- Up to 40% of adults with ID have comorbid mental health issues.

Economic impact
- Estimated average lifetime cost in the US is $1,014,000 per affected individual.

Mount Sinai Expert Guides: Psychiatry, First Edition. Edited by Asher B. Simon, Antonia S. New, and Wayne K. Goodman.
© 2017 John Wiley & Sons, Ltd. Published 2017 by John Wiley & Sons, Ltd.
Companion website: www.mountsinaiexpertguides.com/psychiatry

Etiology

- Prenatal: chromosomal disorders, specific genetic syndromes, errors of metabolism, intrauterine growth restriction, disorders of brain formation, environmental exposures/toxins, intrauterine infections.
- Perinatal: hypoxia, infections, pregnancy complications.
- Postnatal: head injuries, infections, seizure disorders, toxic-metabolic disorders, environmental deprivation, malnutrition.

Pathophysiology

- Specific syndromes may lead to ID through disruption of specific pathways involved in proper CNS development (details are beyond the scope of this chapter).

Predictive/risk factors

- Family history (e.g., chromosomal defects).
- Alcohol and substance use during pregnancy.
- Infection during pregnancy (e.g., varicella).
- Maternal diseases (e.g., hypertension).
- Teratogenic drug use or toxin exposure during pregnancy (e.g., phenytoin).
- Abnormal labor/delivery (e.g., anoxic brain injuries).
- Neonatal disorders (e.g., intracranial hemorrhage).
- Environmental deprivation.
- Malnutrution (maternal and childhood).

BOTTOM LINE/CLINICAL PEARLS
- The prevention of ID to be addressed by the obstetrician and pediatrician, as well as public health measures, as most of the initial risk factors for ID are not modifiable by the time the patient presents for psychiatric treatment.
- Nonetheless, it is important to assess and review each of the risk factors listed above to understand the patient's pathophysiology and prognosis, tailor treatment accordingly, and work to prevent further worsening.
- It is also important to review this information with the patient's family, not only to help the family conceptualize the disease process, but also to reduce ongoing risk factors (i.e., refractory seizures, head injuries) and address risks to potential future siblings (i.e., mother has another pregnancy).

Prevention

Screening

- To be determined by obstetrician and pediatrician as needed.
- Pediatrician will follow early developmental milestones.

Secondary (and primary) prevention

- Early identification of developmental delays and prompt referral to social services (e.g., early intervention, special education, parent training) may improve the patient's potential functioning and quality of life.
- Early identification allows for recognition of possible psychiatric and behavioral problems as well as treatment to prevent further worsening in functioning.

Diagnosis

> **BOTTOM LINE/CLINICAL PEARLS**
> - Requires neuropsychological testing showing deficits in intellectual (IQ testing) *and* adaptive functioning (typically assessed via the Vineland Adaptive Behavioral Scales), described as approximately two standard deviations below the population norm.
> - Onset during childhood.

Differential diagnosis

Diagnosis	Features
Autism Spectrum	Deficits in social communication and repetitive and stereotyped behaviors/interests; may have normal IQ or co-occur with ID
Traumatic Brain Injury	Behavioral/cognitive disturbances absent prior to injury
Hearing Impairment	Abnormal findings on audiology testing; may co-occur with ID
Dementia	Onset later than 18
Communication Disorders (e.g., language disorder)	Overall IQ >70 and adaptive functioning intact
Lack of adequate education	Apparent through psychiatric history

Typical presentation

The patient will not present for treatment of the intellectual disability, *per se*, but for symptoms of psychiatric comorbidity including the following:
- DSM-5 syndromes (e.g., MDD, anxiety disorders, ADHD);
- verbal/physical aggression towards self/others/objects;
- self-injury (head banging, finger biting);
- oppositionality, irritablility;
- neurovegetative symptoms (e.g., hyperactivity, sleep/eating disturbances);
- repetitive and interfering behaviors (e.g., motor/verbal stereotypies).

Clinical diagnosis

History
- Must determine the patient's *baseline* temperament/behavior.
- Clarify the actual problematic behavior in terms of frequency, intensity, antecedents, and consequences.
- Gather collateral information from parents/guardians, agency staff, teachers, etc.
- Note any recent or abrupt changes in physical/medical symptoms, delayed progression or loss of previously acquired language/motor functioning, environmental context, or stressors.
- Look for any symptom clusters that could map onto typical DSM-5 diagnoses.
  - Although presentation of psychiatric syndromes may look different in patients with ID (given cognitive impairment and frequent behavioral manifestations of distress), taking a syndromal view may help clarify and guide treatment approaches.
- Common medical conditions (e.g., ear infections, urinary tract infection, fever, pain, gastrointestinal discomfort) frequently manifest as changes in behavior.

Physical and mental status exams

- Thorough physical exam for any patient with ID who presents with behavior change or new psychiatric symptoms.
- On mental status exam it is important to assess for attention, ability to cooperate/follow directions, aggressiveness, tics, gait, repetitive movements/stereotypies, social relatedness/reciprocity, use of gestures, stuttering, speech fluency, odd intonations or monotony, circumscribed interests, concreteness, basic reading and arithmetic, impulse control.

Disease severity classification

Severity levels are based upon the level of functional impairment and the need for supports, but IQ is included as it is often information available to the clinician.

Mild (significant majority)

- IQ approximately 55–70, with verbal language ability.
- May be able to live independently.
- Academic skills up to 6th grade level.
- Social/emotional immaturity, especially at times of stress/transition.

Moderate (~10%)

- IQ approximately 35–55.
- Language skills can range from simple conversations to communicating only basic needs.
- Limited self-care and motor skills.
- Comorbid neurological conditions and structural abnormalities common.

Severe to profound (4–6%)

- IQ approximately 20–35 (severe) or <20 (profound).
- Expressive language is very limited or absent.
- Variable degrees of receptive language comprehension (may be higher than expressive).
- Comorbid neurological conditions and structural abnormalities common.
- Need to live in highly supervised settings as adults and lack independent ability to perform activities of daily living (ADLs).

Laboratory diagnosis

List of diagnostic tests

- There is no laboratory test that can determine ID, although genetic syndromes will have a certain genetic profile on testing.
  - Refer to colleagues with developmental expertise to consider further work-up.
- If ID is not yet diagnosed, refer to neuropsychologist for IQ/adaptive testing.
  - Wechsler Intelligence Scale for Children-III.
  - Leiter International Performance Scale: non-verbal measure of intelligence.
  - Vineland Adaptive Behavioral Scales: measure global adaptive and social behavior, communication, and daily living skills.
  - If concern for autism spectrum disorder, may use the Autism Diagnostic Observation Schedule (ADOS) or the Autism Diagnostic Interview-Revised (ADIR).
    - Additionally, the Autism Mental Status Exam, developed at the Icahn School of Medicine at Mount Sinai by David Grodberg, MD, is a brief and easily used instrument to screen for symptoms of autism during the clinical interview; it is available for free online at http://www.autismva.org/content/autism-mental-status-examination.

Lists of imaging techniques

Algorithm 26.1 Diagnostic algorithm for assessing psychiatric symptoms and comorbidities in patients with ID

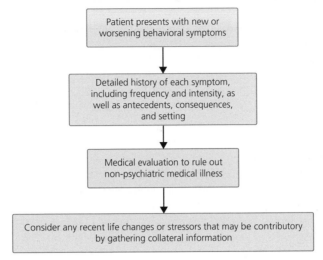

Patient presents with new or worsening behavioral symptoms

Detailed history of each symptom, including frequency and intensity, as well as antecedents, consequences, and setting

Medical evaluation to rule out non-psychiatric medical illness

Consider any recent life changes or stressors that may be contributory by gathering collateral information

- Consider head imaging if not previously done for individuals with physical findings (e.g., microcephaly, cerebral palsy) or abnormal neurologic exam.

Potential pitfalls/common errors made regarding diagnosis of disease
- ID influences symptom presentation and may contribute to under- and over-diagnosis.
  - *Diagnostic overshadowing*: misattributing symptoms to ID instead of considering them part of a psychiatric syndrome (e.g., behavioral outbursts may indicate an acute anxiety disorder).
  - Inappropriately diagnosing psychiatric symptoms (e.g., psychosis) in ID patients who, because of their developmental and language levels, may have different ways of expressing distress as part of their disability (e.g., talking to an imaginary friend or self-talking may not be psychotic).
- Missing medical comorbidities by attributing behavior change to psychiatric issues (medical issues may present as behavior changes in individuals with intellectual and developmental disabilities).
- Clinician inexperience in and anxiety about assessing and treating patients with limited verbal skills.
- Difficulty in noticing and defining the multiple developmental contributors to current presentation (e.g. ID, language disorder, motor disorder, autistic symptoms, etc.).

Treatment
Treatment rationale
Since ID is a pervasive disorder with many phenotypes and no specific "cure" per se, this section will focus on treatment of comorbid psychiatric or behavioral disorders as well as interventions to improve quality of life.
- First, treat any medical comorbidities that may be worsening mental status or behavior.

- If the patient presents with a clear DSM-5 diagnosis, treat using psychotherapy (if possible, given language/cognitive abilities) and/or psychopharmacology as indicated for the diagnosis.
- Strongly consider doing a functional behavioral analysis if problematic behaviors persist to explore the function of the behavior (e.g., attention, self-stimulation, access to tangibles, escape/avoidance, etc.).
  - Once a target behavior is identified, obtain a description of behavior, setting events (e.g., patient was hungry, tired, etc.), antecedent events (what happened before the behavior), and consequences (what happened after).
  - When the purpose(s) of the behavior becomes clear, develop a behavior plan to reinforce adaptive behaviors, teach new adaptive skills (e.g., better ways to communicate), and decrease reinforcements for problem behaviors.
  - If behavioral approaches do not address the behavior, or if the patient is very aggressive, consider psychopharmacologic interventions.

When to hospitalize
- Imminent risk of harm to self or others.
- Ongoing aggressive behaviors despite complicated medication regimen, possibly requiring a medication "wash-out" and new medication trial(s).
- Inability of family to cope and no option of higher intensity outpatient care available.

Managing the hospitalized patient
- Management as above.
- Work with family and/or agency around discharge planning to ensure adequate outpatient services and wrap-around social services.

Table of treatment

Device-based • Communication devices for non-verbal patients (e.g., assistive communication device)	
Psychological • Functional behavioral analysis	• Behavioral techniques should be considered before medications • Explore the function of the behavior and develop a behavioral plan that might include a point system, behavior chart, scheduled rewards; teach more adaptive social/communication skills
• Psychotherapy • CBT: self-monitoring, problem-solving, decision-making, anger management, relaxation skills, and social skills	• Use role modeling, shorter and more frequent sessions, give information at a slower pace, minimize distractions, involve caregivers
Medical General points	• Psychopharmacology should be considered if behavioral interventions and/or psychotherapy are insufficient • Patients with ID are at an *increased risk for side effects* from medications

(Continued)

(Continued)

Depressive symptoms • SSRIs at usual dosages • TCAs	• Side effects include increased agitation, aggression, hypomanic-like behavior • Greater risk for anticholinergic/antihistaminic responses; decreased seizure threshold
ADHD • Stimulants (methylphenidate formulations or mixed salts of amphetamine/dextroamphetamine) • Clonidine (0.1–0.4 mg daily) in single or divided doses	• Stimulants work similarly as in normotypically developing individuals but may have less robust response and greater likelihood of side effects • Better response if IQ >50; side effects include social withdrawal and/or motor tics • Side effects include drowsiness or hypotension; rebound hypertension if stopped abruptly
Aggressive behavior • Risperidone (0.25–1 mg bid) and other second-generation antipsychotics • Clonidine (0.1–0.4 mg daily) • SSRIs	• Widely used in ID for self-injurious/aggressive/destructive behaviors; side effects include extrapyramidal symptoms, sedation, increased appetite/weight gain, and metabolic syndrome
Repetitive behaviors/stereotypies • SSRIs • Atypical antipsychotics	
Self-injurious behaviors - • SSRIs Second-generation antipsychotics	

Prevention/management of complications

- Because patients with ID are at increased risk of developing side effects to medications, start at the lowest possible dose and increase slowly; monitor frequently and educate caregivers on possible side effects. Discontinue medications that are ineffective rather than just adding a new medication.

Management/treatment algorithm (Algorithm 26.2)

Algorithm 26.2 Management of comorbid psychiatric or behavioral disorders in the patient with ID

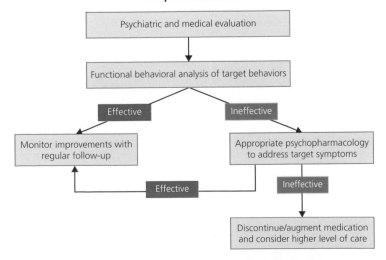

> **CLINICAL PEARLS**
> - Remember that in a patient with limited verbal skills, a variety of underlying symptoms may be manifested by problem behaviors.
> - Do not miss common and often undiagnosed non-psychiatric medical illnesses (e.g., urinary tract infection, ear infections, fever, pain, gastrointestinal discomfort).
> - Examine the psychosocial context that may be contributing to symptom exacerbation.
> - A patient's presentation may be more understandable and easier to treat if you find a major cause for problem behaviors (e.g., basic medical issue, change in environment, move to a new home, etc.).
> - Always consider behavioral techniques and psychotherapy prior to psychopharmacology.

Special populations
Pregnancy
- Persons with ID may be sexually active, and appropriate birth control should be discussed. Often-used medications are pregnancy class C.

Prognosis

> **BOTTOM LINE/CLINICAL PEARLS**
> - Appropriate and early educational interventions are *critical* to optimal development.
> - Social, educational, and language/motor functioning may be profoundly helped if patient and caregivers are engaged in treatment and provide a structured and supportive environment.
> - In adulthood, functional capability (e.g., ability to care for self, ADLs) and language have important prognostic implications.
>   - Employed adults with mild ID have a better prognosis.
>   - Access to social services and resources (e.g., vocational training, residential home) is critical and may scaffold limitations in independence and functioning and improve overall quality of life. (Resources vary by state, and it is important to be familiar with those available in your state.)

Reading list

Agarwal V, Sitholey P, Kumar S, Prasad M. Double-blind, placebo-controlled trial of clonidine in hyperactive children with mental retardation. Ment Retard 2001;39(4):259–67.

Bouras N, Drummond C. Behaviour and psychiatric disorders or people with mental handicaps living in the community. J Intellect Disabil Res 1992;36 (Pt 4):349–57.

Braddock D, Parish SL. An institutional history of disability. In: Braddock D (ed.) Disability at the Dawn of the 21st Century and the State of the States. Washington, DC: American Association on Mental Retardation, 2002.

Centers for Disease Control and Prevention (CDC). Economic costs associated with mental retardation, cerebral palsy, hearing loss, and vision impairment – United States, 2003. MMWR Morb Mortal Wkly Rep 2004;53(3):57–9.

Cipani E, Schock KM. Functional Behavioral Assessment, Diagnosis, and Treatment: A Complete System for Education and Mental Health Settings, 2nd edn. New York, NY: Springer, 2010.

Harris JC. Intellectual Disability: Understanding its Development, Causes, Classification, Evaluation, and Treatment. New York: Oxford University Press, 2006.

Filho AGC, Bodanese R, Silva TL, Alvares JP, Aman M, Rohde LA. Comparison of risperidone and methylphenidate for reducing ADHD symptoms in children and adolescents with moderate mental retardation. J Am Acad Child Adolesc Psychiatry 2005;44(8):748–55.

Handen BL, Hardan AY. Open-label, prospective trial of olanzapine in adolescents with subaverage intelligence and disruptive behavior disorders. J Am Acad Child Adolesc Psychiatry 2006;45(8):928–35.

Suggested websites

American Association on Intellectual and Developmental Disabilities (formerly AAMR – American
Association on Mental Retardation). http://www.aaidd.org

First Signs (dedicated to educating parents and professionals about autism and related disorders).
http://www.firstsigns.org

National Association for the Dually Diagnosed (ID and mental illness). http://thenadd.org

Guidelines
National society guidelines

Title	Source	Weblink
Diagnostic Manual – Intellectual Disability (DM-ID)	National Association for the Dually Diagnosed (NADD), 2007	http://www. dmid.org

Evidence

Type of evidence	Title and comment	Weblink
Review of six randomized controlled trials	Efficacy of atypical antipsychotic medication in the management of behavior problems in children with intellectual disabilities and borderline intelligence: a systematic review. **Comment:** Risperidone vs placebo for aggressive behavioral outbursts; significant improvement with risperidone (average 1–3 mg/day) but also increased overall weight gain (average 5 lb) and somnolence vs placebo group.	http://www.ncbi. nlm.nih.gov/ pubmed/21856116
Single-blind, parallel-group trial	Comparison of risperidone and methylphenidate for reducing ADHD symptoms in children and adolescents with moderate mental retardation. **Comment:** n = 45; risperidone led to greater reductions in ADHD total score but was accompanied by weight gain; recommend stimulants as first-line treatment given side effect profiles.	http://www.ncbi. nlm.nih.gov/ pubmed/16034276
Prospective, ABA design, double-blind crossover study	Weight gain in a controlled study of risperidone in children, adolescents and adults with mental retardation and autism. **Comment:** n = 19; significantly greater weight gain with risperidone; rate of weight gain diminished rapidly when drug tapered and discontinued.	http://www.ncbi. nlm.nih.gov/ pubmed/11642473

Additional material for this chapter can be found online at:
www.mountsinaiexpertguides.com/psychiatry

This includes advice for patients, a case study, ICD codes, and multiple choice questions.

CHAPTER 27

Child and Adolescent Anxiety Disorders

Thomas J. DePrima and Vilma Gabbay

Icahn School of Medicine at Mount Sinai, New York, NY, USA

OVERALL BOTTOM LINE

- Anxiety disorders are among the most common psychiatric disorders diagnosed in childhood, often going undiagnosed/untreated and persisting/worsening with time.
- Impairment primarily stems from avoidance behaviors which result from excessive anxiety.
- Anxiety disorders are differentiated from one another by the specific context eliciting the fear/anxiety/avoidance.
- It is essential to differentiate developmentally and culturally appropriate fear/anxiety behaviors from pathology.
- Psychiatric comorbidity is common, within the anxiety spectrum and with childhood attention deficit hyperactivity disorder (ADHD) and mood disorders.
- Mild cases may be treated with psychotherapy alone, and moderate–severe cases benefit from adding medications.
  - Cognitive behavioral therapy (CBT) and serotonin-selective reuptake inhibitors (SSRIs) are first line.

Background
Definition of disease

According to DSM-5, anxiety disorders share "features of excessive fear and anxiety and related behavioral disturbances," and the disorders differ from one another based on "the type of objects or situations that induce fear, anxiety, or avoidance behavior, and the associated cognitive ideation."

- Generalized Anxiety Disorder (GAD): anxiety/worry about a number of different events/activities.
- Panic Disorder (PD): recurrent/unexpected panic attacks and avoidant behavior.
- Social Anxiety Disorder (Social Phobia) (SAD): fear/anxiety about social situations.
- Specific Phobia (SP): fear/anxiety about a specific object.
- Separation Anxiety: developmentally inappropriate fear/anxiety about separation from attachment figures.
- Selective Mutism: inability to speak in certain situations.

Incidence/prevalence

For all anxiety disorders in children/adolescents, 6- to 12-month prevalence = 10–20%.
- GAD: 0.9–3% prevalence in adolescents.
- PD: 0.6–5% in adolescents.
- SAD: 7% in children/adolescents.

Mount Sinai Expert Guides: Psychiatry, First Edition. Edited by Asher B. Simon, Antonia S. New, and Wayne K. Goodman.
© 2017 John Wiley & Sons, Ltd. Published 2017 by John Wiley & Sons, Ltd.
Companion website: www.mountsinaiexpertguides.com/psychiatry

- SP: 6–9.1% in children/adolescents.
- Separation Anxiety: decreases with age; 4% in children 6–12 months old; 1.6% in adolescents.
- Selective Mutism: 0.3–0.8%.

Economic impact

A 1999 review showed that anxiety disorders represented approximately one-third of the total mental health spending in the US. This figure only goes up when accounting for costs associated with treatment of somatic symptoms related to anxiety. However this was not limited to child/adolescent patients, and research needs to assess accurately the economic burden specific to this age group.

Etiology

- All show some heritability; trait anxiety – a relatively stable and highly heritable component of personality – is associated with the development of anxiety disorders.
- Environmental factors are also influential and may include parenting styles (including attachment styles which play an important role in how children perceive and cope with stressors) and traumatic life events (e.g., loss of a loved one, separation from parental figures, moving to another location, natural disasters, bullying/rejection).

Pathophysiology

- Neural network abnormalities are in line with similar findings in adults, including abnormal connections in amygdala-based networks with medial prefrontal cortex (mPFC), insula, superior temporal gyrus, and cerebellum.
  - Children with anxiety disorders show greater amygdala and ventrolateral prefrontal cortex (vlPFC) activation when exposed to fearful stimuli.
- Connection between CO_2 hypersensitivity and anxiety disorders, both in children/adolescents and adults.

Predictive/risk factors

- Genetics.
- Parental anxiety disorder.
- Overprotective/controlling parenting style.
- Insecure attachment with parent.
- Traumatic childhood experiences.

Prevention

> **BOTTOM LINE/CLINICAL PEARLS**
> - Impairment resulting from avoidant behaviors tends to increase with age, so early detection can help prevent progression of symptoms.
> - Early interventions aimed at prevention include screening, parent skills training, and psychoeducation.

Screening

- Any initial mental health assessment should include screening questions targeting anxiety symptoms.
- Self-report rating scales can be helpful in establishing baseline severity of symptoms and in gauging response to treatment:
  - Multidimensional Anxiety Scale for Children (MASC);
  - Screen for Child Anxiety Related Emotional Disorders (SCARED).

Secondary (and primary) prevention
- Early intervention is key if there is high suspicion for child/adolescent anxiety disorder.
- Appropriate treatment (listed below) and follow-up are essential, including the crucial inclusion of psychoeducation of patient/parents/teachers/others.

Diagnosis
Differential diagnosis

BOTTOM LINE/CLINICAL PEARLS
- DSM-5 uses mostly the same diagnostic criteria for childhood and adult anxiety disorders.
- Anxiety disorders may often be mistaken for ADHD, learning disabilities, or mood disorders.
- Differentiating between anxiety disorders requires a careful clinical interview along with collateral information from multiple sources (family, school, other providers).
- It is important to rule out whether symptoms result from underlying medical conditions or from medication/illicit substance use.

Differential diagnosis	Features
ADHD	Hyperactivity, inattention, academic struggles
Major Depressive Disorder	Low mood, poor concentration, poor sleep
Bipolar Disorder	Irritability, insomnia, restlessness
Psychotic Disorder	Agitation, restlessness, social withdrawal
Learning disorders	Worries regarding poor academic performance
Hyperthyroidism	Irritability/nervousness, poor sleep, fatigue, increased appetite, weight loss
Side effects from medications/substances	Anxiety-like symptoms can arise from SSRIs, antipsychotics, anti-asthmatics, steroids, sympathomimetics, illicit substances

Typical presentation
Children/adolescents with anxiety disorders may not realize that their fear or worry is excessive, and parents may not recognize that it is developmentally inappropriate. Conversely, parents may present children with developmentally-appropriate fears or worries thinking that something is wrong. Alternatively, anxiety may not be the chief complaint: often the child will present with somatic complaints (e.g., gastrointestinal, headaches); concentration problems may lead to academic issues; mood lability (e.g., irritability, crying) and behavioral outbursts may be misinterpreted as oppositionality; children may also express fear/anxiety by tantrums, freezing, clinging, shrinking, failing to speak, etc. When anxiety is not the chief complaint, investigating the context and timing of the somatic and behavioral symptoms can help bring to light the presence of an underlying anxiety disorder.

Clinical diagnosis
History
- For diagnosis, impairment in functioning must result (typically from avoidant behavior).
- The symptoms must not be attributable to another psychiatric disorder, medical condition, or effects of a substance (including medication).

GAD:
- Excessive and difficult-to-control anxiety/worry (and associated symptoms) occurring more days than not for ≥6 months about a number of events or activities.
- Associated with ≥1 of the following (note this is different from the adult criteria in which 3 symptoms are required): restlessness, easily fatigued, difficulty concentrating, irritability, muscle tension, sleep disturbance.

SAD:
- Marked disproportionate anxiety about ≥1 social situations in which exposure to possible scrutiny by others (e.g., social interactions, being observed, eating/drinking/performing) provokes fears of humiliation, embarrassment, rejection, causing offense, etc.
- The social situations are either avoided or are endured with intense anxiety.
- Must occur in peer settings and not just when interacting with adults.
- Typically lasts ≥6 months.

Specific Phobia:
- Marked disproportionate fear about a specific object or situation, leading to active avoidance or endurance but with intense fear.
- Typically lasts ≥6 months.

Separation Anxiety Disorder:
- Developmentally inappropriate and excessive anxiety evidenced by the recurrence/persistence of ≥3 of the following:
  - distress with actual or anticipated separation from home or major attachment figures;
  - worry about harm coming to or losing attachment figures;
  - worry about experiencing an untoward event (e.g., getting lost, being kidnapped, having an accident) that causes separation;
  - reluctance/refusal to go out (including to school) because of fear of separation;
  - fear of or reluctance about being without attachment figures at home or in other settings;
  - reluctance/refusal to sleep away from home or to go to sleep without being near attachment figure;
  - nightmares involving themes of separation;
  - physical symptoms (e.g., headache, gastrointestinal pain, nausea, vomiting) with anticipated or actual separation.
- Lasts ≥4 weeks.

PD: identical criteria to those for adults.

Selective Mutism:
- Consistent failure to speak in specific social situations despite ability to speak.
- Interferes with education or social communication.
- Lasts ≥1 month and not limited to the first month of school.
- Does not result from lack of fluency with the language.
- Not better explained by a communication disorder (e.g., language disorder) and does not occur exclusively during the course of an autism spectrum disorder or psychotic disorder.

Physical and mental status exams
- Thorough review of systems and physical exam.
- Further medical work-up as necessary.
- Establish a documented baseline of somatic complaints before initiating treatment to prevent attributing ongoing somatic complaints to adverse effects of medications.
- Findings on exam can include tremor, rapid heart rate or breathing, sweaty palms, restlessness.

Diagnostic algorithm (Algorithm 27.1)

Algorithm 27.1 Diagnostic algorithm for child/adolescent anxiety disorders

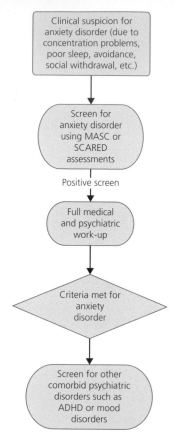

Clinical suspicion for anxiety disorder (due to concentration problems, poor sleep, avoidance, social withdrawal, etc.)

↓

Screen for anxiety disorder using MASC or SCARED assessments

Positive screen

↓

Full medical and psychiatric work-up

↓

Criteria met for anxiety disorder

↓

Screen for other comorbid psychiatric disorders such as ADHD or mood disorders

Potential pitfalls/common errors made regarding diagnosis of disease
- Failing to differentiate developmentally or culturally appropriate worry from pathology.
- Failing to differentiate anxiety disorders from other psychiatric disorders that can present with similar symptoms (e.g., ADHD, developmental disorders, mood disorders).
- Failing to diagnose a comorbid psychiatric disorder in addition to anxiety disorder.

Treatment
Treatment rationale
- Always take into account the patient's age, disease severity, comorbid disorders, psychosocial stressors, attitudes of the patient/family regarding different interventions, and access to and affordability of different interventions.
- All treatment should include psychoeducation for patient, family, primary care providers, and school.
- Psychotherapy is first line for mild cases:
  - CBT has the most empiric evidence for efficacy.
  - Involve the family both at the onset of treatment and throughout the process; can be especially helpful when parents have anxiety disorders or when some aspect of the parent–child relationship has contributed to the patient's disorder.

- Indications for medication:
  - partial response to psychotherapy alone;
  - moderate to severe cases;
  - existence of comorbid disorder requiring medication.
- While no medication has FDA indication for childhood anxiety disorders, three SSRIs are approved for childhood obsessive-compulsive disorder (fluoxetine, fluvoxamine, sertraline), and SSRIs are safe, effective, and generally considered first-line medications.
  - There is no evidence for superiority of a particular SSRI; choice is typically driven by side effect profile, duration of action, and known response by a first-degree relative.
  - There are no specific dosing guidelines in children; we advise following the principle of starting low and slowly titrating.
  - Safety and efficacy of other agents are less studied, although tricyclic antidepressants (TCAs), serotonin–norepinephrine reuptake inhibitors (SNRIs), buspirone, and benzodiazepines have all been suggested as alternative or adjunct treatments.
    - Benzodiazepines should be used judiciously, given abuse potential; they may be most appropriate for short-term rapid reduction of symptoms, often to allow for initiation of more long-term treatment (such as SSRI or CBT).
- Combined treatment with CBT and SSRI is more effective than treatment with either alone.
- Presence of unaddressed comorbid disorders can lead to poor or incomplete treatment response; their identification can help guide treatment choices (e.g., including an SSRI when treating both anxiety disorder and major depressive disorder).

When to hospitalize

- Very rarely do anxiety symptoms become so severe as to require hospitalization; the most common causes are suicidality, behavioral dyscontrol, or severe comorbid illness. Anxiety does increase risk for suicide.

Managing the hospitalized patient

- Treat the primary condition, any comorbid conditions, and engage family in treatment, possibly including a higher level of care post discharge.

Table of treatment

Medications	
SSRIs	• Safety and efficacy have not been established for meds other than SSRIs
• Fluoxetine	
• Sertraline	
• Paroxetine	
• Fluvoxamine	
TCAs	• TCAs are rarely used, due to safety concerns
• Imipramine	
• Clomipramine	
Benzodiazepines	• Benzodiazepines primarily for short-term adjunct rapid treatment while longer-term treatments take effect
• Alprazolam	
• Lorazepam	• Data are limited with regard to medication combinations
• Clonazepam	• Comorbid diagnoses can help guide choice of medication
Others	
• Buspirone	
• Venlafaxine	

(Continued)

(Continued)

Psychotherapy	
• CBT • Psychodynamic • Family therapy	• Consider therapy alone for mild cases • Combine with medications for moderate to severe cases • CBT has the most evidence

Prevention/management of complications

- Black box warning for antidepressants: possible increase in suicidal thoughts and behaviors during treatment initiation for patients aged 24 and under.
  - Monitor closely for worsening depression, agitation, or suicidality; could signal a need for change in level of care (e.g., hospitalization), change in medication choice, or adjuvant safety precautions.
- Before starting an antidepressant, screen patients for past or current symptoms of mania or family history of bipolar disorder; during treatment, closely monitor for emergence of manic symptoms.

Management/treatment algorithm (Algorithm 27.2)

Algorithm 27.2 Management of the child/adolescent with anxiety disorder

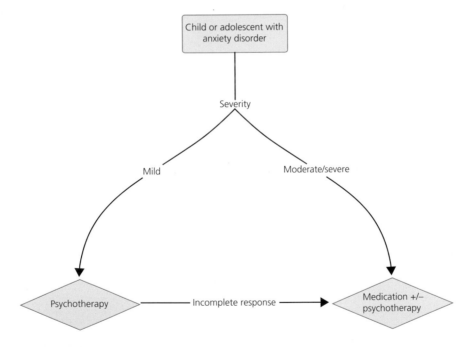

Prognosis

> **CLINICAL PEARLS**
> - Part of treatment includes managing parents' concerns/anxiety.
> - Must address avoidance symptoms.
> - Mild cases can be treated with psychotherapy alone; moderate to severe cases often require addition of medication.
> - CBT and SSRIs have the most evidence and are first line.
> - Presence of comorbid disorders can help guide treatment choices.

> **BOTTOM LINE/CLINICAL PEARLS**
> * Poorly controlled illness may lead to psychiatric, psychosocial, and medical complications.
> * Anxiety often continues into adulthood.
> * Proper treatment may improve prognosis.

Natural history of untreated disease
* Ongoing symptoms, with complications:
  * frequent absences from school and higher dropout rates;
  * higher medical costs, including more ER visits;
  * limited participation in extracurricular activities;
  * higher rates of substance abuse;
  * higher rates of adult pathology (anxiety and depression).
* Symptoms often wax and wane. Some patients no longer meet criteria for any disorder as they age. Many end up maintaining their diagnosis and/or meeting criteria for a different anxiety disorder.

Prognosis for treated patients
* Can be very good, especially if treatment targets avoidance symptoms (i.e., not homeschooling a child with social phobia as this would only reinforce the avoidant behavior).

Follow-up tests and monitoring
* Monitor symptoms, level of functioning.

Reading list

American Psychiatric Publishing. Diagnostic and Statistical Manual of Mental Disorders, 5th edn. Washington, DC: American Psychiatric Publishing, 2013.

Connolly SD, Bernstein GA; Work Group on Quality Issues. Practice parameter for the assessment and treatment of children and adolescents with anxiety disorders. J Am Acad Child Adolesc Psychiatry 2007;46(2):267–83.

Dulcan MK (ed.). Dulcan's Textbook of Child and Adolescent Psychiatry. Washington, DC: American Psychiatric Publishing, 2010.

Ginsburg GS, Kendall PC, Sakolsky D, et al. Remission after acute treatment in children and adolescents with anxiety disorders: findings from the CAMS. J Consult Clin Psychol 2011;79(6):806–13.

In-Albon T, Schneider S. Psychotherapy of childhood anxiety disorders: A meta-analysis. Psychother Psychosom 2007;76(1):15–24.

Ipser JC, Stein DJ, Hawkridge S, Hoppe L. Pharmacotherapy for anxiety disorders in children and adolescents. Cochrane Database Syst Rev 2009;(3):CD005170.

Suggested websites
American Academy of Child & Adolescent Psychiatry. http://www.aacap.org

American Academy of Pediatrics. http://www.aap.org

National Alliance on Mental Illness. http://www.nami.org

Guidelines
National society guidelines

Title	Source	Weblink
Practice Parameter on Child and Adolescent Mental Health Care in Community Systems of Care	American Academy of Child and Adolescent Psychiatry (AACAP), 2007	http://psychiatry.unm. edu/centers/crcbh/docs/ aacapcommunity.pdf

Evidence

Type of evidence	Title and comment	Weblink
Systematic review	Pharmacotherapy for anxiety disorders in children and adolescents. **Comment:** Summarizes evidence base; evidence for efficacy of SSRIs but not other med classes.	http://www.ncbi.nlm.nih.gov/pubmed/19588367
Systematic review	Psychotherapy of childhood anxiety disorders: A meta-analysis. **Comment:** Summarizes evidence base; efficacy for CBT; randomized controlled trials for other modalities are lacking.	http://www.ncbi.nlm.nih.gov/pubmed/17170560
Randomized controlled trial	Remission after acute treatment in children and adolescents with anxiety disorders: Findings from the CAMS. **Comment:** Combination of CBT and sertraline was most effective; CBT alone and sertraline alone were less effective but still more effective than placebo.	http://www.ncbi.nlm.nih.gov/pubmed/22122292

Additional material for this chapter can be found online at:
www.mountsinaiexpertguides.com/psychiatry

This includes advice for patients, a case study, ICD codes, and multiple choice questions.

CHAPTER 28

Attention-Deficit/Hyperactivity Disorder

Jeffrey H. Newcorn[1], Laura Powers[1], and Stacy McAllister[2]
[1] Icahn School of Medicine at Mount Sinai, New York, NY, USA
[2] Children's Hospital of Philadelphia, Philadelphia, PA, USA

OVERALL BOTTOM LINE

- Attention deficit/hyperactivity disorder (ADHD) symptoms reflect impairments in inattention and/or hyperactivity-impulsivity. Symptoms by definition present during childhood, but the disorder frequently persists into adulthood.
- Etiology includes genetic and environmental factors; family and psychosocial factors may exacerbate or reduce impairment.
- Evidence-based pharmacologic and non-pharmacologic treatments are available.
- Treatment decreases levels of core symptoms, impairments, and associated features, but impact on long-term outcome is controversial.

Background

Definition of disease

Persistent pattern of inattention and/or hyperactivity-impulsivity which causes impairment and is present in multiple settings.

Disease classification

- DSM-5 includes ADHD in the new overarching category of "Neurodevelopmental Disorders."

Incidence/prevalence

- Prevalence: 2% of preschoolers, 4–12% of school-age children, 6% of adolescents, 4.5% of adults.
- Males have a 2- to 4-fold higher prevalence, partially but not fully accounted for by "gender bias" (boys are typically more disruptive than girls).

Economic impact

- The estimated cost of childhood ADHD is $46–52 billion annually.

Etiology

- Mean heritability coefficient = 0.76.
- Several genes regulating catecholaminergic function have replicable but small effects.
- Pre- and perinatal exposures to alcohol, nicotine, cocaine, and other drugs, as well as lead, mercury, and neurotoxic substances; often there is shared genetic risk and environmental risk (e.g., mothers with ADHD are at increased risk for substance abuse).

Mount Sinai Expert Guides: Psychiatry, First Edition. Edited by Asher B. Simon, Antonia S. New, and Wayne K. Goodman.
© 2017 John Wiley & Sons, Ltd. Published 2017 by John Wiley & Sons, Ltd.
Companion website: www.mountsinaiexpertguides.com/psychiatry

- Social factors – including maladaptive parenting strategies – may interact with the above to enhance risk.

Pathophysiology

- Neuropsychological:
  - Historically, the focus was on deficits in sustained attention and inhibitory control.
  - Current research suggests a more heterogeneous profile of deficits in executive function, time perception, reward sensitivity, and delay aversion.
- Neurobiological:
  - Disturbances in catecholaminergic function are considered central.
  - One leading hypothesis posits a hypodopaminergic state affecting attention and reward neural circuitry.
  - Neuroimaging studies document abnormalities in fronto-striatal-cerebellar, limbic, and default mode activity.

Predictive/risk factors

- Family history.
- Prenatal exposure to substances of abuse.
- Low birth weight.
- Perinatal distress.
- Electronic media (controversial).
- Diet (minimal impact).

Prevention

> **BOTTOM LINE/CLINICAL PEARLS**
> - High heritability mitigates potential for primary prevention.
> - Good prenatal care, consistent limit-setting, positive parent–child interactions and absence of environmental stress minimize risk.

Screening

- WHO-sanctioned ADHD Self-report Scale (6-item screen) and/or broad-based rating scales.

Secondary (and primary) prevention

- Primary prevention: good prenatal care, abstinence from alcohol/drugs during pregnancy.
- Secondary prevention: consistent limit-setting, positive parent–child interactions, absence of environmental stress, good sleep hygiene, restricted access to television and other "screens."

Diagnosis

> **BOTTOM LINE/CLINICAL PEARLS**
> - Pervasive, impairing, and developmentally inappropriate inattention and/or hyperactivity/impulsivity.
> - According to DSM-5 symptoms begin by age 12, but ADHD is diagnosable at any age.
> - Comorbidity with mood, anxiety, substance use, and other behavior disorders is common.
> - Collateral information is critical; standardized rating scales should be used.
> - Neuropsychological testing can identify associated learning problems.

Differential diagnosis

Differential diagnosis	Features
Oppositional Defiant Disorder/Conduct Disorder	Negativity, defiance, and hostility should be differentiated from the task aversion in ADHD (related to difficulty focusing or remembering instructions)
Depressive disorders	Poor concentration and anhedonia may mimic ADHD, but only occur during depressive states
Anxiety disorders	Poor concentration, fidgetiness, and irritability occur only when anxious
Specific learning disorders	Inattention to and avoidance of academic work specific to the learning disability
Autism Spectrum Disorder	Hyperactivity and inattention to salient stimuli co-occur with repetitive/stereotyped behaviors and significant impairments in socialization

Typical presentation
- Often presents with behavioral problems or academic or occupational under-attainment.
- Typologies:
  - combined (most common subtype);
  - predominantly inattentive (common in girls and adults);
  - predominantly hyperactive/impulsive (generally seen in young children only).

Clinical diagnosis
History
- Clinical interview of the child is insufficient to make the diagnosis.
- Collateral information is critical, because:
  - individuals with ADHD are notoriously bad reporters of symptoms and function;
  - symptoms must begin, by definition, by age 12, and retrospective recall is problematic;
  - symptoms may not manifest in the clinician's office;
  - symptoms and impairment must be documented in multiple settings;
  - standardized rating scales facilitate systematic data collection and longitudinal monitoring (see further on).
- Changes to diagnostic criteria:
  - Core symptoms are unchanged.
  - Several symptoms must be present before age 12 (DSM-5) rather than impairment before age 7 (DSM-IV).
  - In adults and adolescents 17 years and older, 5 (rather than 6) symptoms are required for diagnosis.
  - ADHD and autistic spectrum disorder can now be diagnosed concurrently.

Physical and mental status exams
- Mental status exam: inattention, distractibility, hyperactivity, and impulsivity may be present, but their absence does not preclude the diagnosis.
- No pathognomonic findings on physical exam.

Laboratory diagnosis
List of diagnostic tests
- Neuropsychological tests are used to document learning disabilities as well as cognitive strengths/limitations but are not essential to diagnose ADHD.

Lists of imaging techniques

- MRI, fMRI, diffusion tensor imaging (DTI), and positron emission tomography (PET) are used in research but are not required for clinical assessment.

Diagnostic algorithm (Algorithm 28.1)

Algorithm 28.1 Diagnosis of ADHD

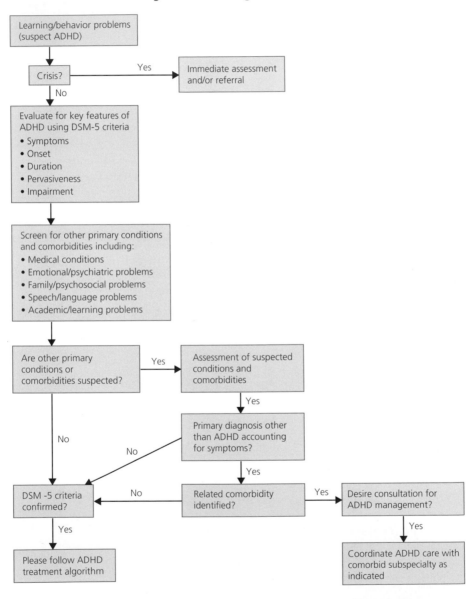

Source: http://www.guideline.gov, Dobie C, Donald WB, Hanson M, et al. Institute for Clinical Systems Improvement (ICSI). Diagnosis and management of attention deficit hyperactivity disorder in primary care for school-age children and adolescents. Bloomington (MN): Institute for Clinical Systems Improvement (ICSI); 2012 Mar. 79 p.

Potential pitfalls/common errors made regarding diagnosis of disease

- ADHD symptoms must be distinguished from those of mood, anxiety, and behavior disorders, but these conditions also often co-occur.
- Inattentive subtype often goes undiagnosed, as symptoms do not result in overtly disruptive behavior. Children with academic difficulties should be screened for ADHD.

Treatment
Treatment rationale

- For core symptoms, medication is often superior to psychosocial treatment.
- Psychostimulants are first-line agents.
  - Two stimulant classes (methylphenidate and amphetamine); each has extended-release (ER) and immediate-release (IR) formulations.
    - Lower abuse potential with ER.
- Non-stimulants are second-line (although they may be first-line for some).
  - Decreased abuse potential and longer duration of action.
  - Atomoxetine (a norepinephrine reuptake inhibitor) is FDA approved for children and adults; it may be especially helpful in patients with comorbid anxiety, substance use, or tic disorders.
  - ER formulations of clonidine and guanfacine (alpha-2-adrenergic agonists) are approved as monotherapy or adjunctive to stimulants in children and adolescents; they may be useful in patients with over-arousal/aggression, comorbid tic disorders, and/or substance abuse.
- Off-label medication treatments:
  - Bupropion: mixed norepinephrine and dopamine reuptake inhibitor – positive data from controlled multisite studies in children and adults.
  - Modafinil/armodafinil – FDA approved in narcolepsy for children and adults; extensive controlled data for modafinil in youth with ADHD.
  - Noradrenergic tricyclic antidepressants and monoamine oxidase inhibitors (MAOIs): seldom used.
  - Serotonin–norepinephrine reuptake inhibitors (SNRIs): several options, but most have low noradrenergic activity except at high doses.
- For most patients with ADHD, combined treatment (including psychotherapy) is often superior to unimodal treatment.

When to hospitalize

- ADHD alone is not an indication for hospitalization in the absence of aggression or mood dysregulation.
- In youth with depression, comorbid ADHD confers increased risk for suicidal behavior.

Managing the hospitalized patient

- Comorbid aggression often declines when ADHD treatment is optimized.
- Identifying ADHD in inpatients with other disorders can aid in treatment and disposition planning (e.g., educational and/or occupational placement, remedial services).

Table of treatment

Medication	Side effects
Stimulants	**For all stimulants**
Methylphenidates	Dry mouth, headache, insomnia, abdominal pain, appetite suppression, weight loss, edginess/irritability, anxiety, mood changes, increased HR and BP
• Ritalin immediate release (5–20 mg bid–tid); Ritalin LA (20–40 mg qAM);	
• Ritalin SR (20–60 mg/day daily)	
• Concerta (18–72 mg qAM)	Rarely: tics, psychosis, mania, severe mood disturbance, severe cardiovascular side effects (risks not higher than in general population, screen for family or personal history of cardiac symptoms)
• Daytrana (transdermal patch) (10–30 mg/9 hr patch/once daily)	
• Metadate CD (20–60 mg qAM)	
• Focalin immediate release (5–15 mg bid); Focalin XR (5–30 mg qAM)	
• Quillivant XR (liquid) (20–60 mg qAM)	
Amphetamines	
• Adderall immediate release (5–40 mg/day divided bid–tid), Adderall XR (10–40 mg qAM)	
• Vyvanse (20–70 mg qAM)	
• Dexedrine immediate release (5–40 mg/day divided bid–tid)	
• Dexedrine Spansule (5–40 mg) administered qd–bid (in divided doses)	
Titrate using sequential dose escalation to best tolerated dose; increase every 3–7 days	
Non-stimulants	Strattera (atomoxetine):
• Strattera (atomoxetine) (0.5 mg/kg to start; target 1.2 mg/kg. Maximum dose 1.4 mg/kg. Dosed bid or daily)	Dry mouth, headache, sedation in children, insomnia in adults, nausea/vomiting, increased HR and BP
	Rarely: Raynaud's syndrome, tics, sexual side effects (older males), depressed mood, hypomania, suicidal behavior, liver toxicity
	Caution in patients with hypertension, tachycardia, cardiovascular or cerebrovascular disease
Alpha-2 agonists	**For all alpha-2 agonists**
• Clonidine immediate release (0.1–0.4 mg daily, divided bid–qid)	Sedation, fatigue, decrease in HR/BP, orthostatic hypotension, syncope, mood changes, rebound hypertension
• Kapvay (clonidine XR) (0.1–0.4 mg daily, divided bid)	Rarely: severe hypotension, syncope, increased or decreased cardiovascular indices (though risk not as severe as once suspected)
• Clonidine transdermal (0.1–0.3 mg/24 hr patch weekly)	
• Guanfacine IR (1–4 mg daily, divided bid–tid)	
• Intuniv (guanfacine XR) (1–4 mg daily)	
Psychosocial	
Psychoeducational intervention	Target populations
• Education about symptoms, impairments, and treatment	All patients and their families can benefit Implemented by teachers/parents. CBT is evidence-based in adults. Organizational training now evidence-based in youth
• Accommodations at home, work, school, lifestyle	
• Goal-setting by patient and family	
Behavioral therapy	
• Behavior management training	
• Cognitive behavioral therapy (adults)	
• Organizational training	
• Social skills training	

* Note: Brand names are used to distinguish among the various stimulant formulations.

Prevention/management of complications

- Cardiovascular risk (stimulants and atomoxetine): screen for cardiac history, family history of premature cardiac disease, and other medications. Obtain physical exam; monitor HR/BP. Obtain ECG or additional cardiac tests if risk factors are present.
- Growth delay [stimulants, atomoxetine (less so)]: monitor height, weight. Obtain family growth history. If possible, offer medication holidays on weekends or over the summer.
- Misuse/abuse/diversion (stimulants): obtain history of substance use/abuse; counsel patients regarding diversion; monitor prescriptions. Use extended-release, long-acting formulations, or preferably non-stimulants.
- Suicidality (atomoxetine): risk of 0.38% in clinical trials; all were prepubertal children and almost all had drug ingestions of uncertain intent. Observe for irritability and mental status changes.

Management/treatment algorithm (Algorithm 28.2)

Algorithm 28.2 Management of ADHD

Source: the Texas algorithm and AACAP guidelines.

> **CLINICAL PEARLS**
> - Stimulants are the most effective and frequently prescribed treatments.
> - Non-stimulants may be recommended for stimulant non-responders or individuals with certain comorbidities (e.g., substance abuse, anxiety, tics, ASD).
> - Long-acting formulations (stimulant and non-stimulant) are preferable.
> - Adherence to treatment is notoriously poor and compromises response.
> - Optimal management often involves both medication and evidence-based psychosocial treatments.

Special populations

Pregnancy
- Avoid ADHD medications; rather, employ psychosocial treatment (CBT).

Others
- **Comorbid oppositional defiant disorder/conduct disorder (ODD/CD):** stimulants are effective for ODD and impulsive aggression. Alpha-2 agonists improve behavioral over-arousal and aggression. Psychosocial intervention is almost always indicated.
- **Comorbid anxiety disorders:** Although anxiety is a labeled contraindication, stimulants may be safe and effective in some cases. Atomoxetine decreases anxiety as well as ADHD symptoms.
- **Comorbid tic disorder:** Although tic disorders are a relative contraindication, stimulants are safe and effective in some cases. Alpha-2 agonists are effective for tic disorders. Atomoxetine does not exacerbate tics and may treat severe tic disorders.
- **Comorbid substance abuse:** non-stimulants are preferred. In cases with past history but no active use, it may be safe to use extended-duration stimulants.
- **Comorbid ASD:** stimulants may be useful but often provoke irritability; keep doses low. Non-stimulants (e.g., atomoxetine) have been used with some success and may be better tolerated.
- **Comorbid learning disorders:** all treatments can be used, but they generally do not improve learning if ADHD is absent.

Prognosis

> **BOTTOM LINE/CLINICAL PEARLS**
> - Outcome is moderated by constitutional, socio-demographic, and treatment factors.
> - Early treatment of functional consequences of ADHD can have positive effects on academic and emotional function.
> - Early treatment may decrease risk for emergence of other psychiatric disorders.
> - Robust, acute efficacy of stimulant medication has not necessarily translated into improved long-term outcome in observational studies.

Natural history of untreated disease
- Approximately two-thirds of children with ADHD continue to have symptoms in adulthood.
- There is increased risk for poor academic and/or occupational attainment, lower earning potential, interpersonal conflict, and other psychiatric disorders, including mood and anxiety, substance abuse, and personality disorders.

Prognosis for treated patients

- Early positive response to treatment is associated with improved symptom trajectory and improved cognitive, behavioral, and social functioning.
- Ongoing treatment is often required, even in the best responders.
- Successful treatment in childhood does not guarantee good long-term outcome.

Follow-up tests and monitoring

- Clinical interviews with parent and teacher and/or patient; parent and/or patient rating scales; teacher ratings (as indicated). Neuropsychological testing if indicated. HR/BP measurement. No other cardiovascular work-up or laboratory tests required unless indicated. Monitor trajectory of growth.

Reading list

Atkinson M, Hollis C. NICE guideline: attention deficit hyperactivity disorder. Arch Dis Child Educ Pract Ed 2010;95(1):24–7.

Cooper WO, Habel LA, Sox CM, et al. ADHD drugs and serious cardiovascular events in children and young adults. N Engl J Med 2011;365(20):1896–904.

Fabiano GA, Pelham WE Jr, Coles EK, Gnagy EM, Chronis-Tuscano A, O'Connor BC. A meta-analysis of behavioral treatments for attention-deficit/hyperactivity disorder. Clin Psychol Rev 2009; 29(2):129–40.

Humphreys KL, Eng T, Lee SS. Stimulant medication and substance use outcomes: a meta-analysis. JAMA Psychiatry 2013;70(7):740–9.

Molina BS, Hinshaw SP, Swanson JM, et al.; MTA Cooperative Group. The MTA at 8 years: prospective follow-up of children treated for combined-type ADHD in a multisite study. J Am Acad Child Adolesc Psychiatry 2009;48(5):484–500.

Pliszka S; AACAP Work Group on Quality Issues. Practice parameter for the assessment and treatment of children and adolescents with attention-deficit/hyperactivity disorder. J Am Acad Child Adolesc Psychiatry 2007;46(7):894–921.

Pliszka SR, Crismon ML, Hughes CW, et al.; Texas Consensus Conference Panel on Pharmacotherapy of Childhood Attention Deficit Hyperactivity Disorder. The Texas Children's Medication Algorithm Project: revision of the algorithm for pharmacotherapy of attention deficit/hyperactivity disorder. J Am Acad Child Adolesc Psychiatry 2006;45(6):642–57.

Subcommittee on Attention-Deficit/Hyperactivity Disorder; Steering Committee on Quality Improvement and Management, Wolraich M, Brown L, Brown RT, et al. ADHD: clinical practice guideline for the diagnosis, evaluation, and treatment of attention-deficit/hyperactivity disorder in children and adolescents. Pediatrics 2011;128(5):1007–22.

The MTA Cooperative Group. Multimodal Treatment Study of Children with ADHD. A 14-month randomized clinical trial of treatment strategies for attention-deficit/hyperactivity disorder. Arch Gen Psychiatry 1999;56(12):1073–86.

Suggested websites

American Academy of Pediatrics sponsored rating scale to assess ADHD and related conditions. Free download. http://www.nichq.org/childrens-health/adhd/resources/vanderbilt-assessment-scales

Centers for Disease Control and Prevention: consumer-oriented information about prevalence, presentation, and diagnosis of ADHD. http://www.cdc.gov/ncbddd/adhd

CHADD (national advocacy group). http://www.chadd.org

National Institute of Mental Health: consumer-oriented information about ADHD diagnosis and treatment. http://www.nimh.nih.gov/health/publications/attention-deficit-hyperactivity-disorder/index.shtml

NICE guideline: full text. https://www.nice.org.uk/guidance/cg72?unlid=55501660920152752236

Guidelines
National society guidelines

Title	Source	Weblink
Practice parameter for the assessment and treatment of children and adolescents with attention-deficit/hyperactivity disorder	American Academy of Child and Adolescent Psychiatry (AACAP), 2007	http://www.jaacap.com/content/pracparam
ADHD: clinical practice guideline for the diagnosis, evaluation, and treatment of attention-deficit/hyperactivity disorder in children and adolescents	American Academy of Pediatrics (AAP), 2011	http://pediatrics.aappublications.org/content/early/2011/10/14/peds.2011-2654
Texas Consensus Conference Panel on Pharmacotherapy of Childhood Attention Deficit Hyperactivity Disorder. The Texas Children's Medication Algorithm Project: revision of the algorithm for pharmacotherapy of attention-deficit/hyperactivity disorder	Texas Department of Mental Health and Mental Retardation, 2006	http://dx.doi.org/10.1097/01.chi.0000215326.51175.eb

International society guidelines

Title	Source	Weblink
The NICE Guideline on Diagnosis and Management of ADHD in Children, Young People and Adults	National Institute for Health and Care Excellence [formerly National Institute for Health and Clinical Excellence (NICE)], 2008	https://www.nice.org.uk/guidance/cg72?unlid=55501660920152752236

Evidence

Type of evidence	Title and comment	Weblink
Multisite randomized comparison study	A 14-month randomized clinical trial of treatment strategies for attention-deficit/hyperactivity disorder. **Comment:** Demonstrated robust efficacy of acute stimulant treatment of ADHD, with larger effects for medication treatment than behavior therapy.	http://www.ncbi.nlm.nih.gov/pubmed/10591283

(Continued)

(Continued)

Type of evidence	Title and comment	Weblink
Multisite follow-up study; both randomized and naturalistic	The MTA at 8 years: prospective follow-up of children treated for combined-type ADHD in a multisite study. **Comment:** Type or intensity of initial treatment in childhood did not predict functioning 6–8 years later. Early ADHD symptom trajectory was prognostic, regardless of treatment type.	http://www.ncbi.nlm.nih.gov/pubmed/19318991
Meta-analysis	A meta-analysis of behavioral treatments for attention-deficit/hyperactivity disorder. **Comment:** Documents the utility of behavioral interventions in children with ADHD.	http://www.ncbi.nlm.nih.gov/pubmed/19131150
Retrospective cohort study (health system databases)	ADHD drugs and serious cardiovascular events in children and young adults. **Comment:** No evidence that ADHD drug treatment is associated with increased risk of serious cardiovascular events.	http://www.nejm.org/doi/full/10.1056/NEJMoa1110212
Meta-analysis	Stimulant medication and substance use outcomes; a meta-analysis. **Comment:** Indicates that stimulant treatment neither protects from nor increases substance abuse risk.	http://www.ncbi.nlm.nih.gov/pubmed/23754458

Additional material for this chapter can be found online at:
www.mountsinaiexpertguides.com/psychiatry

This includes advice for patients, a case study, ICD codes, and multiple choice questions.

CHAPTER 29

Child and Adolescent Disruptive, Impulse Control, and Conduct Disorders

Iliyan Ivanov[1], Robert J. Jaffe[1], and John Leikauf[2]

[1] Icahn School of Medicine at Mount Sinai, New York, NY, USA
[2] Stanford University School of Medicine, Palo Alto, CA, USA

OVERALL BOTTOM LINE

- Both Oppositional Defiant Disorder (ODD) and Conduct Disorder (CD) may have a sizable impact on child development and social functioning.
- Preventive treatment approaches for ODD and CD have been shown to have the best effect on children's function and family interactions.
- Use of both behavioral and pharmacological treatments may significantly reduce symptom severity and may lead to behavioral improvement on a short-term basis.

Background
Definition of disease

ODD and CD, along with Unspecified Disruptive, Impulse-Control, and Conduct Disorder, are characterized by oppositional, disruptive, aggressive, and destructive behaviors in children and adolescents. They are often conceived of as existing on a spectrum progressing from ODD to CD to antisocial personality disorder (ASPD), although only approximately one-third will progress from ODD to CD and another one-third progress from CD to ASPD. Additionally, not all children with CD will have previously met criteria for ODD.

Disease classification

ODD, CD, and Impulse Control Disorders are now classified in the DSM-5 section titled Disruptive, Impulse-Control, and Conduct Disorders. ODD and CD have been separated from ADHD for the new edition.

Incidence/prevalence

- Community prevalence estimates of ODD vary from 1 to 16%.
- Prevalence of CD is estimated to range from 1.5 to 3.4%.

Economic impact

- The economic impacts of conduct and antisocial behaviors are difficult to calculate, but studies suggest that the costs to society are massive, likely in the range of hundreds of billions of dollars annually in the US.
- Major contributors to the economic costs of these disorders include the costs of incarceration and loss of productivity.

Mount Sinai Expert Guides: Psychiatry, First Edition. Edited by Asher B. Simon, Antonia S. New, and Wayne K. Goodman.
© 2017 John Wiley & Sons, Ltd. Published 2017 by John Wiley & Sons, Ltd.
Companion website: www.mountsinaiexpertguides.com/psychiatry

Etiology

- These psychiatric disorders are defined by symptom clusters in DSM-5 but cannot be classified by etiology and pathogenesis.
- Nevertheless, many experts believe that biological factors are important in the development of ODD and CD as familial aggregation suggests a genetic susceptibility. Much of the genetic risk for CD may be attributable to callous-unemotional traits as heritability among this subgroup may be as high as 0.81, but only 0.3 among those without the trait.

Pathology/pathogenesis

- The full pathogenesis of disruptive behavior disorders is unknown.
- Low socioeconomic status confers risk, with some investigators finding that risk varies neighborhood by neighborhood.
- Attachment theory posits that insecure attachment style plays a role. Oppositional behavior is conceptualized as a signal to gain the attention of an unresponsive parent.
- Male sex is a risk factor for CD, with boys at a 3- to 5-fold greater risk than girls.
- Family characteristics including coercive family process, lack of parental supervision, inconsistent discipline, and physical or sexual abuse predispose to disruptive behaviors and CD.
- Peer relationships can reinforce oppositional or antisocial behaviors, and association with deviant peers is linked to the initiation of these behaviors in boys.

Prevention

> **BOTTOM LINE/CLINICAL PEARLS**
> - Prevention is generally regarded as the key intervention, and prevention methods overlap with treatment methods.

Screening

ODD and CD are probably the most common reason for referral to mental health services among adolescents.

Primary prevention

- A combination of universal prevention measures (e.g., community policing) and targeted interventions (substance abuse resistance) is recommended.
- Parent management strategies have the most empiric support from randomized, controlled trials.
  - Programs focus on school-age children and their families and school environments with conflict resolution and anger management strategies, based on the rationale that oppositional behaviors are learned and sustained by maladaptive parent–child interactions.
  - Programs focusing on children alone have not been found to be as effective.

Secondary prevention

- Interventions typically reduce the severity of the behaviors, and may decrease prevalence of delinquent behaviors and progression to CD or ASPD.

Diagnosis

> **BOTTOM LINE/CLINICAL PEARLS**
> - Diagnoses of ODD and CD are established by thorough psychiatric evaluation, using DSM-5 criteria as guidelines.
> - There are no confirmatory laboratory tests.
> - Rating scales are available and may be helpful, but do not substitute for clinical diagnosis.

Differential diagnosis

Differential diagnosis	Features
Attention-Deficit/Hyperactivity Disorder (ADHD)	• Significant overlap and comorbidity. • ADHD is thought to hasten onset of ODD or CD
Anxiety Disorders	• Oppositional behaviors can be used to manage anxiety • Careful clinical history with attention to timing of symptom onset is key • Comorbidity is high (14% or greater) and both disorders should be diagnosed if present
Mood Disorders	• Mood disorders, especially depressive disorders, are common among children with ODD and CD • History taking is again key
Pervasive Development Disorders	• These disorders may present with oppositionality
Language and Learning Disorders	• These are often precursors to and comorbid with ODD and CD
Pyromania	• Deliberate fire-setting without full CD symptoms • Often with tension or arousal before the act and pleasure/gratification afterwards
Kleptomania	• Deliberate stealing without full CD symptoms, often items of nominal value • Often with tension or arousal before the act and pleasure/gratification afterward
Intermittent Explosive Disorder	• Discrete episodes of impulsive, affective aggression with little or no prodrome • Frequently distressing to the child

Typical presentation

ODD and CD present with recurrent, negativistic, hostile, and defiant behaviors which cause functional impairment *for at least 6 months*. ODD presents with angry and vindictive behavior and problems with temper control, but excludes the major antisocial violations of the rights of others or age-appropriate societal norms that are criteria of CD and ASPD. Behaviors must be impairing and outside the normal range for the developmental stage of the child.

Clinical diagnosis

History

- Clinical interview should focus on identifying the behaviors listed in the DSM-5 criteria.
- Collateral informants are crucial. Youth with this disorder often lack insight and are likely to deceive treatment providers.

- Clinicians should rule in or out commonly comorbid conditions (see above).
- DSM-5 has changed the diagnostic criteria of ODD and CD relatively little:
  - The exclusion criterion for CD has been removed from the definition of ODD.
  - Severity ratings have been added to ODD.
  - A specifier has been added to CD for patients who present with a callous and unemotional style in multiple settings.

Physical and mental status exams
Mental status exam findings are nonspecific but may include lack of insight and an uncooperative or hostile attitude.

Disease severity classification
- ODD is classified as mild, moderate, or severe if symptoms are present in 1, 2, or 3 or more settings, respectively.
- CD is classified as mild if few symptoms are present and they cause relatively minor harm to others, and severe if many symptoms are present and cause significant harm to others. The moderate specifier is used for intermediate number and severity of symptoms.

Potential pitfalls/common errors made regarding diagnosis of disease
- Externalizing behaviors (e.g., fighting, stealing, cursing, running away from home) can result from mood problems or trauma.
- Normal oppositional behaviors may be pathologized if criteria are not used carefully.

Treatment
Treatment rationale
- For CD and ODD, primary prevention is often considered the gold standard and should involve the home, school, and community.
- Programs should focus on the child as well as parents and family, peers, and the school.
- Treatment should be frequent (daily–weekly), last for years, be skill-focused, begin at an early age, and be collaborative.
- Parents should be educated about behavioral reinforcement.
- Multisystemic treatment (MST) and multidimensional treatment foster care (MTFC) may help adolescent patients.
- Pharmacological interventions are considered adjuncts to target symptoms; most frequently used are mood stabilizers and atypical antipsychotics for aggression.
- Treatment of comorbid affective disorders or anxiety using antidepressants (e.g., serotonin-selective reuptake inhibitors; SSRIs), and comorbid ADHD using both stimulant and non-stimulant agents, has shown to be effective in controlling some of the symptoms related to ODD/CD.
- Studies for impulse control disorders are limited. There is some evidence for lithium, anti-convulsants, and antipsychotics for aggression. However, high-dose antipsychotics are not recommended given their lack of specificity and side effect profile. SSRIs and opioid antagonists are areas of exploration with mixed results to date. CBT may be useful as well.

When to hospitalize
- The least restrictive level of intervention that helps the patient should be sought.
- Hospitalization should be considered when the patient is felt to represent an imminent danger to himself or others, or there is a marked change from the patient's baseline.
- Suicidal, self-injurious, homicidal, or aggressive behaviors are likely indications.

Managing the hospitalized patient

- For CD and ODD, hospitalization should involve a therapeutic milieu with interventions focused on managing any acute risk. There should be continued psychosocial and psychoeducational interventions, and collaboration with community resources.
- Family involvement is recommended.
- Screening and treating any comorbid conditions contributing to hospitalization should also be considered.

Table of treatment

Medical Mood stabilizers, atypical antipsychotics for aggression in CD and ODD. Stimulants for comorbid ADHD	Monitor therapeutic levels for valproic acid, lithium, carbamazepine, as well as metabolic monitoring for atypical antipsychotics. EKG may be considered for certain antipsychotics (e.g. ziprasidone)
Psychological Psychoeducational, psychosocial, and community services. Behavioral reinforcement education in families. CBT for some types of impulse control disorders	Treatment should be delivered consistently and booster therapy sessions should be considered over time; interventions should be started as soon as diagnoses of CD and ODD are established
Complementary Further research needs to be done	

Prevention/management of complications

- Regular monitoring every 3–6 months of lipid profile, hemoglobin A1c, fasting glucose, and weight for patients on atypical antipsychotics, lithium, and valproic acid.
- Therapeutic levels of valproic acid (50–125 µg/mL) and lithium (0.6–1.2 mmol/L) have to be monitored for chronic treatment.
- Valproic acid reduces metabolism of lamotrigine, and therefore doses for the latter should be reduced if used concomitantly.
- Carbamazepine may reduce valproic acid levels.
- LFTs and CBC should be monitored for patients on valproic acid.
- Renal and thyroid function should be monitored for patients on lithium, as well as EKG in patients over 50.
- Slow titration for lamotrigine and careful monitoring for Stevens–Johnson syndrome by monitoring for rash development.

Management/treatment algorithm

Early intervention involves parents, peers, the school, and the community. Medication is considered adjunctive and should target specific symptoms or comorbid conditions (e.g., impulsivity, irritability, inattention, mood changes).

CLINICAL PEARLS
- Frequent and collaborative intervention is key.
- Screen for comorbid disorders.
- Impulse control disorders is a broad category and the available research differs for specific subtypes.

Special populations
Pregnancy
- Medications are considered adjunctive. Should psychopharmacological treatment be deemed necessary, mood stabilizers associated with birth defects (e.g. valproic acid, lithium) should be avoided.

Prognosis

> **BOTTOM LINE/CLINICAL PEARLS**
> - Established behaviors tend to persist over time.
> - Comorbid ADHD is a risk for more serious adverse behavior.
> - About 30% of boys with ODD will progress to CD, 40% of whom will then progress to ASPD; 10% of children with ODD will progress to ASPD.
> - 60–70% of children with ODD will no longer carry the diagnosis in 3 years.

Natural history of untreated disease
- Untreated CD may progress to a worsening of aggressive behavior and potentially more serious antisocial behavior.
- Early onset and severity of symptoms carry a greater likelihood of progression.

Prognosis for treated patients
- Treatment has been shown to prevent the worsening of aggression and behavioral problems.
- MST and MTFC may reduce arrest rates in severely aggressive adolescents.

Reading list
Burke JD, Loeber R, Birmaher B. Oppositional defiant disorder and conduct disorder: a review of the past 10 years, part II. J Am Acad Child Adolesc Psychiatry 2002;41(11):1275–93.

Connor D, Disruptive behavior disorders. In: Sadock BJ, Sadock VA, Ruiz P (eds). Kaplan & Sadock's Comprehensive Textbook of Psychiatry, 9th edn. Philadelphia, PA: Wolters Kluwer Health/Lippincott Williams & Wilkins, 2009.

Donovan SJ. Childhood conduct disorder and the antisocial spectrum. In: Hollander E, Stein DJ (eds). Clinical Manual of Impulse-Control Disorders. Arlington, VA: American Psychiatric Publishing, 2006, pp. 39–62.

Doshi JA, Hodgkins P, Kahle J, et al. Economic impact of childhood and adult attention-deficit/hyperactivity disorder in the United States. J Am Acad Child Adolesc Psychiatry 2012;51(10):990–1002.

Kimonis ER, Frick PJ. Oppositional defiant disorder and conduct disorder grown-up. J Dev Behav Pediatr 2010;31(3):244–254.

Steiner H, Dunne JE. Practice parameters for the assessment and treatment of children and adolescents with conduct disorder. J Am Acad Child Adolesc Psychiatry 1997;36(10):1482–5.

Steiner H, Remsing L; Work Group on Quality Issues. Practice parameter for the assessment and treatment of children and adolescents with oppositional defiant disorder. Am Acad Child Adolesc Psychiatry 2007;46(1):126–41.

Viding E, McCrory EJ. Genetic and neurocognitive contributions to the development of psychopathy. Dev Psychopathol 2012;24(3):969–83.

Guidelines
National society guidelines

Title	Source	Weblink
Practice Parameter for the Assessment and Treatment of Children and Adolescents With Oppositional Defiant Disorder	American Academy of Child and Adolescent Psychiatry (AACAP), 2007	http://www.ncbi.nlm.nih.gov/pubmed/17195736
Practice Parameters for the Assessment and Treatment of Children and Adolescents With Conduct Disorder	American Academy of Child and Adolescent Psychiatry (AACAP), 1997	https://www.aacap.org/App_Themes/AACAP/docs/practice_parameters/conduct_disorder_practice_parameter.pdf

Evidence

Type of evidence	Title and comment	Weblink
Review	Perspectives on oppositional defiant disorder, conduct disorder, and psychopathic features. **Comment:** Review of ODD, CD, and the controversial subject of so-called psychopathic features.	http://www.ncbi.nlm.nih.gov/pubmed/19220596
Meta-analysis	Atypical antipsychotics for disruptive behaviour disorders in children and youths. **Comment:** Cochrane Review of pharmacologic interventions for CD and ODD, finding some evidence of efficacy of risperidone reducing aggression and conduct problems in children aged 5–18 with disruptive behavior disorders in the short term.	http://www.ncbi.nlm.nih.gov/pubmed/22972123

Additional material for this chapter can be found online at:
www.mountsinaiexpertguides.com/psychiatry

This includes advice for patients, a case study, ICD codes, and multiple choice questions.

CHAPTER 30

Mood Disorders in Childhood and Adolescence

Brandon D. Johnson, Anne F. Bird, and Vilma Gabbay
Icahn School of Medicine at Mount Sinai, New York, NY, USA

OVERALL BOTTOM LINE
- Mood disorders in childhood are associated with significant morbidity and mortality, including impaired growth and development, family and peer relationships, and school performance, as well as suicide.
- They confer an increased risk for comorbid substance use and anxiety disorders as well as adult psychopathologies.
- Appropriate diagnosis and treatment provide the best opportunity to improve outcomes.
- This chapter focuses on major depressive disorder (MDD) and bipolar disorders (BD).

Background
Definition of disease
Major depressive disorder (MDD)
- Psychiatric disorder marked by anhedonia, sadness, worthlessness, irritability, and additional cognitive, emotional, and behavioral symptoms.
- Differs from normal distress in that symptoms persist longer than 2 weeks and cause impairment in social or school functioning.

Bipolar disorders (BD)
- A group of psychiatric disorders marked by alternating and often distinct depressive and manic/hypomanic (e.g., irritability, elation, poor judgment) episodes causing social/school impairment.

Disease classification
- Mood disorders.

Incidence/prevalence
- **MDD**:
  - Point prevalence = 2% children; 5–8% adolescents.
  - Male:female = 1:1 children; 1:2 adolescents.
  - Lifetime prevalence for adolescents = 7.7% (M); 18.2% (F).
- **BD**: prevalence = 2.9% adolescents.

Mount Sinai Expert Guides: Psychiatry, First Edition. Edited by Asher B. Simon, Antonia S. New, and Wayne K. Goodman.
© 2017 John Wiley & Sons, Ltd. Published 2017 by John Wiley & Sons, Ltd.
Companion website: www.mountsinaiexpertguides.com/psychiatry

Economic impact

- Significant inasmuch as childhood MDD predicts adult MDD, and childhood BD persists into adulthood; both are substantial causes of disability.

Etiology/pathophysiology

- Exact etiologies are unknown; multiple environmental, biological, and genetic mechanisms have been implicated.

	MDD	BD
Neurotransmitters	Serotonin, dopamine, norepinephrine, glutamate, GABA	
Brain circuitry	Prefrontal cortex, striatum, anterior cingulate cortex	
Other	HPA axis and immune system dysfunction	
Genetics	Most predictive factor: 2–4× increased risk if one parent has MDD; more if both parents affected	May account for 80%: 25× increased risk if parent has BD

Predictive/risk factors

MDD

- Family history of MDD or BD.
- Environmental stressors (e.g., loss, abuse, neglect, ongoing conflicts).
- Comorbid disorders (e.g., anxiety, substance abuse, ADHD, medical illness).

BD

- Family history of BD or schizophrenia.
- High income.

Prevention

> **BOTTOM LINE/CLINICAL PEARLS**
> - There are no known interventions to prevent the development of childhood mood disorders.

Screening

	Clinician-administered	Youth- and parent-administered
MDD	- Children's Depression Rating Scale-Revised (CDRS-R)	- Beck Depression Inventory (BDI) - Childhood Depression Inventory (CDI) - Suicidal Ideation Questionnaire (SIQ)
BD	- Young Mania Rating Scale (YMRS) - Kiddie Schedule for Affective Disorders and Schizophrenia, Mania Rating Scale (KSADS-MRS)	- General Behavioral Inventory (GBI) - Young Mania Rating Scale – parent version (YMRS-P) - Child Behavior Checklist (CBCL)

Mood timelines and diaries are completed by parents and youth for MDD and BD.

Secondary (and primary) prevention

- Screen youth with multiple risk factors.
- Limited data regarding secondary prevention, although maintenance treatment may limit recurrence of MDD and BD.
- Successful treatment of depressed mothers has been shown to decrease rates of depression in children.

Diagnosis

BOTTOM LINE/CLINICAL PEARLS

MDD
- Often manifests with irritability, somatic complaints, social withdrawal, and academic failures.
  - In youth, irritability can present as a core symptom (unusual in adults).
- Symptoms include depressed/irritable mood, loss of interest/pleasure, change in appetite, change in sleep, psychomotor agitation/retardation, loss of energy, feelings of worthlessness or guilt, poor concentration, suicidal ideation.
- Always assess suicide and substance abuse.

BD
- BD-1 = ≥1 manic episode.
- BD-2 = hypomanic and depressive episodes.
- First presentation of either may be a depressive episode.
- Very difficult to diagnose, given overlap with ADHD, ODD, and DMDD.
  - Look for clear departures from baseline mood/behaviors.
  - Adolescent mania looks like adult mania.
  - Childhood mania tends to have more erratic/labile mood, irritability, belligerence, and mixed presentations, with high rates of rapid cycling.
  - BD diagnosis is not validated in children <6.

Differential diagnosis

Diagnosis	Features
MDD	
Persistent Depressive Disorder	- New to DSM-5; reflects consolidation of DSM-IV's dysthymic and chronic depressive disorders - Depressed/irritable mood for most of the day, more days than not, for ≥1 year in children and adolescents; also ≥2 of changes in sleep, appetite, low energy, low self-esteem, poor concentration, or hopelessness. Child must not be free of symptoms for ≥2 consecutive months
Seasonal Affective Disorder	Occurs in fall/winter; depressed mood, low energy, carb cravings; responds to light therapy
Adjustment Disorder with depressed mood	Occurs in response to a stressor; does not meet full criteria for MDD
Bipolar Disorder	- May present similarly to depressive episode with primarily irritable mood; more likely BD if psychotic symptoms or family history of BD - DSM-5 allows for the presence of co-occurring manic symptoms during a depressive episode as long as they do not meet full criteria for mania

(Continued)

(Continued)

Diagnosis	Features
ADHD	Chronic distractibility and low frustration tolerance with irritable mood should be distinguished from episodic MDD, although they can co-occur
Substance Abuse	Intoxication or withdrawal; check urine toxicology
Non-psychiatric medical conditions	E.g., mononucleosis, anemia, autoimmune disease, hypothyroidism, some cancers
BD	
ADHD, ODD, Conduct Disorder (CD)	More constant symptoms and not associated with change in mood
Disruptive Mood Dysregulation Disorder (DMDD)	• New to DSM-5; persistently irritable mood with frequent tantrums rather than discrete mood episodes • Chronic, severe irritability with verbal or behavioral outbursts (≥3/week) in multiple settings and out of proportion to the situation. Mood between tantrums is persistently irritable or angry most of the day, every day, and present for ≥12 months • Must be inconsistent with developmental level; only diagnose between ages 6 and 18; initial onset of symptoms must be before age 10 • 6- to 12-month prevalence is 2–5%. More common in pre-adolescents, as opposed to BD, which increases from adolescence into adulthood • Rates of DMDD converting to episodic bipolar disorder are reportedly low
Cyclothymia	• ≥1 year of persistent alternating sub-threshold hypomanic and depressive symptoms present most days, with no symptom-free periods longer than 2 consecutive months • Requires that patients have never met criteria for a major depressive, manic, or hypomanic episode
MDD	Isolated depression episode with possible sub-threshold manic/hypomanic symptoms
Substance Abuse	Intoxication or withdrawal; check urine toxicology
Medication reaction	SSRIs can induce a disinhibition distinct from mania (giddiness, silliness, poor attention) that resolves when medication is reduced/stopped; corticosteroids
Non-psychiatric medical conditions	e.g., head trauma, brain tumor, hyperthyroidism

Typical presentation

MDD

MDD most often emerges in adolescence with symptoms of irritability, decreased concentration, social withdrawal, and a noticeable change from prior functioning. In younger children depression often presents with anger outbursts, social withdrawal, and somatic complaints rather than depressed mood. Unlike in adults, irritability often presents as the core mood symptom in pediatric depression. Depressed youth often present very tired, with inability to get out of bed to go to school.

BD

Mood symptoms often have an abrupt onset (as opposed to their slower onset in MDD). Adolescent mania presents as elation, grandiosity, rapid thinking/speech, distractibility, decreased need for sleep, increased energy, hypersexuality, increased activity, agitation, and risky behavior, and is frequently associated with psychotic symptoms (grandiose delusions, paranoia, auditory hallucinations), labile moods, and mixed manic/depressive symptoms. However, patients may first present with a depressive episode. Non-adolescent children with BD frequently show labile/irritable mood with mixed manic and depressive symptoms, rather than with euphoria, as well as higher rates of rapid cycling and lower rates of inter-episode recovery. Belligerence and behavioral disruption are common, and disruptive behavior disorders are often comorbid.

Clinical diagnosis
History
MDD
- ≥5 symptoms for ≥2 weeks, causing impairment:
  - Depressed/irritable mood and/or loss of interest/pleasure (i.e., anhedonia) must account for at least one of the symptoms.
  - Others: change in appetite, insomnia/hypersomnia, psychomotor agitation/retardation, loss of energy, feelings of worthlessness or guilt, poor concentration or indecisiveness, suicidal ideation.
- Inquire about level of functioning in different situations (home, school, with peers).
- Perform thorough evaluation of suicidality: content of suicidal thoughts, passive versus active, and presence of intent or plan.

BD
- **Bipolar I Disorder (BD-1):** diagnosed by a single manic episode although usually character-ized by recurrent mania and depression.
  - Mania: persistently elevated, expansive, or irritable mood along with increased energy and ≥3 symptoms for ≥7 days (or less if requires hospitalization):
    - Inflated self-esteem or grandiosity, decreased need for sleep, pressured speech, flight of ideas, distractibility, increased goal-directed behavior or psychomotor agitation, excessive involvement in risky behaviors.
    - Unlike hypomania, mania causes marked impairment in functioning, may necessitate hos-pitalization, and may involve psychotic symptoms.
- **Bipolar II Disorder (BD-2):** recurrent hypomania and depression; hypomania alone is insuffi-cient for diagnosis.
  - Hypomania: same criteria as mania but requires only ≥4 days and not severe enough to necessitate hospitalization.
- Rapid cycling = ≥4 mood episodes in a 12-month period.
- Mood episodes must be discrete events.
  - Chronic irritability or short/frequent mood swings/tantrums are reclassified under Disruptive Mood Dysregulation Disorder (DMDD).
- May use clinician-administered rating scales to limit subjectivity and maximize inter-rater reliability.
- In the first episode of MDD, consider BD if family history, if pharmacologically-induced mania/hypomania, or if psychosis.
- Perform thorough evaluation of suicidality: content of suicidal thoughts, passive versus active, and presence of intent or plan.
  - Risk is heightened due to mood lability, psychomotor agitation, impulsivity.

Physical and mental status exams
- Indicative features must represent a departure from patient's baseline.

	MDD	BD
Appearance	Poor hygiene, disheveled	Disheveled, odd dress
Behavior	Psychomotor retardation, poor eye contact	Psychomotor agitation, goal-directed behavior
Attention	Distractible, apathetic	Distractible
Attitude	Irritable, cooperative or uncooperative, despondent, disengaged	Irritable and uncooperative
Speech	Monotonous, latency, slow rate, quiet; may be mute	Rapid, pressured, may be disorganized
Mood/affect	Dysphoric, blunted, decreased reactivity; may be irritable or labile	Euphoric, grandiose, irritable, labile
Thought process	Slowed, but may be linear and goal directed	Flight of ideas, may be tangential
Thought content	Negative/guilty ruminations, hopeless/helpless; may have paranoid delusions; may have suicidal ideation	May have grandiose delusions or paranoia; may have suicidal or homicidal ideation
Perceptions	May have hallucinations (most commonly auditory and mood congruent)	May have hallucinations (most commonly auditory)
Insight/judgment	Insight usually intact	Often impaired insight with poor impulse control

Disease severity classification
- A particular mood episode (manic or depressed, but not hypomanic) may be distinguished as mild, moderate, or severe with/without psychotic features.

Laboratory diagnosis
List of diagnostic tests
- No confirmatory test.
- Rule out non-psychiatric causes: CBC, serum chemistries, liver function, TSH, RPR, B_{12}, lead levels.
- If clinically indicated, consider urine toxicology, alcohol level, and Lyme titers.
  - For MDD, also consider ESR, EBV, CMV.
  - For BD, also consider anti-NMDA receptor antibodies; 24-hour EEG for mania to rule out seizures.

Lists of imaging techniques
- **MDD**: before ordering CT or MRI, use clinical judgment to determine the likelihood of an intracranial finding (e.g., neurologic signs/symptoms, history of head trauma, psychosis, etc.).
- **BD**: CT or MRI is generally indicated for a first manic episode, particularly when accompanied by psychotic features.

Potential pitfalls/common errors made regarding diagnosis of disease
- **MDD**: comorbid psychiatric disorders may cloud diagnosis (e.g., anxiety, ADHD, behavioral disorders, OCD, substance abuse, eating disorders).

- Always consider BD, in which the first mood episode often presents as depression; risk factors include family history of BD, presence of psychotic symptoms, and previous hypomania.
- **BD**: due to symptomatic overlap with DMDD, ODD, and ADHD, the diagnosis of childhood BD must adhere to criteria specifying discrete episodes of identified duration.

Treatment
Treatment rationale

MDD
- Moderate depression may respond to psychotherapy alone.
  - Cognitive behavioral therapy (CBT) and interpersonal therapy (IPT) have the most evidence.
- Severe cases (e.g., chronic/recurrent, serious impairment, suicidal ideation) may require antidepressants.
  - Treatment for Adolescents with Depression Study (TADS): CBT + fluoxetine outperformed either alone.
  - Treatment Resistant Depression In Adolescents (TORDIA) study: if no response to initial SSRI, switching to another antidepressant and adding CBT provided the best outcome; adding a mood stabilizer increased remission rates if initiated in the first 12 weeks of treatment.
- Of the SSRIs, only fluoxetine and escitalopram are FDA-approved for treating pediatric MDD (escitalopram only in adolescents), although many others are commonly used in practice (e.g., sertraline and fluvoxamine are FDA-approved for treating childhood OCD, so safety profiles may be extrapolated).
  - An adequate medication trial is approximately 8–12 weeks.
  - Treatment of an uncomplicated first episode should continue for 6–12 months after remission. Longer treatment/prophylaxis is appropriate for more chronic or recurrent depression.
- For MDD with psychotic features, use the combination of an antipsychotic and antidepressant.

BD
- Family history of response to a particular medication may predict patient response.
- Consider side effect profile.
- **Acute pediatric mania:**
  - FDA-approved for children (ages):
    - aripiprazole, quetiapine, risperidone, asenapine: ≥10;
    - lithium: ≥12;
    - olanzapine: ≥13.
  - Approved in adults but often used off-label in children: valproate, ziprasidone.
  - Benzodiazepines (especially clonazepam) may be effective, but consider risk of paradoxical disinhibition.
- **Maintenance treatment:**
  - No FDA-approved agent for use in children.
  - Approved in adults but often used off-label in children: aripiprazole, olanzapine, quetiapine, ziprasidone, lamotrigine, lithium.
- **Bipolar depression:**
  - Approved in adults but may be used off-label in children: quetiapine, olanzapine/fluoxetine combination.
  - Antidepressants should only be prescribed concurrently with a mood stabilizer.

- **Approach to patients with comorbidities and associated symptoms:**
  - Psychosis: include antipsychotic in regimen.
  - Suicidal ideation: may require hospitalization; lithium has been shown to decrease suicidal ideation in adults with BD.
  - ADHD: can safely use stimulants when mood symptoms are adequately controlled.
  - Anxiety disorders: can use SSRIs if concurrently with a mood-stabilizing agent; CBT is also very effective for anxiety and may be used first line if SSRI contraindicated.

When to hospitalize

- Acute risk for suicide.
  - Distinguish between passive and active suicidality, and inquire about plan and intent. Impulsivity is a major risk factor for completion.
- Disorganization in thoughts/behavior, aggression, or severe impulsivity may also make one unsafe in the community.

Managing the hospitalized patient

- Use medications to stabilize the patient as quickly and as safely as possible.
- Observe the patient with appropriate frequency, given severity of presentation.
- Involve the family throughout the process to approve medication recommendations and receive psychoeducation.

Table of treatment

Medical	
Major depressive disorder	
FDA-approved antidepressants	
• Fluoxetine: start at 10 mg/day; increase by 10 mg/dose every 7 days; target dose 10–20 mg/day • Escitalopram (adolescents): start at 10 mg/day; may increase by 10 mg/dose after 3 weeks; target dose 10–20 mg/day	Suicidal ideation or events may increase during early treatment. Side effects may include restlessness, irritability, disinhibition, or worsening of depression
Others frequently used	
• Citalopram • Sertraline • Venlafaxine (adolescents) • Bupropion	
Bipolar disorder	
Acute mania	
• Lithium: start 15–40 mg/kg/day divided bid–qid, may increase by 5–10 mg/kg/day every 5 days; max 60 mg/kg/day	Lithium: follow creatinine, thyroid function, drug levels (0.8–1.2 mEq/L for acute mania, 0.6–1.2 mEq/L for maintenance, >1.5 mEq/L is toxic level)
• Aripiprazole: start 2 mg daily × 2 days, then 5 mg daily × 2 days, then may increase in increments of 5 mg with max dose 30 mg/day • Olanzapine: start 2.5–5 mg daily, may adjust in 2.5–5 mg increments with max dose 20 mg/day	Antipsychotics: observe for metabolic syndrome indicators; follow EKG for QTc prolongation Lamotrigine: risk of Stevens–Johnson syndrome is higher in children
• Risperidone: start 0.5 mg daily, may increase in 0.5–1 mg/day increments in daily or bid dosing with max 6 mg/day (doses >2.5 mg/day rarely more effective)	Pregnancy test is essential for all females of child-bearing age

(Continued)

(Continued)

• Quetiapine: start 25 mg × 1 day, then 50 mg × 1 day, then may increase by 100 mg/day up to 200 mg/day by day 5, then may increase by 50–100 mg/day as needed for max of 600 mg/day • Valproate • Clonazepam **Maintenance** • Lithium: see above • Aripiprazole: see above • Olanzapine: see above • Quetiapine: see above • Ziprasidone • Lamotrigine **Bipolar depression** • Olanzapine + fluoxetine • Quetiapine: see above • Lamotrigine **Device-based** • Electroconvulsive therapy (ECT)	 • MDD: non-controlled reports suggest may be useful for depressed psychotic adolescents • BD: considered only for patients with severe and well-delineated symptoms that have not responded to medications
Psychological • CBT, IPT, family therapy, psychodynamic psychotherapy, supportive psychotherapy	Focus on psychoeducation, relapse prevention, and social and family functioning
Community consultation • Schools, juvenile justice system, social welfare programs, intensive community-based services	Individual education plans may be necessary for a patient to function well in school; various community resources may aid in continued stabilization

Prevention/management of complications
MDD
• AACAP guidelines: after starting an antidepressant for a child/adolescent patient, the clinician should meet with the patient weekly for one month and every other week for three subsequent months to assess for treatment-emergent suicidal ideation. Discontinuation of antidepressant may be necessary in these cases.
• Development of akathisia, irritability, behavioral activation, or worsening of depression may require a dosage decrease or discontinuation.

BD
• Lithium levels must be monitored regularly. Changes in hydration status or concomitant use of medications that affect renal function (NSAIDs, etc.) may lead to toxicity (dizziness, weakness, nausea/vomiting, tremor, ataxia, slurred speech).
• Patients with pre-existing heart conditions (especially conduction problems) should be monitored for QTc prolongation if prescribed second-generation antipsychotics.

CLINICAL PEARLS

MDD
- Psychotherapy alone is often effective in treating mild to moderate cases.
- Fluoxetine and escitalopram are the only FDA-approved antidepressants for the treatment of MDD in youth, although others are often used.
- An adequate medication trial is approximately 8–12 weeks.
- After remission, continue antidepressants for 6–12 months (longer if episodes are recurrent or more serious).
- FDA black box warning states that antidepressants may increase the risk of suicidal ideation; requires close clinical monitoring.

BD
- Mood stabilizers (anticonvulsants and second-generation antipsychotics) are the mainstays of treatment.
- An adequate medication trial is approximately 6–8 weeks.
- After remission of an acute mood episode, continue treatment for 12–24 months to prevent relapse; may reduce doses of meds to limit side effects after acute episode subsides.
- Antidepressants should only be used in patients with BD alongside concomitant mood stabilizers.

Prognosis

BOTTOM LINE/CLINICAL PEARLS
- **MDD**: depressive syndrome is episodic in nature, with natural remission given enough time; treatment shortens duration of episode and may help prevent recurrence.
  - 20–40% of adolescents with MDD will develop BD-1 within 5 years.
- **BD**: relapse is very common, especially without maintenance therapy.
  - Patients with rapid cycling tend to have earlier onset and poorer prognosis.
  - Return to functional baseline between episodes is common, but functional recovery tends to lag behind symptom remission.
  - Impairments on cognitive tests may persist during interval euthymic periods.

Natural history of untreated disease
- **MDD**: average duration of episode = 4–8 months.
  - ~90% of episodes remit after 1½–2 years.
  - Recurrence rate = 20–60% by 1–2 years; 70% by 5 years.
- **BD**:
  - Mania leads to recurrent mood episodes in >90% patients.
  - ~60% of manic episodes are immediately followed by a depressive episode.

Prognosis for treated patients
- Reduced relapse rates.
- **MDD**:
  - psychotherapy effect size = modest (0.29);
  - SSRI response rate = 40–70%.
- **BD**: with maintenance lithium, in one study 37.5% relapsed during 18-month follow-up.

Follow-up tests and monitoring

- Initial weekly visits to monitor drug effects and side effects.
- Follow regularly and closely to assess mood state and symptoms and continued need for appropriate medication.
- With lithium, monitor levels, renal and thyroid function, and urinalysis every 3–6 months.
- With second-generation antipsychotics, monitor metabolic indices.

Reading list

American Psychiatric Association. Diagnostic and Statistical Manual for Mental Disorders, 5th edn. Arlington, VA: American Psychiatric Publishing, 2013.

Emslie GJ, Mayes T, Porta G, et al. Treatment of Resistant Depression in Adolescents (TORDIA): week 24 outcomes. Am J Psychiatry 2010;167(7):782–91.

Goldstein BI, Sassi R, Diler RS. Pharmacologic treatment of bipolar disorder in children and adolescents. Child Adolesc Psychiatr Clin N Am 2012;21:911–39.

March J, Silva S, Petrycki S, et al.; Treatment for Adolescents With Depression Study (TADS) Team. Fluoxetine, cognitive-behavioral therapy, and their combination for adolescents with depression: Treatment for Adolescents With Depression Study (TADS) randomized controlled trial. JAMA 2004;292(7):807–20.

McClellan J, Kowatch R, Findling RL; Work Group on Quality Issues. Practice Parameter for the Assessment and Treatment of Children and Adolescents with Bipolar Disorder. J Am Acad Child Adolesc Psychiatry 2007;46(1):107–25.

Suggested websites

American Academy of Child and Adolescent Psychiatry. http://www.aacap.org

Brain & Behavior Research Foundation. https://bbrfoundation.org

National Alliance on Mental Illness (NAMI). https://www.nami.org

Guidelines
National society guidelines

Title	Source	Weblink
Practice Parameter for the Assessment and Treatment of Children and Adolescents with Depressive Disorders	American Academy of Child and Adolescent Psychiatry (AACAP), 2007	http://www.ncbi.nlm.nih.gov/pubmed/18049300
Practice Parameter for the Assessment and Treatment of Children and Adolescents with Bipolar Disorder	American Academy of Child and Adolescent Psychiatry (AACAP), 2007	http://www.ncbi.nlm.nih.gov/pubmed/17195735

Evidence

Type of evidence	Title and comment	Weblink
Randomized controlled trial (RCT)	Fluoxetine, cognitive-behavioral therapy, and their combination for adolescents with depression: Treatment for Adolescents With Depression Study (TADS) randomized controlled trial. **Comment:** Combination CBT+fluoxetine, and fluoxetine alone had faster response than CBT alone. Outcomes from all treatment arms converged at 36-week endpoint.	http://www.ncbi.nlm.nih.gov/pubmed/15315995

(Continued)

(Continued)

Type of evidence	Title and comment	Weblink
RCT	Treatment of Resistant Depression in Adolescents (TORDIA): week 24 outcomes. **Comment:** CBT + medication (SSRI or venlafaxine) was superior to medication switch in treatment-resistant depression. Switch from SSRI to venlafaxine or vice versa showed similar response rates.	http://www.ncbi.nlm.nih.gov/pubmed/20478877
Meta-analysis	Performance of evidence-based youth psychotherapies compared with usual clinical care: a multilevel meta-analysis. **Comment:** Evidence-based psychotherapies outperform usual care, but effect sizes were modest (mean 0.29).	http://www.ncbi.nlm.nih.gov/pubmed/23754332
Review	Pharmacologic treatment of bipolar disorder in children and adolescents. **Comment:** Review of data.	http://www.ncbi.nlm.nih.gov/pubmed/23040907

**Additional material for this chapter can be found online at:
www.mountsinaiexpertguides.com/psychiatry**

This includes advice for patients, a case study, ICD codes, and multiple choice questions.

CHAPTER 31

Tics and Other Motor Disorders

Amy L. Egolf[1], Paul A. Mitrani[2], and Barbara J. Coffey[1]
[1] Icahn School of Medicine at Mount Sinai, New York, NY, USA
[2] Stony Brook University School of Medicine, Stony Brook, NY, USA

OVERALL BOTTOM LINE
- Tics include both motor and vocal symptoms.
- Treatment is indicated if tics cause distress or impairment.
- Most tics attenuate by late adolescence, but some adults may have persistent disabling tics.
- Comorbid psychiatric disorders, particularly Attention-Deficit/Hyperactivity Disorder (ADHD) and Obsessive-Compulsive Disorder (OCD), are highly prevalent and need to be disentangled.
- Treatment includes both cognitive behavioral interventions and medication management.

Background
Definition of disease
Tics, defined as sudden, rapid, recurrent, non-rhythmic motor movements or vocalizations, are categorized in DSM-5 among the neurodevelopmental disorders. These childhood onset disorders include Provisional Tic Disorder (tics present for less than a year), Persistent (chronic) Motor or Vocal Tic Disorder (motor or vocal tics present for greater than one year), and Tourette's Disorder (TD; multiple motor and at least one vocal tic present for greater than one year).

Disease classification
Tics typically involve one muscle or a group of muscles and are classified by anatomical location, number, frequency, duration, and complexity. Simple tics are of short duration (milliseconds) and typically involve one muscle (e.g., eye blinking or shoulder shrugging) or sound (e.g., throat clearing or grunting); complex tics are of longer duration (seconds), can be a combination of simple tics, and may appear purposeful due to the involvement of multiple muscle groups (e.g., touching objects or rotating) or multiple sounds (e.g., repeating words or phrases).

Incidence/prevalence
- Provisional tic disorder is the most common: up to 20% prevalence in school-age children.
- TD prevalence of 0.3–1% in children age 6–17.
  - Some community samples report up to 3%.
  - More common in males (2–4:1) and white, non-Hispanic children (2:1).

Mount Sinai Expert Guides: Psychiatry, First Edition. Edited by Asher B. Simon, Antonia S. New, and Wayne K. Goodman.
© 2017 John Wiley & Sons, Ltd. Published 2017 by John Wiley & Sons, Ltd.
Companion website: www.mountsinaiexpertguides.com/psychiatry

Economic impact

- Quality of life and productivity can be negatively impacted in patients with TD, particularly when comorbid with other psychiatric disorders.
  - Poorer psychosocial outcomes and their resultant economic costs are associated with greater tic, ADHD, and OCD severity.

Etiology

- While etiology remains unknown, growing evidence suggests involvement of cortico-striato-thalamo-cortical pathways in the basal ganglia, striatum, and frontal lobes.
- Although no unique genetic locus has been identified for TD or other tic disorders, tic disorders do cluster in families, with twin studies showing concordance rates of:
  - 50–90% (monozygotic);
  - ~20% (dizygotic).

Pathophysiology

- Neurotransmitters, including dopamine, GABA, serotonin, and histamine, and other neuro-modulators play a role in the abnormal activity of motor pathways in tic disorders.

Risk factors

- Family history (first-degree relatives have a higher frequency of TD, chronic tics, and OCD).
- Male.
- Comorbid psychiatric disorders.
  - ADHD: 50–75% of TD patients meet criteria; up to 30% of patients with ADHD meet criteria for a tic disorder.
  - OCD: 20–40% of TD patients meet full criteria, and up to 90% have sub-threshold symptoms; up to 30% of patients with OCD meet criteria for a tic disorder.
  - Other mood and anxiety disorders.
- Stress, anxiety, and excitement.
- Certain environmental risks (an individual with a tic disorder may observe and then repeat a gesture or sound made by another person).
- Obstetrical complications, low birth weight, and maternal smoking during pregnancy.

Prevention

> **BOTTOM LINE/CLINICAL PEARLS**
> - No intervention has been shown to prevent the development of tic disorders.

Screening

- Screen based on the presence of risk factors, such as family history or comorbid disorders.

Secondary (and primary) prevention

- Tic severity can fluctuate with treatment and mitigation of modifiable risk factors. Most childhood onset tics remit, and the majority of children with TD experience a significant attenuation of tics in later adolescence or young adulthood.

Diagnosis

> **BOTTOM LINE/CLINICAL PEARLS**
> - Diagnosis requires a comprehensive history from parents and other reliable sources.
> - Absence of tics on mental status exam does not rule out the diagnosis as tics may be suppressed during initial interviews.
> - No laboratory test is confirmatory of TD.

Differential diagnosis

Diagnosis	Features
Dystonia	Sustained contracture of both agonist and antagonist muscles; may follow neuroleptic use
Myoclonus	Sudden and involuntary movement, single or multiple muscle jerks, not suppressible; no premonitory urge
Choreiform movements	Rapid, random, continual, abrupt, irregular, unpredictable, non-stereotyped actions that are usually bilateral and affect all parts of the body (i.e., face, trunk, and limbs). Sydenham's chorea develops weeks to months after *Streptococcus* infection
Compulsions in OCD	Occur in response to an obsession or according to rigidly applied rules
Stereotypic Movement Disorder, or stereotypies in Autism Spectrum Disorder	Non-functional, usually rhythmic, seemingly-driven behaviors that are generally more complex than tics
Pediatric autoimmune neuropsychiatric disorders associated with streptococcal infections (PANDAS)/pediatric acute-onset neuropsychiatric syndrome (PANS)	Tics and/or OCD with dramatic onset following Group A streptococcal infection or other infectious agent; associated with other neuropsychiatric symptoms
Allergies	Allergic rhinitis and conjunctivitis may present with sniffing, eye blinking, and other facial tic-like symptoms
Cough variant asthma	Chronic cough associated with exposure to allergens or following resolution of an upper respiratory infection may have a similar presentation

Typical presentation

Onset of tics and TD generally occurs between ages 4 and 8. Onset of motor tics generally precedes that of vocal tics, and simple tics precede complex tics. Tics usually occur in bouts and wax and wane in severity. Many patients report premonitory urges or sensations before their tics, which are relieved by tic occurrence. Tics generally peak around ages 10–12. Severity begins to decline in adolescence, and tics usually attenuate by adulthood.

Clinical diagnosis

History

- It is essential to obtain a comprehensive, detailed history from caregivers, as the natural course of tics is to wax and wane, and tics may not be observable during initial visits.
- Evaluate for presence or history of common psychiatric comorbidities (ADHD, OCD, mood/anxiety disorders).
- Obtain a comprehensive family history, as tics often run in families.
- Changes in DSM-5:
  - Tic disorders are now categorized as neurodevelopmental disorders.
  - Transient tic disorder (DSM-IV-TR) is now provisional tic disorder.
  - Chronic tic (motor or vocal) disorders are now persistent tic disorders.
  - TD remains essentially the same.
  - Tic Disorder Not Otherwise Specified is now Unspecified Tic Disorder.
- Tic severity rating scales are not used for diagnosis.

Physical and mental status exams

- Neurological exam to differentiate tics from other movement disorders; pay careful attention to findings such as unilateral tics or staring spells that may suggest seizures.
- Cases that are atypical in nature warrant further medical work-up.
- Mental status exam can be completely normal in TD.

Disease severity classification

- Mild, moderate, or severe based on tics' interference with daily functioning.
- Yale Global Tic Severity Scale (YGTSS) is gold standard for assessment of tic severity and treatment response over time.

Laboratory diagnosis

- None.

Lists of imaging techniques

- Imaging is not needed for diagnosis.
- CT or MRI of brain only if another neurological disorder is suspected.
- EEG only if seizure activity is in the differential.

Potential pitfalls/common errors made regarding diagnosis of disease

- Some tics, such as throat clearing and sniffing, may be mistaken for allergies or asthma, although these disorders can be comorbid; eye blinking may be mistaken for ophthalmological problems.

Treatment

Treatment rationale

- Treatment of comorbid psychiatric disorders may alleviate tics.
- Mild tics that do not cause distress or interfere with daily functioning do not need to be treated. Educate patient and family to alleviate concerns.
- Moderate or severe tics that interfere with functioning should be treated.
- First-line approach is evidence-based behavior therapy:
  - Comprehensive behavioral intervention for tics (CBIT) and habit reversal therapy (HRT).
- If behavior therapy alone is unsuccessful, second-line approach involves adding medication:
  - Although haloperidol, aripiprazole and pimozide carry the only FDA approval for tics, initial pharmacotherapy should be with an alpha-adrenergic agonist (clonidine or guanfacine).
  - If unsuccessful, the next step is a second-generation antipsychotic, specifically aripiprazole.
- Third-line combines a second-generation antipsychotic with an alpha agonist.

Table of treatment

Medical
 • Alpha-adrenergic agonists
   • Clonidine, 0.025–0.4 mg daily
   • Guanfacine, 0.25–4 mg daily
	Alpha-adrenergic side effects include sedation, headache, hypotension, and stomach upset

• Second-generation antipsychotics
   • Aripiprazole, 1–15 mg daily
   • Risperidone, 0.125–3 mg daily
	Second-generation antipsychotics: monitor metabolic side effects; baseline height/weight, hemoglobin A1c, lipid panel

• Pimozide or haloperidol
   • Haloperidol, 0.25–4 mg daily
   • Pimozide, 0.5–8 mg daily
	Pimozide/haloperidol: monitor extrapyramidal symptoms

Psychological • CBIT • HRT	First-line treatment, with evidence of sustained response
Complementary • Omega-3 fatty acids	Has not shown tic reduction, but may reduce tic-related impairment
Other • Botulinum toxin injection	May be beneficial for isolated motor tics (eye blinking) and decreases premonitory urge

Prevention/management of complications

- To reduce short- and long-term adverse effects, use the lowest effective dose of medication.
  - Haloperidol and pimozide should be avoided if possible.

Management/treatment algorithm (Algorithm 31.1)

Algorithm 31.1 Management of tic disorder

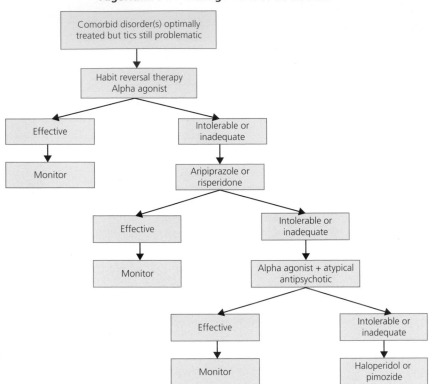

CLINICAL PEARLS
- Given the high prevalence of psychiatric comorbidity, the clinician must make it a priority to disentangle and diagnose.
  - Treatment of co-occurring psychiatric disorders may improve tics.
- Tics do not need to be treated if they do not cause distress or impair functioning.
- Behavior therapy is first-line treatment, followed by pharmacological interventions.

Special populations
- Young children whose symptoms remit should be re-evaluated in late adolescence.
- All patients should have active monitoring during times of stress or developmental changes.
- If effective medications are to be discontinued (in context of the natural waxing and waning course), recommend slow taper to reduce risk of rebound tics.
- Caution is advised when using stimulants in patients with ADHD and comorbid tics, but there is no contraindications for use.

Prognosis

- Tics tend to stabilize over time; severity usually peaks during early adolescence, with a trend toward significant reduction by the end of adolescence.
- Assessment of treatment response can vary depending on when treatment starts, due to the natural fluctuating course of tics.
- Increased severity or persistence of symptoms is associated with increased likelihood of treatment resistance, as well as OCD and ADHD later in life.

Reading list

Bloch MH, Panza KE, Landeros-Weisenberger A, Leckman JF. Meta-analysis: treatment of attention-deficit/ hyperactivity disorder in children with comorbid tic disorders. J Am Acad Child Adolesc Psychiatry 2009;48(9):884–93.

Cohen SC, Mulqueen JM, Ferracioli-Oda E, et al. Meta-Analysis: Risk of tics associated with psychostimulant use in randomized, placebo-controlled trials. J Am Acad Child Adolesc Psychiatry 2015;54(9):728–36.

Lam K, Coffey BJ. Movement disorders: tics and Tourette's disorder. In: Klykylo WM, Kay J (eds).Clinical Child Psychiatry, 3rd edn. Chichester, UK: John Wiley & Sons, 2012.

Leckman JF, Bloch MH, Smith ME, Larabi D, Hampson M. Neurobiological substrates of Tourette's disorder. J Child Adolesc Psychopharmacol 2010;20(4):237–47.

Storch EA, Merlo LJ, Lack C, et al. Quality of life in youth with Tourette's syndrome and chronic tic disorder. J Clin Child Adolesc Psychol 2007;36(2):217–27.

Woods DW, Piacentini JC, Walkup JT (eds). Treating Tourette Syndrome and Tic Disorders: A Guide for Practitioners. New York: The Guildford Press, 2007.

Suggested websites

National Institute of Mental Health. http://www.nimh.nih.gov

National Institute of Neurological Disorders and Stroke, section on TD. http://www.ninds.nih.gov

Tourette Association of America. https://www.tourette.org/

Guidelines
National society guidelines

Title	Source	Weblink
Practice Parameter for the Assessment and Treatment of Children and Adolescents with Tic Disorders	American Academy of Child and Adolescent Psychiatry, 2013	http://www.ncbi.nlm.nih.gov/pubmed/24290467

International society guidelines

Title	Source	Weblink
European clinical guidelines for Tourette syndrome and other tic disorders.	European Child and Adolescent Psychiatry, 2011	http://www.ncbi.nlm.nih.gov/pubmed/21445724
Canadian guidelines for the evidence-based treatment of tic disorders.	Canadian Journal of Psychiatry, 2012	http://www.ncbi.nlm.nih.gov/pubmed/22397999

Evidence

Type of evidence	Title and comment	Weblink
Meta-analysis	**Comment:** Resent review (Cohen et al. 2015) indicates no significant risk of tic increase with stimulants.	http://www.ncbi.nlm.nih.gov/ pubmed/19625978

Additional material for this chapter can be found online at:
www.mountsinaiexpertguides.com/psychiatry

This includes advice for patients, a case study, ICD codes, and multiple choice questions.

PART 4

Geriatric Disorders

CHAPTER 32

Dementia and Other Neurocognitive Disorders

Judith Neugroschl[1], Erica Rapp[2], and Mary Sano[1,3]
[1] Icahn School of Medicine at Mount Sinai, New York, NY, USA
[2] University of Colorado, Aurora, CO, USA
[3] James J. Peters VAMC, Bronx, NY, USA

OVERALL BOTTOM LINE

- Dementia is an acquired cognitive impairment, with interference in social and occupational function.
- Alzheimer's disease (AD) is the most common type of dementia, defined pathologically by brain amyloid plaque and neurofibrillary tau tangles.
- Dementia is associated with behavioral disturbances, worse medical outcomes, and increased medical and custodial costs due to caregiving needs.
- Diagnosis hinges on clarifying the time course of cognitive decline and order of symptom presentation.
  - Acute or subacute time course likely indicates delirium and should trigger an aggressive medical work-up.
  - Early memory, executive, or other cognitive symptoms in the absence of behavioral or movement disorders favor an AD diagnosis.
  - Potentially reversible causes of dementia should be diagnosed and treated (see below).
- In the presence of dementia, amyloid imaging can confirm a diagnosis of AD, although amyloid may still occur in the presence of a mixed dementia and does not direct treatment or management.
- Treatment can provide relief from cognitive symptoms at most stages of the disease but does not arrest the course of the illness.
- For progressive dementias such as AD, vascular dementia, and Lewy body disease, there are no preventions or cures at this time.

Background
Definition of disease

- DSM-5 defines Major and Minor Neurocognitive disorders.
  - Major Neurocognitive disorders involve significant decline in one or more areas of cognition, which interferes with complex instrumental activities of daily living (paying bills, cooking, etc.). These disorders are further classified by severity (mild, moderate, or severe) and as with or without behavioral disturbance (e.g., wandering agitation, aggression, marked apathy, etc.).
  - Mild Neurocognitive disorders, also called Mild Cognitive Impairment (MCI), involve measurable decline that is of concern to the individual and an informant, and are objectively measurable on cognitive testing, but do not interfere with capacity for independent functioning.

Mount Sinai Expert Guides: Psychiatry, First Edition. Edited by Asher B. Simon, Antonia S. New, and Wayne K. Goodman.
© 2017 John Wiley & Sons, Ltd. Published 2017 by John Wiley & Sons, Ltd.
Companion website: www.mountsinaiexpertguides.com/psychiatry

- Diagnosis of AD requires memory impairment and impairment in at least one other cognitive domain, with gradual onset and progressive decline. Cognitive decline must not be due to a general medical condition, psychiatric illness, other neurological illness, or the enduring effects of a substance.

Disease classification
- Dementia is caused by a variety of pathologies, each of which has specific diagnostic criteria, including:
  - Alzheimer's disease;
  - vascular dementia;
  - Parkinson's disease;
  - frontotemporal lobar degeneration;
  - Lewy body dementias;
  - dementia secondary to enduring effects of alcohol or other toxic exposures.

Incidence/prevalence
- The prevalence of dementia increases with age:
  - 1.4–1.6% ages 65–69 years;
  - 16–25% over age 85 years.
- The most common dementia in the US is AD with 5.3 million cases in 2009, expected to rise to 11 to 16 million in 2050.
- Vascular dementia is the second most prevalent dementia.
- 30% of cognitively normal older adults may have positive amyloid scans (presumably representing amyloid plaques), although the significance of this is not known.
- Frontotemporal lobar degeneration is the third most prevalent dementia under age 65, with an incidence of about 3.5/100,000, and a mean age of onset of 58.

Economic impact
The yearly per-person monetary cost attributable to dementia in 2010 was between $41,689 and $56,290, depending on how informal care, i.e., care given by non-paid caregivers, was valued. This suggests a total yearly cost between $157 billion and $215 billion ($11 billion paid by Medicare).

Etiology
- The precise etiologies of most dementias are unclear and are presumed due to a complex interaction between genetics and environment.
- The most consistent finding of genetic risk for AD is the e4 form of the apolipoprotein E gene.
  - This gene has three major alleles, epsilon2, epsilon 3, and epsilon 4, which code for the apo E2, E3, and E4 isoforms, respectively.
  - The E3 allele is the most prevalent, with about 60% of Caucasians homozygous for E3.
  - The E4 allele has been found in up to 50% of AD patients, versus 16% of controls, and is considered a risk gene.
  - The rare E2 allele may be protective.
- Known genetic mutations account for 2% of AD cases, usually seen in early onset (below age 60), and may demonstrate autosomal dominant inheritance. Mutations are in the amyloid precursor protein (APP) gene (chromosome 21), presenilin (PS) 1 (chromosome 14), and presenilin 2 (chromosome 1).

- The genetics of the other common causes of dementia (see above) are complex, although Huntington's is usually autosomal dominant, and frontotemporal lobar degeneration may be autosomal dominant in 10–25% of cases.

   Less common but potentially reversible causes of dementia include syphilis, vitamin deficiencies, and endocrine abnormalities.

Pathophysiology

The etiology of dementia can be thought of as cell loss and synaptic impairment for a variety of reasons. For example, in vascular dementia, it is secondary to cell death from ischemia.

- AD:
  - AD has two key neuropathological components: neurofibrillary tangles formed from hyperphosphorylated tau protein, and accumulation of Aβ either in plaques or soluble oligomers.
  - Hyperphosphorylated tau interferes with microtubule assembly.
  - Neurofibrillary tangles (particularly in the entorhinal cortex) correlate with disease severity.
  - Tangles, plaques, and oligomers may initiate a cascade of events activating microglia, synaptic degeneration, oxidative injury, and apoptosis.
- Diffuse Lewy body dementia (DLBD):
  - Associated with Lewy bodies (insoluble intracytoplasmic inclusions of alpha-synuclein) in deep cortical layers (especially temporal and anterior frontal lobes).
  - Amyloid plaques are also common, although less numerous than in AD, and neuronal loss is seen.
- Frontotemporal lobar degeneration (FTLD) is associated with:
  - neuronal loss;
  - loss of myelin;
  - astrocytic gliosis.
  - Intranuclear or intracytoplasmic inclusions are commonly seen. About 50% have inclusions with hyperphosphorylated tau protein; ubiquitinated DNA binding protein (TDP-43) inclusions are also common.
- Known risk factors for dementia include:
  - increasing age;
  - family history (particularly of early-onset dementia);
  - carrying one or two copies of the ApoE4 allele;
  - poor educational attainment.

Prevention

> **BOTTOM LINE/CLINICAL PEARLS**
> - No intervention has been demonstrated to prevent the development of the disease.
> - Disease Prevalence is lower in developed countries and seems to be negatively associated with higher SES (e.g., education, health status, net worth).
> - Inconclusive evidence exists for physical, social, and intellectual stimulation, as well as reducing cardiovascular risk factors.

Screening

- The U.S. Preventive Services Task Force notes that there is not enough evidence to either recommend or discourage formal screening in patients without suspected cognitive impairment.
- There is no recommended lab or imaging test for screening purposes. Please see: http://www.uspreventiveservicestaskforce.org/uspstf/uspsdeme.htm for further information.

- In 2011, Medicare began to reimburse the detection of cognitive impairment as part of its Annual Wellness benefits.
- The Alzheimer's Association published guidelines in 2013 for screening, suggesting that if annual questioning/observation raises suspicion, it should be followed up with a brief structured assessment (e.g., Mini-Cog, Memory Impairment Screen, AD8, or short version of the Informant Questionnaire on Cognitive Decline in the Elderly), particularly if an informant is not available.

Secondary (and primary) prevention

Many primary and secondary prevention trials have been performed with *negative* results, including NSAIDs, steroids, vitamin E, statins, estrogen, cholinesterase inhibitors, and ginkgo biloba.

Diagnosis

BOTTOM LINE/CLINICAL PEARLS

- Patients' insight into their cognitive changes varies widely and worsens as dementia progresses; corroborative information is essential.
- Prodromal disease states may be detectable via patient complaint even prior to apparent dysfunction. Formal neuropsychological testing can be helpful to assess cognitive changes and potentially to help predict clinical worsening observable over 3–5 years.
- The features of illness onset can help to identify the subtype of dementia.
- Neurological exam may help to classify the etiology.
  - Focality suggests a vascular etiology.
  - Bradykinesia and tremor suggest Parkinson's.
  - Magnetic gait and incontinence suggest normal pressure hydrocephalus (NPH).
- Recommend evaluation to rule out reversible dementias including TSH, B_{12}, folate levels, and RPR. Neuroimaging can characterize vascular dementia.
- AD and other progressive dementias may last for up to 20 years. Individuals may present at any time during the illness course depending on a variety of factors including cultural expectations of aging and cognition, adequate resources, health literacy about dementia and cognitive loss, underlying health status, co-morbid conditions, etc.
- More than one etiology may be present at a time.

Differential diagnosis

Differential diagnosis	Features
Dementia of Alzheimer's type	• Insidious onset and progressive decline with prominent memory symptoms
Delirium	• Difficulty sustaining and shifting attention and memory and other cognitive impairments • Acute or subacute onset • Waxing and waning course • Information from family/informants and extended observations necessary

(Continued)

(Continued)

Differential diagnosis	Features
Dementia due to prion disease	• Rare neurodegenerative diseases, often aggressive once clinical symptoms appear, with rapidly progressive dementia, behavioral changes, and myoclonus with death within a year • E.g., kuru, Creutzfeldt–Jakob disease (CJD), variant CJD (vCJD), Gerstmann–Sträussler–Scheinker syndrome, and fatal familial insomnia • CJD accounts for more than 90% of sporadic prion disease
Dementia due to other general medical condition (e.g., HIV)	• Evidence from history, physical exam, and labs indicating another disease known to cause dementia
Diffuse Lewy body disease	• Early deficits in executive and visuospatial functioning, with memory impairment usually presenting later • Motor symptoms similar to Parkinson's disease (PD), but the cognitive symptoms of DLBD appear early and may precede or be coincident with the motor symptoms • DLBD often associated with well-formed visual hallucinations, marked fluctuations in cognition, REM sleep behavior disorders and neuroleptic sensitivity
Frontotemporal lobar degeneration	• Progressive changes in personality and behavior and/or speech/language disturbance • Motor symptoms including rigidity, apraxia, bradykinesia, and falls • Memory symptoms appear later in the disease
Major Depressive Disorder	• May be associated with complaints of memory impairment, difficulty thinking and concentrating, and overall reduction in intellectual abilities • "Pseudodementia" due to depression more likely to be associated with good premorbid functioning and quick decline in the context of severe depressive symptoms
Mental retardation (MR)	• Developmental onset apparent before age 18 • Associated with impaired intellectual function but not necessarily memory impairment • Dementia may be diagnosed in MR with loss of previous level of functioning due to stroke, head trauma, Alzheimer's, etc. • AD commonly seen neuropathologically in Down syndrome (trisomy 21), as APP gene located on chromosome 21
Normal pressure hydrocephalus	• Classic triad: gait disturbance, urinary incontinence, and memory impairment • Brain imaging: ventricular enlargement out of proportion to sulcal enlargement
Parkinson's disease	• Motor symptoms of low frequency resting tremor ("pill rolling" tremor), bradykinesia, and rigidity • Dementia often a late complication
Progressive supranuclear palsy	• Disturbance of gait resulting in falls • Supranuclear ophthalmoplegia, dysarthria, dysphagia, pseudobulbar palsy, rigidity, cognitive abnormalities, and sleep disturbances • Mean age of onset is 62, male > female • Most patients become dependent within 4 years from presentation, with death in 6–12 years from diagnosis
Substance induced persisting dementia	• Due to effects of substance use, outside acute intoxication or withdrawal • Deficit presumed stable with cessation of toxic exposure

(Continued)

(Continued)

Differential diagnosis	Features
Traumatic brain injury	• Repeated concussions can cause cumulative neuropsychological deficits, mood, behavioral and personality changes, and parkinsonism • Increasing evidence from the football and hockey leagues that multiple concussions are associated with chronic traumatic encephalopathy leading to neurodegenerative changes • Dementia pugilistica long recognized in boxers (~20% in professional boxers) • Current studies evaluating effect of blast-related head injuries in military personnel
Vascular dementia	• Focal neurological signs (e.g., exaggeration of deep tendon reflexes, extensor plantar response) • Laboratory evidence of vascular disease. • Temporal association of clinical stroke with cognitive decline is definitive

Typical presentation
- Dementias typically present with cognitive, behavioral, or functional complaints, noted by the patient particularly at early stages in high-functioning individuals.
- More often, an informant notes the change.
- Motor disturbances with extrapyramidal signs may co-occur.
- Mild cognitive impairment (MCI) (now called "Mild Neurocognitive Disorder" in DSM-5) may precede the clinical diagnosis of AD.
- MCI is characterized by insidious onset of deficits, usually in recent memory, and lasts 1–6 years.
- AD is diagnosed when the patient begins to experience functional impairment. After several years this may be followed by aphasia, apraxia, and/or agnosia.

Clinical diagnosis
History
- Clinicians should inquire about:
  - time course of memory impairment, medical problems that may contribute (vascular disease, hypothyroidism, HIV), substance use, symptoms of depression, and motor symptoms (could indicate Parkinson's or Huntington's disease).
- Discussion of symptoms and progression should be done with an informant, as patients may have poor insight into their symptoms.
- Neuropsychological testing can be extremely helpful in establishing the extent of the person's impairments, particularly with subtle changes, early stage illness, and with teasing out comorbidities.

DSM-IV/5
- DSM-IV defined four different types of dementia: Alzheimer's, vascular, due to a general medical condition, and not otherwise specified. Criteria for each required memory loss with at least one other area of cognitive decline: aphasia, apraxia, agnosia, or executive functioning disturbances.
- DSM-5 changed the nomenclature from "Dementia" to "Major Neurocognitive Disorder," defined as significant cognitive decline in one or more areas of cognition, which interferes with complex instrumental activities of daily living (paying bills, cooking, etc.).
  - Memory impairment is no longer a requirement for a dementia diagnosis, broadening the scope to include, for example, earlier stage frontotemporal dementia where the greatest cognitive changes may be seen in executive function.
- MCI, not included in DSM-IV, is called "Mild Neurocognitive Disorder" in DSM-5.

Physical and mental status exams

- Physical exams are used to evaluate possible etiologies for dementia.
  - Neurologic exam should look for symptoms of parkinsonism, gait changes, and other focal neurological findings.
  - Mild AD is not associated with physical findings.
  - Later stages of AD: extrapyramidal signs, myoclonus, and gait disturbance may occur.
  - A mini mental state exam (MMSE) or a Montreal Cognitive Assessment (MoCA) is used to screen for MCI or more severe impairment in patients with subjective complaints of memory difficulty.
  - MMSE has been the "gold standard" although it may not be sensitive to mild changes in highly educated individuals (24 is considered a cut-off score for normal cognition).

Useful clinical decision rules and calculators

It is important to take any cognitive complaint seriously. An individual may be more sensitive to their difficulties at very mild stages and an informant more sensitive as the disease progresses.

Disease severity classification

Commonly used scales to assess disease stage and progression:

- The Clinical Dementia Rating scale (CDR), scored on a scale of 0–3 or 0–5, with higher scores indicating more impairment, is based on an interview with the patient and a caregiver and assesses functioning in six areas (memory, orientation, judgment and problem solving, community affairs, home and hobbies, personal care). 0 is normal, 0.5 corresponds to questionable dementia or MCI, and 1 is mild stage dementia.
- The Global Deterioration Scale (GDS) is scored on a scale of 1–7 with higher scores indicating later disease stage. Here stage 1 is cognitively intact, whereas 2 corresponds to MCI, and 3 very early stage dementia.

Laboratory diagnosis

List of diagnostic tests

- There is no accepted confirmatory laboratory test for AD.
- Medical conditions such as hypothyroidism, B_{12} and folate deficiencies, and syphilis should be ruled out by obtaining TSH, B_{12} and folate levels, and RPR.
- CSF can be sent for biomarkers (amyloid beta and hyperphosphorylated tau), and can demonstrate patterns that are consistent with AD in the context of cognitive symptoms.

Lists of imaging techniques

- Brain imaging (CT or MRI): in AD structural imaging may show cortical atrophy. In FTD it may show marked atrophy of frontal and temporal lobes.
- Molecular imaging using ligands that bind to amyloid can be used to confirm the diagnosis of AD in the presence of cognitive impairment. In the absence of cognitive impairment it has no value outside of a research setting because cognitively normal elders may have amyloid, and the precise predictive value has not been fully elucidated. New ligands that bind to hyperphospholylated tau proteins are being developed.

Diagnostic algorithm (Algorithm 32.1)

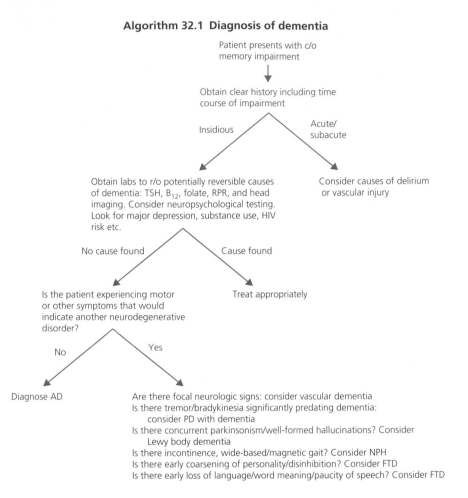

Algorithm 32.1 Diagnosis of dementia

Potential pitfalls/common errors made regarding diagnosis of disease

- The most common error in diagnosis is under-recognition of cognitive deficit and functional decline because of the absence of an adequate informant, a common occurrence in an elderly population.
- Cognitive change may be inappropriately attributed to comorbid conditions and life events without adequate evaluation.
- Non-compliance with medical management may be a sign of cognitive impairment.

Treatment
Treatment rationale
FDA-approved medications to treat AD:
- Four are acetylcholinesterase inhibitors (donepezil, galantamine, rivastigmine, and tacrine) and the fifth is the N-methyl-D-aspartate (NMDA) antagonist memantine.
  - Cholinesterase inhibitors have been found to improve cognitive functioning for up to a year, followed by decline along a parallel path. Approved for all disease stages.

- Stopping treatment tends to put patients back on their original path of decline.
  - Memantine: approved for moderate to severe AD only. Results in a modest improvement in functional measures. May be an additive effect of memantine and a cholinesterase inhibitor.
  - Rivastigmine has an additional indication for dementia of Parkinson's disease.
- Vitamin E 2000 iu daily may be effective in delaying progression of functional decline in all stages of AD, although studies do not show benefit on cognitive testing.
- Memantine and the cholinesterase inhibitors are generally well tolerated.

Approach to the complex patient with behavioral disturbance and medical problems:
- Neuropsychiatric symptoms are very common in dementias, and may affect up to 90% of individuals at some time during their illness. They are as source of caregiver burden and may lead to increased cost, hospitalizations and nursing home placement. Despite this there are no FDA approved medications to treat these symptoms.
- In a patient with behavioral disturbances (wandering, agitation) or psychotic symptoms more psychopharmacological management may be required. Antipsychotics in elderly patients with dementia received a black box warning due to an increase in all-cause mortality; use must weigh risks and benefits for safety and prevention of caregiver burnout.
- A rational approach to behavioral disturbances includes:
  - Identifying and treating physical or medical causes (e.g., urinary tract infection, constipation, pain, skin problems, exacerbation of medical illness).
  - Evaluating psychosocial triggers (e.g., loneliness, frustration re vision, hearing, difficulty chewing/denture problems, embarrassment/modesty concerns, frustration in not being able to complete complex/multistep tasks etc.).
Antipsychotics have greatest evidence base but have most known side effects.
- Metabolic parameters and EKGs should be done to minimize risk for serious adverse events, and patients should be monitored closely for response. There is no evidence regarding how long to continue antipsychotic treatment once the target symptom has resolved, but the patient should be evaluated after 4–6 weeks to assess need for continued treatment and, as clinically appropriate, attempts should be made to taper the medications.
  - Other medications including SSRIs, trazodone, mood stabilizers (gabapentin, lamotrigine) should be considered prior to embarking on an antipsychotic if the behavioral symptoms are not too severe.
  - Targeting symptoms that may be due to anxiety and depression (pacing, irritability, tearfulness) with antidepressants, although they have been associated with increased risk of falls, gastrointestinal disturbance, and hyponatremia.

When to hospitalize
- Behavioral problems leading to dangerous behavior, e.g., wandering at night, significant aggression.
- Psychotic symptoms leading to dangerous behavior (e.g., refusal to eat, accept care, aggression).
- Failure to care for self if no available caretaker.

Managing the hospitalized patient
- Rule out medical problems, medication side effects, and substance use that may be causing or exacerbating symptoms. If the patient is to be started on an antipsychotic medication, obtain a baseline EKG and metabolic labs (hemoglobin A1c, fasting lipids).
- Discuss goals of care with the patient and family.
- Consider nursing home placement if appropriate.
- On discharge, ensure that the patient has adequate care to remain safe in their environment.

Table of treatment

Medications	Clinical pearls
• Donepezil (Aricept), start 5mg qhs, titrate to 10mg. In severe dementia, can be increased to 23mg qhs as tolerated • Galantamine (Razadyne), start 4mg bid, titrate up to 12mg bid as tolerated. This also comes as an oral solution 4mg/mL • Galantamine ER comes in 8mg, 16mg, and 24mg. Target dose is >/=16mg, and titration should be monthly as tolerated • Rivastigmine (Exelon), start 1.5mg bid, titrate to 6mg bid as tolerated • Rivastigmine transdermal system begin at 4.6mg/24 hours after four weeks increase to 9.5mg/24 hours. Further titration can be attempted to 13.3mg/24 hours dose, particularly in severe stage disease • Memantine (Namenda), start 5mg daily, titrate to 10mg bid as tolerated, usually over a month • Memantine XR start at 7mg daily, and increase weekly in 7mg increments to 28mg daily • There is a combo drug containing memantine ER and donepezil (Namzaric) which has an indication for patients with moderate to severe dementia who are already stabilized on the component meds (28mg/10mg)	• Acetylcholinesterase inhibitors: use caution in cardiac patients as has been associated with bradycardia, AV block; may exacerbate reactive airway disease; has been associated rarely with stevens johnson; insomnia, nausea, diarrhea, headache, dizziness, syncope • Cholinesterase inhibitors should be dosage adjusted in moderate renal and hepatic insufficiency. And in severe renal or hepatic disease should not be used • Donepezil 23mg is only approved in severe stage and may have more side effects • Memantine: common adverse effects include dizziness, headache confusion and constipation. Dosage should be lowered in severe renal insufficiency, effect of severe hepatic insufficiency was not studied. Post Marketing associations included CHF, thrombocytopenia, and Stevens Johnson's syndrome
Behavioral interventions	• Ensure that patient has everything needed to function optimally, e.g., glasses, dentures • Break tasks into small component parts • Address problematic behavior using ABCs (define the **A**ctivating event, **B**ehavior, **C**onsequence, and look for places to intervene – e.g., change bath time, change dinner table partner, redirect to other activity, etc.)
Complementary	• There have been trials looking at a variety of complementary interventions including music therapy, exercise, art therapy and aromatherapy • Although evidence is limited, risk for harm is very low and these techniques should be used if patient and/or family seem to enjoy them

Prevention/management of complications
• Safety is the foremost consideration in a patient with advancing dementia:
  • driving;
  • wandering;
  • cooking (patients may burn themselves or leave pots on the stove.)

Algorithm 32.2 Management of dementia

Cognitive impairment in dementia	Behavioral problems in dementia

Cognitive impairment in dementia

Mild impairment → Start acetylcholinesterase inhibitor

Moderate to severe impairment → Add memantine

Behavioral problems in dementia

Rule out delirium or other medical etiology (e.g., pain, exacerbation of medical condition, UTI)

↓

Maximize environmental and behavioral management

↓

Attempt treatment first with medications not known to cause serious harm, e.g., SSRIs, trazodone, gabapentin

↓

Use antipsychotic medications if necessary after discussing risks and benefits with family

Consider hospitalization if patient is at risk of harming self or others or cannot be managed at home

Management/treatment algorithm (Algorithm 32.2)

CLINICAL PEARLS
- For behavioral changes in a cognitively impaired patient, first rule out causes of delirium that may be causing or exacerbating symptoms.
- To treat mild stage AD, use an acetylcholinesterase inhibitor. To treat moderate to severe AD, use or add memantine.
- To treat behavioral disturbances, first maximize environmental and behavioral management, then try medications not known to cause serious harm such as SSRIs, then move to antipsychotic if necessary after discussing risks and benefits with family

Special populations
Others
- Patients with PD or DLBD: rivastigmine is approved for treatment of cognitive impairment in Parkinson's dementia. Other acetylcholinesterase inhibitors and memantine have not been studied.
- Patients with other dementias: there are no FDA-approved treatments, but can try memantine or acetylcholinesterase inhibitor. Treatment for vascular dementia should include treating all modifiable risk factors for strokes, including cholesterol, blood pressure, possible use of medications such as clopidogrel, warfarin, or aspirin in the appropriate circumstances.

Prognosis

> **BOTTOM LINE/CLINICAL PEARLS**
> - AD is a progressive neurodegenerative disorder that leads to death approximately 8–10 years after diagnosis.
> - Other forms of dementia may have a more aggressive course leading to death or disability in shorter periods of time.
> - Medications may afford symptomatic treatment in AD and improve survival.

Natural history of untreated disease
- Patients typically experience gradual cognitive and functional decline leading to death 8–10 years after diagnosis in AD. Other etiologies of dementia may have a more aggressive course.
- Medical comorbidities, age of onset and disease severity of onset also affect the course and duration of the illness.

Prognosis for treated patients
- It is unclear if treatment significantly changes the overall course of the illness, although studies demonstrate better survival and higher performance on cognitive measures and functional scales, with treatment.

Follow-up tests and monitoring
- Monitor MMSE to evaluate response. No follow-up labs or imaging are necessary to follow disease, but remain vigilant for delirium disease progression, and response to treatments.
- If an antipsychotic is used, monitor metabolic labs (hemoglobin A1c, fasting lipids) every 3 months and EKG for QTc prolongation after medication is started.

Reading list
Clark CM, Schneider JA, Bedell BJ, et al. Use of florbetapir-PET for imaging beta-amyloid pathology. JAMA 2011;305(3):275–83.

Daviglus ML, Bell CC, Berrettini W, et al. National Institutes of Health State-of-the-Science Conference statement: preventing Alzheimer disease and cognitive decline. Ann Intern Med 2010;153(3):176–81.

DSM 5: American Psychiatric Association. (2013). Neurocognitive disorders. Diagnostic and statistical manual of mental disorders (5th ed.). Washington, DC.

McKhann GM, Knopman DS, Chertkow H, et al. The diagnosis of dementia due to Alzheimer's disease: recommendations from the National Institute on Aging – Alzheimer's Association workgroups on diagnostic guidelines for Alzheimer's disease. Alzheimer's Dement 2011;7(3):263–9.

Neugroschl J, Wang S. Alzheimer's disease: diagnosis and treatment across the spectrum of disease severity. Mt Sinai J Med 2011;78(4):596–612.

Suggested websites
Alzheimer's Association. http://www.alz.org

National Institute for Health and Care Excellence. http://pathways.nice.org.uk/pathways/dementia

U.S. Preventive Services Task Force. http://www.uspreventiveservicestaskforce.org/uspstf/uspsdeme.htm

Guidelines
National society guidelines

Title	Source	Weblink
Fourth Canadian Consensus Conference on the Diagnosis and Treatment of Dementia	2012 Canadian Consensus Conference on Dementia	http://www.cccdtd.ca/
Clinical practice with anti-dementia drugs: a revised (second) consensus statement from the British Association for Psychopharmacology	British Association for Psychopharmacology, 2011	http://www.ncbi.nlm.nih.gov/pubmed/21088041
Current pharmacologic treatment of dementia: a clinical practice guideline from the American College of Physicians and the American Academy of Family Physicians	American College of Physicians; American Academy of Family Physicians, 2008	https://www.acponline.org/acp_policy/guidelines/dementia_pharmacologic_treatment_guideline_2008.pdf
Alzheimer's disease management guideline: update 2008	California Workgroup on Guidelines for Alzheimer's Disease Management, 2008	http://www.ncbi.nlm.nih.gov/pubmed/21546322
Guideline Summary for Clinicians Detection, Diagnosis, and Management of Dementia	American Academy of Neurology (AAN), multiple guidelines (diagnosis, driving, CJD, MCI, management) updated between 2001 and 2013	http://tools.aan.com/professionals/practice/pdfs/dementia_guideline.pdf
Dementia Guidelines	American Psychiatric Association (APA)	http://psychiatryonline.org/guidelines. aspxhttp://ajp.psychiatryonline.org/doi/pdf/10.1176/appi.ajp.2015.173501and http://psychiatryonline.org/pb/assets/raw/sitewide/practice_guidelines/guidelines/alzheimerwatch.pdf

Evidence

Type of evidence	Title and comment	Weblink
Meta-analysis	Cholinesterase inhibitors for Alzheimer's disease. **Comment:** Meta-analysis and review of efficacy of cholinesterase inhibitors for AD.	http://www.ncbi.nlm.nih.gov/pubmed/16437532
Systematic review	Evolution of the evidence on the effectiveness and cost-effectiveness of acetylcholinesterase inhibitors and memantine for Alzheimer's disease: systematic review and economic model. **Comment:** In the UK, since 2011 the National Health Service has defined these medications and memantine as cost effective given the data on efficacy.	http://www.ncbi.nlm.nih.gov/pubmed/23179169

(Continued)

(Continued)

Type of evidence	Title and comment	Weblink
Systematic review	Screening for cognitive impairment in older adults: A systematic review for the U.S. Preventive Services Task Force. **Comment:** Brief instruments to screen for cognitive impairment but unclear clinical benefit of early detection.	http://www.ncbi.nlm.nih.gov/pubmed/24145578
Meta-analysis	Lack of evidence for the efficacy of memantine in mild Alzheimer disease. **Comment:** Despite its frequent off-label use, evidence is lacking for memantine in mild AD.	http://www.ncbi.nlm.nih.gov/pubmed/21482915
Randomized controlled trial	Donepezil and memantine for moderate-to-severe Alzheimer's disease. **Comment:** In patients with moderate to severe AD, continued treatment with donepezil and/or memantine is associated with significant benefits over 12 months.	http://www.nejm.org/doi/full/10.1056/NEJMoa1106668#t=article

Additional material for this chapter can be found online at:
www.mountsinaiexpertguides.com/psychiatry

This includes advice for patients, ICD codes, and multiple choice questions.

CHAPTER 33

Delirium

Joseph I. Friedman[1] and Devendra S. Thakur[2]
[1] Icahn School of Medicine at Mount Sinai, New York, NY, USA
[2] Geisel School of Medicine at Dartmouth College, Hanover, NH, USA

OVERALL BOTTOM LINE
- Delirium is a reversible state of global cerebral dysfunction caused by many different medical conditions, medications, substance intoxication, or withdrawal.
- Symptoms: disturbance of attention and awareness accompanied by cognitive and behavioral changes which are highly variable in presentation.
- Onset and course: abrupt onset of symptoms with fluctuation in presentation during the course of the day. Symptoms may resolve in hours to days or persist for weeks to months.
- Treatment of delirium involves: (1) identification of the delirium-precipitating etiology, (2) addressing modifiable risk factors for the development of delirium, (3) pharmacological interventions to address distressing behavioral symptoms.

Background
Definition of disease
Delirium, as defined by DSM-5, manifests as abrupt onset of reduced awareness and ability to direct, focus, sustain, and shift attention.
- Additional cognitive disturbances (not accounted for by pre-existing dementia) include:
  - impaired memory;
  - disorientation;
  - language and perceptual disturbances.
- Symptoms fluctuate during the course of the day, and there is evidence that the disturbance is caused by a direct physiologic consequence of a general medical condition, medication use, substance intoxication or withdrawal, or multiple causes.

Disease classification
- Delirium is often subtyped on the basis of motor activity:
  - hyperactive subtype: agitated and hyperalert features;
  - hypoactive subtype: calmer patients with a decreased level of alertness;
  - mixed subtype, with features of both hyperactivity and hypoactivity.
- Although the hypoactive and mixed delirium subtypes predominate, they are the least recognized.

Mount Sinai Expert Guides: Psychiatry, First Edition. Edited by Asher B. Simon, Antonia S. New, and Wayne K. Goodman.
© 2017 John Wiley & Sons, Ltd. Published 2017 by John Wiley & Sons, Ltd.
Companion website: www.mountsinaiexpertguides.com/psychiatry

Incidence/prevalence

- Prevalence rates in medical inpatients at admission range from 10% to 31%.
- Incidence of new delirium post admission ranges from 3% to 29%.
- Prevalence rates vary among different hospital settings with rates as high as 80% in mechanically ventilated patients in intensive care units.

Economic impact

- $64,421 of estimated additional healthcare costs per delirious patient per year.
- Assuming that delirium complicates hospital stays for 20% of the 11.8 million persons 65 years and older who are hospitalized annually, the total direct 1-year healthcare costs attributable to delirium range from $38 billion to $152 billion annually.

Etiology

- Almost any general medical condition, major surgical procedures, substance intoxication or withdrawal, and certain types of medication (i.e., anticholinergics, benzodiazepines, opiates) can precipitate delirium.
- However, delirium is rarely caused by a single factor and is most often multifactorial, involving a complex interplay between risk factors and precipitating factors.
- Certain pre-existing risk factors increase susceptibility to the delirium-inducing effects of a precipitating factor/event.

Predictive/risk factors

Factor	Vulnerability
Age	Older age
Cognitive	Pre-existing dementia, other cognitive impairment, history of delirium
Sensory impairment	Visual and auditory
Functional	Requires assistance with ADLs/IADLs
Medical comorbidity	(1) Greater number of comorbid medical conditions, (2) greater severity of comorbid medical conditions.
Decreased oral intake	(1) Dehydration, (2) malnutrition
Medication and drugs	(1) Use of psychoactive medications, (2) history of recreational drug/alcohol abuse
Mobility	(1) Immobilization, (2) use of physical restraints

Pathophysiology

There is no single ubiquitously accepted pathophysiology underlying delirium. However, a number of mechanisms have been put forward including:

- cholinergic deficiency (supported by the delirogenic effects of anticholinergic medications);
- dopamine excess (supported by the effectiveness of antipsychotics in delirium);
- altered gamma-hydroxybutyric acid activity (supported by the delirogenic effects of benzodiazepines);
- acute inflammatory responses in the brain (microglial, astrocyte, and cytokine activation).

Prevention

Prevention strategies are based upon addressing the modifiable risk factors outlined above:

- Assess for and address visual and hearing deficits: i.e., glasses or visual aids for the visually impaired, hearing aids for the hearing impaired.
- Maintain adequate hydration and nutrititon.
- Early mobilization of inactive patients, including early involvement of physical and occupational therapy in inpatient setting.
- Avoid use of physical restraints when possible.
- Minimize use of indwelling urinary catheters.
- Use orientation boards, clocks, and calendars to keep the patient oriented.
- Maintain/re-establish normal sleep-wake cycle.
- Minimize use of psychoactive medications, especially opiates, anticholinergics and benzodiazepines.
- Provide of cognitive stimulation.

Screening

Several screening tools have been developed for delirium. However, since delirium can occur in almost any patient admitted to the hospital, formal screening of every patient is not feasible.

Secondary (and primary) prevention

Patients with a recent episode of delirium are at high risk of recurrence. Prevention is crucial, and the same strategies utilized in primary prevention apply for secondary prevention.

Diagnosis

BOTTOM LINE/CLINICAL PEARLS
- The diagnosis of delirium is clinical. No laboratory test can diagnose delirium.
- Accurately ascertain the patient's baseline (using corroborative sources for history), and determine if there is an acute change in attention and awareness from baseline.
- Assess for fluctuation of symptoms throughout the day.
- Keep in mind the diversity of psychomotor behavior which presents with delirium (i.e., do not overlook hyperactive or "quiet" delirium).

Differential diagnosis

Differential diagnosis	Features
Dementia	Characterized by slow, progressive cognitive decline that does not fluctuate or affect awareness
Depressive disorders	Delirious patients frequently endorse depressive symptoms, so clinicians need to consider onset (depression does not develop over hours to days), course (delirium-associated symptom fluctuation throughout day vs no fluctuation or diurnal pattern of depression) Impaired awareness not characteristic of depression, and cognitive and attention impairments of delirium vs possible pseudodementia of depression

(Continued)

(Continued)

Differential diagnosis	Features
Mania and psychotic disorders	The hyperactive subtype of delirium is often mistaken for psychosis or mania, given the presence of agitation, psychotic symptoms, and affective lability. Most cases of delirium occur in the geriatric population; thus new-onset psychosis in the elderly is likely delirium, given that schizophrenia and bipolar disorder rarely manifest for the first time after age 50. The administration of benzodiazepines to schizophrenic and manic patients for agitation is effective, whereas delirious patients frequently get worse

Typical presentation

- The abrupt development of impaired attention and awareness with fluctuation in their manifestation throughout the day is the hallmark of delirium.
- The presentation of additional cognitive impairments, psychotic and psychomotor symptoms is highly variable.

Clinical diagnosis

- Determination of the abrupt onset and fluctuating course of core symptoms is essential.
- Frequent superimposition of delirium on pre-existing cognitive impairment necessitates the acquisition of corroborative history from caregivers to establish the patient's baseline and determine if and when there was a change.
- Clinical information from hospital staff to elucidate unappreciated symptoms that may not manifest during formal assessment is also important.

Physical and mental status exams

- Assess the patient's ability to direct, focus, sustain, and shift attention; this may require performing a formal test of attention.
- In addition to the routine mental status examination, a more in-depth cognitive assessment than usual should be performed: i.e., language ability, short-term and long-term memory, orientation in all spheres.
- Physical signs that may be useful in identifying an underlying etiology include:
  - tremors and autonomic instability (suggestive of alcohol withdrawal syndrome);
  - expressive aphasia, facial droop, focal weakness (suggestive of CVA);
  - fever and rigors (suggestive of infection).

Disease severity classification

- Formal severity rating instruments are not practical in the clinical setting.
- Patients presenting with symptoms of delirium not sufficient in quantity or severity to meet criteria for delirium are classified as having sub-syndromal delirium (SSD).
  - Not all patients with SSD progress to "full-blown" delirium, but they are at a greatly increased risk of developing delirium.
  - Identifying SSD in patients should trigger a treatment plan for delirium risk factor reduction and monitoring for progression to "full-blown" delirium.

Laboratory diagnosis

List of diagnostic tests

- There is no single test or collection of pathognomonic laboratory indices for delirium; however, laboratory studies may be helpful in determining the underlying precipitating condition.
- If routine laboratory testing is non-revealing, consider testing for overlooked endocrine disturbances and vitamin deficiencies (TSH and B_{12} for example).
- Combinations of laboratory abnormalities may also be revealing: i.e., elevated mean corpuscular volume and gamma-glutamyl transferase should raise suspicion for chronic alcohol abuse.

Lists of imaging techniques

- There is no standard imaging technique used to diagnose delirium, but imaging may be useful to assess for underlying causes of delirium.
  - CT is a relatively inexpensive and fast method to assess for acute CVAs, subdural hematomas, and other masses.
  - Diffuse generalized slowing on EEG is nonspecific to delirium and also observed in other conditions such as moderate–severe dementia, limiting its use in the assessment of delirium.

Potential pitfalls/common errors made regarding diagnosis of disease

- A patient with delirium superimposed on dementia is presumed to be at his/her "baseline" level of impairment.
- Hyperactive or mixed delirium is often mistaken for psychosis or mania.
- Hypoactive delirium is often mistaken for depression or is ignored by clinical staff because these patients are not disruptive.

Treatment

Treatment rationale

- First-line treatment for the delirious patient is *identification and treatment of the underlying precipitant* (e.g., acute medical condition, alcohol withdrawal, use of delirogenic medication).
- Address modifiable risk factors outlined in "Prevention," above.
- Antipsychotics are recommended for the management of agitation and psychosis, the QTc interval permitting.

When to hospitalize

As delirium is the result of an underlying medical cause determining if the cause is acute and severe is crucial to determine the need for hospitalization. Alcohol-withdrawal delirium warrants hospitalization because of the high mortality risk.

Prevention/management of complications

- Delirium is associated with increased rates of:
  - pressure ulcers;
  - falls;
  - requirement of ICU;
  - hospital re-admission;
  - death.

- Delay to diagnosis and/or intervention increases the risk of these complications.
- If using antipsychotics, monitor QTc interval to avoid arrhythmias.
- Physical restraints can cause nerve damage and asphyxia. Their use should be minimized and the patient closely monitored when used.

CLINICAL PEARLS
- Primary treatment goal: identify and treat the underlying delirium precipitant(s).
- Address modifiable delirium risk factors in patients with delirium and with SSD.

Prognosis

BOTTOM LINE/CLINICAL PEARLS
- Delirium resolves completely within several days in most patients; however, delirium can persist for weeks to months.
- Delirium is associated with higher rates of nursing home placement, long-term cognitive impairment, and functional decline post hospitalization.
- The longer the duration and the more severe the delirium episode, the greater the long-term cognitive and functional impairments.

Reading list

Cole M, McCusker J, Dendukuri N, Han L. The prognostic significance of subsyndromal delirium in elderly medical inpatients. J Am Geriatr Soc 2003;51(6):754–60.

Cole MG, McCusker J, Voyer P, et al. Subsyndromal delirium in older long-term care residents: incidence, risk factors, and outcomes. J Am Geriatr Soc 2011;59(10):1829–36.

Dasgupta M, Dumbrell AC. Preoperative risk assessment for delirium after noncardiac surgery: a systematic review. J Am Geriatr Soc 2006;54:1578–89.

Elie M, Cole MG, Primeau FJ, Bellavance F. Delirium risk factors in elderly hospitalized patients. J Gen Intern Med 1998;13:204–12.

Farrell KR, Ganzini L. Misdiagnosing delirium as depression in medically ill elderly patients. Arch Intern Med 1995;155(22):2459–64.

Flaherty JH, Rudolph J, Shay K, et al. Delirium is a serious and under-recognized problem: why assessment of mental status should be the sixth vital sign. J Am Med Dir Assoc 2007;8(5):273–5.

Inouye SK, Charpentier PA. Precipitating factors for delirium in hospitalized elderly persons. Predictive model and interrelationship with baseline vulnerability. JAMA 1996;275(11):852–7.

Lawlor P, Gagnon B, Mancini IL, Pereira J, Bruera E. Phenomenology of delirium and its subtypes in advanced cancer patients: a prospective study. Palliat Care 1998;14:106.

Pisani MA, Murphy TE, Araujo KL, et al. Benzodiazepine and opioid use and the duration of intensive care unit delirium in an older population. Crit Care Med 2009;37:177–83.

van den Boogaard M, Schoonhoven L, Evers AW, et al. Delirium in critically ill patients: impact on long-term health-related quality of life and cognitive functioning. Crit Care Med 2012;40:112–18.

Suggested websites

Vanderbilt University Medical Center, ICU Delirium and Cognitive Impairment Study Group. http://www.mc.vanderbilt.edu/icudelirium/

Guidelines
National society guidelines

Title	Source	Weblink
Practice Guideline for the Treatment of Patients With Delirium	American Psychiatric Association (APA), 1999	http://psychiatryonline.org/pb/assets/raw/sitewide/practice_guidelines/guidelines/delirium.pdf
Clinical practice guidelines for the management of pain, agitation, and delirium in adult patients in the intensive care unit	American College of Critical Care Medicine, 2013	http://www.learnicu.org/SiteCollectionDocuments/Pain,%20Agitation,%20Delirium.pdf

International society guidelines

Title	Source	Weblink
Delirium: Diagnosis, Prevention and Management	National Institute for Health and Care Excellence (NICE), 2010	https://www.nice.org.uk/guidance/cg103/chapter/1-Guidance

Additional material for this chapter can be found online at:
www.mountsinaiexpertguides.com/psychiatry

This includes advice for patients, a case study, and ICD codes.

CHAPTER 34

Late-Life Depression

Samuel P. Greenstein[1], Daniel McGonigle[2], and Charles H. Kellner[2]
[1] University of Cincinnati College of Medicine, Cincinnati, OH, USA
[2] Icahn School of Medicine at Mount Sinai, New York, NY, USA

OVERALL BOTTOM LINE

- Late-life depression is often undetected, undertreated, and associated with a poor quality of life, worsening of chronic medical problems, and increased morbidity and mortality.
- In screening for geriatric depression, clinicians should recognize symptomatology other than depressed mood (e.g., cognitive impairment, physical complaints).
- Psychopharmacology, psychotherapy, and electroconvulsive therapy (ECT) are effective treatments.

Background
Definition of disease
- Broadly defined: severe depressive illness occurring in elderly patients.
- Certain authorities restrict the definition to those whose first onset of depressive illness occurs after age 65.

Disease classification
- Not-yet-categorized subtype of DSM-5 depressive disorder.

Incidence/prevalence
- Incidence: 7 per 1000 person-years.
- Prevalence:
  - Major Depression: 1.8%;
  - Minor Depression: 9.8%;
  - Depressive syndromes: 13.5%.

Economic impact
- Total costs, including ambulatory medical care and inpatient hospitalizations, are ~ 50% higher in depressed versus non-depressed elderly.

Mount Sinai Expert Guides: Psychiatry, First Edition. Edited by Asher B. Simon, Antonia S. New, and Wayne K. Goodman.
© 2017 John Wiley & Sons, Ltd. Published 2017 by John Wiley & Sons, Ltd.
Companion website: www.mountsinaiexpertguides.com/psychiatry

Etiology
- Exact etiology unknown, although genetic factors are less significant in late-onset depressive illness.
- Vascular risk factors may play a role.

Pathophysiology
- Pathogenesis not completely understood.
- Certain subtypes may implicate damage to frontal subcortical circuitry (i.e., striato-pallido-thalamo-cortical pathways).
  - Subclinical cerebrovascular lesions affecting subcortical and periventricular regions, as well as cerebral atrophy, are implicated in susceptibility to and/or expression of the vascular depression subtype.

Predictive/risk factors
- Female.
- Social isolation.
- Single (widowed, divorced, separated).
- Comorbid medical conditions.
- Lower socioeconomic status.
- Insomnia.
- Cognitive and/or functional impairment.

Prevention

> **BOTTOM LINE/CLINICAL PEARLS**
> - Risk for vascular depression is reduced by managing cardiac risk (e.g., hypertension, hypercholesterolemia, diabetes).

Screening
- Geriatric Depression Scale (GDS): self-administered; takes ~7 minutes; emphasizes cognitive function more than do traditional depression screening instruments used in general adult populations.
- Patient Health Questionnaire (PHQ-9): designed to assist primary care physicians in quickly and comprehensively assessing for depression and treatment effectiveness; 9 items.
- Cornell Scale for Depression in Dementia (CSDD): use in patients with concomitant cognitive impairment.

Secondary (and primary) prevention
- Reduction of modifiable risk factors.
- Initiation/continuation of pharmacotherapy, psychotherapy, and/or ECT.

Diagnosis

BOTTOM LINE/CLINICAL PEARLS
- Presenting symptoms may differ from those of general adult depressive illness.
  - Cognitive impairment, physical complaints, social withdrawal, impairment in activities of daily living (change in grooming can be an early symptom).
- Complete neurological exam, including assessing cognition (using either the mini mental status exam or Montreal Cognitive Assessment).
- Labs to rule out non-psychiatric etiology are critical.
- Consider neuroimaging to rule out structural lesions or vascular disease.

Differential diagnosis

Differential diagnosis	Features
Low mood associated with bereavement	Milder symptoms, generally of shorter duration, and not associated with feelings of worthlessness or psychosis
Dementia	More prominent apathy, as opposed to dysphoria
Bipolar depression	History of mania
Pharmacologically induced depression	Recent treatment with corticosteroids, beta-blockers, anticonvulsants
Depression associated with medical illness	Thyroid disease, anemia, cancer, nutritional deficiencies

Typical presentation

Late-life depression often does not present with the cluster of symptoms characterizing depression in a younger cohort (i.e., usual complaints of low mood, neurovegetative symptoms, anhedonia). Patients with late-life depression often present to primary care providers due to unexplained physical complaints (low energy, chronic generalized pain, constipation, diarrhea, nausea, abdominal pain). Medical work-up is frequently unrevealing. Family members often report that listlessness and lack of motivation are the primary changes occurring in the patient.

Clinical diagnosis

History
- In addition to standard DSM-5 symptoms of Major Depressive Disorder, assess for impaired ADLs, cognitive impairment, and general physical complaints.
- Geriatric Depression Scale may be helpful.
- The bereavement exclusion in DSM-IV (depressive syndromes within 2 months of a death) has been omitted from DSM-5, due to a greater appreciation that severe depressive illness occurring after the death of a partner can have serious adverse effects on medical health and is deserving of aggressive treatment.

Physical and mental status exams

- Appearance: Disheveled, malodorous? Underweight/overweight?
- Attention/behavior/motor: Appropriateness? Slow moving? Poor concentration? Able to pay attention to the conversation?
- Mood/affect: Does content match demeanor/affect?
- Cognition: Oriented and alert? Able to stay with flow of conversation?
- Thought content: What is the patient saying? Impoverished? 1- to 2-word answers? Under-detailed and uninformative responses are often one of the major indicators of depression in the elderly.

Disease severity classification

- Persistent Depressive Disorder.
- Unspecified Depressive Disorder.
- Major Depressive Disorder, Mild, Moderate, Severe.
- Major Depressive Disorder, Severe with Psychotic Features.

Laboratory diagnosis

List of diagnostic tests

- There is no confirmatory test.
- Tests to rule out other conditions:
  - thyroid function (TSH, T_4, T_3);
  - vitamin B_{12} and folate levels;
  - CBC.

Lists of imaging techniques

- MRI of brain ± contrast to rule out tumors, strokes, and structural lesions.

Potential pitfalls/common errors made regarding diagnosis of disease

- Patients presenting with cognitive decline and an inability to carry out formerly manageable tasks of daily living may lead clinicians to make a cursory diagnosis of dementia, without fully appreciating that depressive illness has a primary role in the functional decline.
- Healthcare providers may miss the presence of a depressive illness by narrowly assessing only mood, while failing to recognize that somatic complaints and behavioral withdrawal are often the most significant harbingers of late-life depression.

Diagnostic algorithm (Algorithm 34.1)

Algorithm 34.1 Diagnosis of late-life depression

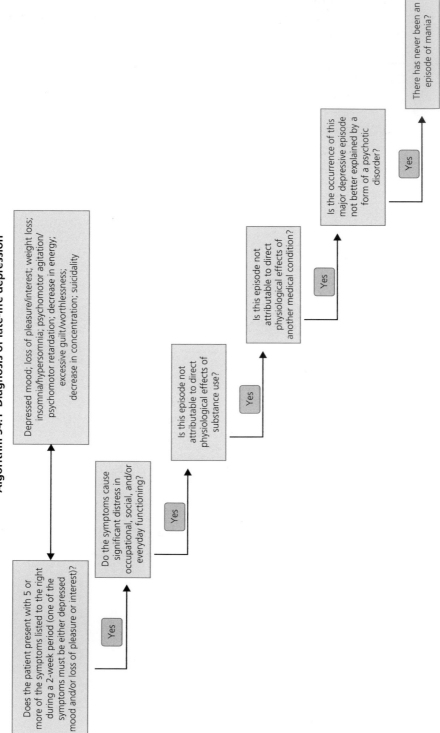

Treatment
Treatment rationale
- SSRI for 6–12 months is usually first-line treatment, although depending on comorbid symptoms may instead consider:
  - Mirtazapine (if poor sleep/appetite).
  - SNRI (if severe psychomotor retardation).
  - Well-validated psychotherapy: CBT, problem-solving therapy, interpersonal psychotherapy; alone or in combination with medications.
    - The decision to begin with medication or psychotherapy should be informed by assessment of illness severity, medical comorbidities, treatment history, and patient preference.
  - Side effect profile should generally guide medication choice.
  - Rule is "start low and go slow, but go," so as to minimize side effects, but final target dose for remission may be no different from general adult populations.
- If initial medication is ineffective after reaching therapeutic dose and after a fair time trial, change medication.
  - If second medication is ineffective, consider adjunctive medications with different mechanisms of action (e.g., bupropion, although literature supporting its efficacy as an augmenting strategy in geriatric patients is limited).
  - Methylphenidate can also be a second- or third-line treatment strategy.
- ECT is effective for treatment-refractory depression or depression with psychotic features, and is treatment of choice in patients with severe weight loss and profound anorexia.
  - Standard course: 6–12 treatments over 2–4 weeks, followed by maintenance antidepressant treatment with possible continuation of ECT.
- Low doses of benzodiazepines are often useful for comorbid anxiety; use caution in patients with unsteady gait and cognitive impairment as side effects include falls and confusion.
- Most experts advocate maintenance pharmacotherapy for 6–12 months following remission. Some evidence shows lower relapse rates with pharmacotherapy plus psychotherapy for 2 years. For recurrent late-life depression requiring hospitalization, continuation of pharmacotherapy for 3 years or life-long treatment may help sustain remission.

When to hospitalize
- Patients who pose a danger to themselves because of suicidal thinking or behavior.
- Patients who pose a danger to others due to aggression or agitation.
- Poor self-care leading to malnutrition and dehydration.

Managing the hospitalized patient
- Ensure the patient is not a danger to self or others.
- Titrate medications appropriately.
- For patients who have had multiple medication trials, consider ECT.
- Arrange for appropriate outpatient treatment, including referral to comprehensive psychosocial services and medical consultants if appropriate.

Table of treatment

Medication
• Fluoxetine
  10–40 mg daily
• Sertraline
  100–200 mg daily
• Paroxetine
  10–40 mg nightly
• Citalopram
  10–40 mg daily
• Escitalopram
  10–20 mg daily
• Mirtazapine
  7.5–45 mg nightly
• Venlafaxine
  150–300 mg daily
• Duloxetine
  20–120 mg daily
• Bupropion
  75–300 mg daily in
  divided doses
• Nortriptyline
  10–125 mg nightly
• Desipramine
  25–200 mg daily
• Methylphenidate
  5–20 mg daily
	• Many can cause nausea, tremor, insomnia, fatigue
	• SSRIs can cause platelet disaggregation; caution in patients on anticoagulants
	• Citalopram can lead to prolonged QTc at ≥40 mg
	• Venlafaxine may cause increased blood pressure at higher doses; monitor BP
	• Duloxetine should be used with caution in patients with liver disease
	• Bupropion should not be used in patients with seizure disorders
	• Tricyclics are contraindicated in patients with cardiac arrhythmias, recent myocardial infarction, glaucoma, urinary retention, benign prostatic hyperplasia, or cognitive impairment
	• Methylphenidate may cause increased anxiety, restlessness, and tachycardia

	• Methylphenidate may cause increased anxiety, restlessness, and tachycardia. Should not be used in patients with seizure disorder, cardiac arrhythmias and patients with family history of sudden cardiac arrest
ECT	• May cause temporary anterograde and retrograde amnesia
Psychotherapy • CBT • Interpersonal psychotherapy	

Prevention/management of complications
- SSRIs/SNRIs can cause syndrome of inappropriate antidiuretic hormone secretion (SIADH); monitor sodium for hyponatremia.
- Tricyclic antidepressants: monitor for cardiac abnormalities and anticholinergic effects.
- ECT: monitor for memory impairment in the immediate post-treatment period. Consider decreasing frequency of treatments if cognitive impairment is problematic.

Management/treatment algorithm (Algorithm 34.2)

Algorithm 34.2 Management of late-life depression

```
┌──────────────────────┐       ┌──────────────────────┐
│ Does patient also    │◄─────►│ Does the patient meet│
│ present with         │       │ criteria for         │
│ psychotic features?  │       │ late-life depression?│
└──────────────────────┘       └──────────────────────┘
         │ Yes                          │ Yes
         ▼                              ▼
┌──────────────────────┐       ┌──────────────────────┐       ┌──────────────────────┐
│ Start adjunctive     │       │ Start SSRI and titrate│◄────►│ Add psychotherapy    │
│ antipsychotic        │       │ to theraputic dose   │       │ (CBT, IPT, PST)      │
└──────────────────────┘       └──────────────────────┘       └──────────────────────┘
                                          │
                           No             ▼            Yes
                        ┌─────── Is there remission of symptoms? ───────┐
                        ▼                                               ▼
┌──────────────────────────────┐                         ┌──────────────────────┐
│ Switch SSRI agents, consider │                         │ Continue maintenance │
│ atypical agents if there are │                         │ therapy (6–12 months)│
│ other comorbidities, consider│                         └──────────────────────┘
│ adding adjunctive            │                                    │
│ antidepressant such as       │                                    │
│ bupropion                    │                                    │
└──────────────────────────────┘                                    │
          │                                                          │
          └───────── Does the patient stay in remission? ───────────┘
                                    │ No
                                    ▼
┌──────────────────────────────┐
│ Consider antidepressant for  │◄── No
│ 3 year–lifetime duration     │
│ (depending on severity of    │
│ number of relapses)          │
└──────────────────────────────┘
          │
          └───────── Does the patient stay in remission?
                                    │ No
                                    ▼
┌──────────────────────────────┐
│ Consider ECT                 │◄── No
└──────────────────────────────┘
```

CLINICAL PEARLS

- With medications, "start low and go slow, but go."
- Inadequate treatment can lead to poor outcomes and frequent relapses.
- Advise patients/families that full benefit of antidepressants may not be apparent until 12 weeks after initiation of treatment.
- Treatment failure with one medication does not necessarily mean the patient will not respond to another medication in the same class.
- Combined psychotherapy and psychopharmacology is effective treatment for late-life depression.
- ECT is the treatment of choice for treatment-refractory depression, psychotic depression, and depression with severe weight loss and anorexia.

Prognosis

BOTTOM LINE/CLINICAL PEARLS
- Relapse/recurrence rates (50–90% over 2–3 years) are higher in late-life than in general adult depression.
- Relapse may be prevented by maintenance antidepressant treatment.

Natural history of untreated disease
- Multiple recurrences, with increased risk of suicide, medical comorbidities, and disability.

Prognosis for treated patients
- Approximately 50% of patients receiving adequate medication(s) achieve full response or remission.
- A recently published meta-analysis demonstrated that geriatric patients with a longer duration of depression receive greater benefit from antidepressants than do those with a shorter duration of illness.
- Older age seems to positively influence robustness of response to ECT.

Follow-up tests and monitoring
- Monitor for symptoms after remission.
- Rating scales are efficient and can be used in primary care settings.
- Patients whose illness requires hospitalization, ECT, or complicated psychopharmacological regimens should be monitored by specialists in geriatric psychiatry.

Reading list
Andreescu C, Roynolds CF 3rd. Late-life depression: evidenced-based treatment and promising new directions for research and clinical practice. Psychiatr Clin North Am 2011;34(2):335–55.

Ellison JM, Kyomen HH, Harper DG. Depression in later life: an overview with treatment recommendations. Psychiatr Clin North Am 2012;35(1):203–29.

Kastenschmidt EK, Kennedy GJ. Depression and anxiety in late life: diagnostic insights and therapeutic options. Mt Sinai J Med 2011;78(4):527–45.

Nelson JC, Delucchi KL, Schneider LS. Moderators of outcome in late-life depression: a patient level meta-analysis. Am J Psychiatry 2013;170(6):651–9.

Unutzer J. Late-life depression. N Engl J Med 2007;357:22.

van der Wurff FB, Stek ML, Hoogendijk WJ, Beekman AT. The efficacy and safety of ECT in depressed older adults: a literature review. Int J Geriatr Psychiatry 2003;18(10):894–904.

Suggested websites
UpToDate®. http://www.uptodate.com

American Association for Geriatric Psychiatry. http://www.aagponline.org

Guidelines
National society guidelines

Title	Source	Weblink
Pharmacotherapy for late-life depression	Journal of Clinical Psychiatry, 2011	http://www.ncbi.nlm.nih.gov/pubmed/21272511
Pharmacotherapy of depression in older patients: a summary of the expert consensus guidelines	Journal of Psychiatric Practice, 2001	http://www.ncbi.nlm.nih.gov/pubmed/15990550

International society guidelines

Title	Source	Weblink
Guideline for the management of late-life depression in primary care	International Journal of Geriatric Psychiatry, 2003	http://www.ncbi.nlm.nih.gov/pubmed/12949851

Evidence

Type of evidence	Title and comment	Weblink
Cochrane Review	Antidepressants for depressed elderly (Review). **Comment:** TCAs and SSRIs have similar efficacy, although TCAs have greater side effect and withdrawal profile.	http://www.ncbi.nlm.nih.gov/pubmed/16437456
Randomized controlled trial (RCT)	Maintenance treatment of major depression in old age. **Comment:** Depressed patients ≥70 years who responded to initial treatment with paroxetine and interpersonal psychotherapy were less likely to have recurrence if they received additional 2 years of maintenance paroxetine.	http://www.ncbi.nlm.nih.gov/pubmed/16540613
Literature review	The efficacy and safety of ECT in depressed older adults: a literature review. **Comment:** ECT is effective and generally considered safe. More studies need to be performed regarding long-term efficacy, morbidity, and mortality of ECT vs antidepressants.	http://www.ncbi.nlm.nih.gov/pubmed/14533122
Meta-analysis	Moderators of outcome in late-life depression: a patient level meta-analysis. **Comment:** Older patients with a long duration of moderate–severe depression benefit from antidepressants.	http://www.ncbi.nlm.nih.gov/pubmed/23598969

Additional material for this chapter can be found online at:
www.mountsinaiexpertguides.com/psychiatry

This includes advice for patients, a case study, ICD codes, and multiple choice questions.

CHAPTER 35

Late-Life Psychosis

Matthew F. Majeske[1], Violeta Nistor[2], and Charles H. Kellner[1]

[1] Icahn School of Medicine at Mount Sinai, New York, NY, USA
[2] Western Carolina Psychiatric Associates, Greenwood, SC, USA

OVERALL BOTTOM LINE

- The most common diagnoses associated with psychosis in geriatric patients are, in order, major neurocognitive disorder (dementia) and major depressive disorder (MDD).
- Visual hallucinations may reflect delirium or neurocognitive disorder (NCD) due to Lewy body disease.
- MDD with psychotic features responds robustly to electroconvulsive therapy (ECT), which should be considered a first-line treatment.
- When prescribing antipsychotics, start with low doses, titrate slowly, and frequently reassess. Geriatric patients may be at greater risk of side effects. If the patient stabilizes after several months, attempt a slow taper.
- In this chapter we will limit discussion to non-schizophrenic late-life psychosis.

Background
Definition of disease
- Psychosis is a gross impairment of reality testing, often manifest by hallucinations or delusions.
- In elderly patients, psychotic symptoms are frequently a complicating feature of an underlying psychiatric, neurological, or medical disorder.

Disease classification
- Psychotic symptoms can be an inherent aspect of an illness (so-called primary, e.g., schizophrenia, MDD with psychotic features) or a secondary complicating factor (e.g., dementia, substances, medications, medical conditions, delirium).

Incidence/prevalence
- 0.2–4.7% in community samples.
- 10% in nursing homes.
- 63% in NCD due to Alzheimer's disease (AD).

Economic impact
- Medical treatment of the illness (medications, hospitalization, worsened physical health status, etc.) carries substantial costs.
- Severe functional disability affects the surrounding environment and worsens caregiver stress, leading to reduced productivity beyond that of the patient.

Mount Sinai Expert Guides: Psychiatry, First Edition. Edited by Asher B. Simon, Antonia S. New, and Wayne K. Goodman.
© 2017 John Wiley & Sons, Ltd. Published 2017 by John Wiley & Sons, Ltd.
Companion website: www.mountsinaiexpertguides.com/psychiatry

Etiology

- Earlier-onset/primary psychotic disorders – schizophrenia and related disorders, bipolar disorder with psychotic features – often extend into old age.
- Late-life psychosis most often occurs secondary to NCD (dementia), MDD, delirium, medications (e.g., dopaminergic agents, steroids), and medical conditions.
  - Several interconnecting mechanisms may lead to psychosis in these patients:
    - limited cognitive reserve; frailty; increased vulnerability to the effects of stressors and poor ability to adapt; aberrant neurotransmitters controlling cognitive function, behavior, mood, and perception; social isolation; genetics.

Pathophysiology

- The aging brain shows a disproportion in the synthesis, discharge, and inactivation of noradrenergic, serotonergic, and dopaminergic neurons, loss of resilience, and loss of cognitive reserve, all increasing the risk for psychosis developing as a complication of an underlying pathology.
- Psychosis in dementia is correlated with decreased serotonin in the cerebral cortex and enhanced catecholamine responsiveness.

Predictive/risk factors

- Moderate to severe neurocognitive impairment.
- Depression.
- Polypharmacy.
- Multiple medical problems.

Prevention

> **BOTTOM LINE/CLINICAL PEARLS**
> - Maintain good overall mental and physical health.
> - In patients with NCD, provide environmental orienting cues (e.g., lighting according to a normal circadian rhythm, adequate intellectual and environmental stimulation, limit isolation).
> - Limit polypharmacy in patients with NCD.

Screening

- Patients with first episode late-onset psychosis.
- General Health Questionnaire (GHQ): 5 items; first step to screen psychiatric symptoms.
- Mental status exam (MSE).
- Brief Psychiatric Rating Scale (BPRS): can target psychotic symptoms.
- Neuropsychiatric Inventory (NPI): for behavioral disturbances in patients with dementia.

Secondary (and primary) prevention

- Maintain good nutrition.
- Avoid medical illness.
- Avoid vitamin-deficiency states.
- Avoid substances and other toxic exposures (alcohol, cannabis, heavy metals).
- Maintenance treatment with antipsychotics if needed.
- Person-centered care may reduce agitation in demented elderly.
- Caregiver education and support.

Diagnosis

> **BOTTOM LINE/CLINICAL PEARLS**
> - Inquire about history of hallucinations or delusions; ask patient and family.
> - Consider whether symptoms occur in the context of cognitive impairment, mood disturbance, or medical illness.
> - In the MSE, explore unusual sensory experiences (visual, auditory) and idiosyncratic/odd beliefs.
> - Consider metabolic panel, CBC, thyroid function, vitamin levels, neuroimaging, and neuropsychological testing.

Differential diagnosis

Differential diagnosis	Features
NCD	Moderate to severe cognitive impairment (psychosis may be a complication)
Delirium	Altered sensorium, medical illness, intoxication (psychosis may be a complication)
Depression	Low mood, guilt, suicidality (psychosis may be a complication)
Mania	Elated/irritable mood, hyperactivity, pressured speech (psychosis may be a complication)
Schizophrenia	History of psychosis antecedes old age
Delusional disorder	Retained functionality

Typical presentation
- Psychosis complicating dementia typically presents in patients >65 with medical comorbidities. The patient is usually brought in by family who report that he or she is behaving in an increasingly strange manner (e.g., inactive/withdrawn; smiling/laughing for no apparent reason; whispering when alone; incoherence).
- Elderly patients with psychotic depression are usually brought in by family who report that the patient has been more withdrawn and slowed down. Further inquiry reveals that the patient has seemed or has mentioned feeling sad and helpless and has been worrying excessively about finances and health problems. Usual depressive symptoms complete the picture, although elderly patients may manifest more complaints of physical symptoms (e.g., pain, gastrointestinal problems). Psychotic symptoms are often mood-congruent (e.g., delusions of guilt or punishment, nihilistic delusions, persecutory voices).

Clinical diagnosis
History
- Delusions, hallucinations, disorganized behavior, abnormal motor behavior (including catatonia), negative symptoms (apathy, social withdrawal, alogia).
- Assess for impaired cognition, depression, and mania.
- Corroborating information from family and caregivers is crucial, as patients may not share relevant information due to paranoia, memory impairment, etc.
- The context, presumed etiology, and severity of psychotic symptoms guide diagnosis, treatment, and prognosis.

- Persecutory delusions with cognitive impairment in elderly patients may suggest NCD.
- Psychosis with depression suggests major depression with psychotic features.
- Prominent negative symptoms are characteristic of schizophrenia.
- Recent or sudden onset of psychotic symptoms in the context of medical illness or polypharmacy may indicate delirium.

Physical and mental status exams
- Delusions and formal thought disorder are best elicited by open-ended questions:
  - "Has anything been troubling you lately?"
  - "How is your relationship with your spouse?"
  - "Has anyone been playing games on you?"
  - When responses are difficult to comprehend, incoherent, impoverished, or devoid of content, this can be indicative of loosening of associations, tangentiality, or poverty of speech or content of speech.
- Hallucinations are elicited by asking about sensory experiences:
  - "Do you see things no one else sees?"
  - "Do you hear people talking when no one else is around?"
  - "Do you ever hear your thoughts out loud?"
- Evaluate the patient's level of alertness when considering delirium.

Useful clinical decision rules
- Brief Psychiatric Rating Scale (BPRS) can be useful across multiple domains (psychotic and mood symptoms).
- Mini mental state exam (MMSE) is a rapid and useful gauge of cognitive function.

Disease severity classification
- "Clinician Rated Dimensions of Psychosis Symptom Severity" in DSM-5 provides assessment of multiple factors on a scale of 0–4.

Laboratory diagnosis
List of diagnostic tests
- Consider metabolic panel, CBC, B$_{12}$, folate, thyroid function, RPR, and urinalysis to rule out possible medical causes (e.g., infection, electrolyte abnormality, endocrinopathy, metabolic disturbance, vitamin deficiency, etc.).
- EEG if seizures suspected.
- Lumbar puncture if CNS infection suspected.

Lists of imaging techniques
- Consider a CT or MRI of the brain to rule out a mass lesion for a sudden onset of psychotic symptoms in a previously healthy individual.

Diagnostic algorithm (Algorithm 35.1)

Potential pitfalls/common errors made regarding diagnosis of disease
- Failure to rule out medical causes.
- Failure to identify cognitive impairment or mood disturbance.

Algorithm 35.1 Diagnosis of late-life psychosis

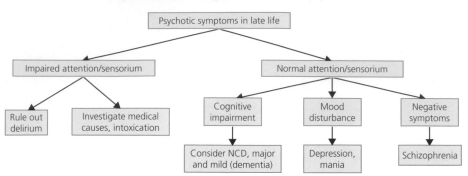

Treatment
Treatment rationale
- Antipsychotics pose special risks in the elderly.
  - Higher risk of extrapyramidal symptoms (EPS).
  - Increased risk of stroke and mortality from all causes.
  - In patients with NCD, clinical benefit may be modest.
- Start with low doses and titrate slowly.
  - Frequently reassess target symptoms and toxicity.
  - Avoid polypharmacy; several drug trials may be necessary to find an effective agent.
  - First-generation antipsychotics (e.g., haloperidol) have greater EPS.
  - Second-generation antipsychotics (e.g., risperidone, olanzapine) have greater metabolic side effects (e.g., weight gain, hyperglycemia).
  - After 3–6 months of symptom remission, attempt taper and discontinue.
- Patients with schizophrenia may require higher doses than patients with other psychoses.
- ECT has a robust effect in elderly patients and should be considered first-line in patients with psychotic mood disorders.
- When psychosis occurs in the context of delirium, identify and treat the underlying cause.
  - Short-term use of high-potency and low-anticholinergic antipsychotics may be used to control symptoms.

When to hospitalize
- Suicidality.
- Severe malnutrition or failure to care for self.
- Violence.
- Severe caregiver stress.

Managing the hospitalized patient
- Same medication principles as outpatient.
- Geriatric medicine evaluation to address underlying medical illness.
- ECT consultation if mood symptoms predominate.

Table of treatment

Medical • Aripiprazole 2–15 mg daily • Risperidone 0.5–2 mg once to twice daily • Quetiapine 25–600 mg once to twice daily • Olanzapine 2.5–10 mg once daily • Haloperidol 0.5–2 mg two to three times daily • Clozapine 25–400 mg once to twice daily	• Moderate sedation, occasional akathisia • Moderate EPS, metabolic side effects • Greater sedation; best choice for psychosis in Parkinson's disease due to low antidopaminergic effects • Greater metabolic and anticholinergic side effects • Greater EPS • Treatment-resistant schizophrenia; use in psychosis in Parkinson's disease due to low EPS
Device-based • ECT	• Excellent efficacy in mood disorders; may cause memory disturbance
Other • Orienting the patient, maintaining regular routines and activities (including sleep), interpersonal and independent skills training as well as programs and interventions aimed to improve coping skills and reduce stress	

Prevention/management of complications
- From antipsychotics:
  - EPS: treat very judiciously with anticholinergics (benztropine 0.5–2 mg daily).
  - Akathisia: attempt dose reduction; propranolol 10–20 mg bid.
  - Weight gain, hyperglycemia: cross taper to another agent.
  - Increased risk of stroke or death: after period of stability, attempt slow taper of drug.
- From ECT:
  - Confusion, memory impairment: pause or discontinue treatments.

Management/treatment algorithm (Algorithm 35.2)

Algorithm 35.2 Management of late-life psychosis

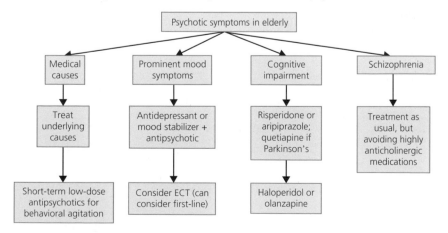

CLINICAL PEARLS
- Use low doses of antipsychotics and titrate slowly.
- Choose antipsychotic based on side-effect profile.
- Consider taper after 3–6 months of symptom control.
- ECT has unparalleled efficacy in mood disorders with psychotic features.

Prognosis

BOTTOM LINE/CLINICAL PEARLS
- In dementia, psychotic symptoms have a fluctuating course and may give way to apathy or aggression as the disease progresses.
- In mood disorders, psychotic symptoms may improve and remit along with the mood symptoms.
- In delirium, psychotic symptoms tend to wax and wane.

Reading list

Chenoweth L, King MT, Jeon YH, et al. Caring for Aged Dementia Care Resident Study (CADRES) of person-centred care, dementia-care mapping, and usual care in dementia: a cluster-randomised trial. Lancet Neurol 2009;8(4):317–25.

Devanand DP. Psychosis. In: Coffey CE, Cummings JL (eds). Textbook of Geriatric Neuropsychiatry, 3rd edn. Washington, DC: American Psychiatric Publishing, 2011, pp. 517–535.

Holroyd S, Laurie S. Correlates of psychotic symptoms among elderly outpatients. Int J Geriatr Psychiatry 1999;14(5):379–84.

Schneider LS, Tariot PN, Dagerman KS, et al.; CATIE-AD Study Group. Effectiveness of atypical antipsychotic drugs in patients with Alzheimer's disease. N Engl J Med 2006;355(15):1525–38.

Solai L. Late-life psychosis. In: Miller MD, Solai LK (eds). Geriatric Psychiatry. New York: Oxford University Press, 2013, pp. 237–53.

Zayas EM, Grossberg GT. The treatment of psychosis in late life. J Clin Psychiatry 1998;59 Suppl 1:5–10.

Suggested websites

American Geriatrics Society (AGS). http://www.americangeriatrics.org

American Psychiatric Association. http://www.psychiatry.org

Guidelines
National society guidelines

Title	Source	Weblink
Practice Guideline on the Use of Antipsychotics to Treat Agitation or Psychosis in Patients with Dementia	American Psychiatric Association (APA), 2016	http://dx.doi.org/10.1176/appi.books.9780890426807

Evidence

Type of evidence	Title and comment	Weblink
Meta-analysis	Efficacy and adverse effects of atypical antipsychotics for dementia: meta-analysis of randomized, placebo-controlled trials. **Comment:** Modest efficacy of atypical antipsychotics for treatment of behavioral symptoms in Alzheimer's dementia.	http://www.ncbi.nlm.nih.gov/pubmed/16505124
Systematic review and meta-analysis	Early interventions to prevent psychosis: systematic review and meta-analysis. **Comment:** Individual cognitive behavioral therapy (CBT), with or without family CBT, could be used as a first-line treatment for people at a high risk of developing psychosis.	http://www.ncbi.nlm.nih.gov/pubmedhealth/PMH0051983/

Additional material for this chapter can be found online at: www.mountsinaiexpertguides.com/psychiatry

This includes advice for patients, a case study, ICD codes, and multiple choice questions.

PART 5

Special Topics

CHAPTER 36

Approach to the Violent, Aggressive, and Agitated Patient

Nelly Alia-Klein[1], Amy L. Johnson[2], Naomi Schmelzer[3], and Antonia S. New[1]

[1] Icahn School of Medicine at Mount Sinai, New York, NY, USA
[2] Weill Cornell Medical College, New York, NY, USA
[3] Brigham and Women's Hospital, Boston, MA, USA

OVERALL BOTTOM LINE
- Agitation, aggression, and violent behaviors can be found across many psychiatric disorders but there are a few diagnoses where these behaviors are core features.
- Aggressive behaviors start in childhood with genetic and environmental contributions and are amenable to primary prevention, such as anti-bullying education.
- Staff acute management of immediate threat by the agitated patient is paramount and includes behavioral and pharmacological intervention and clear environmental controls.
- Chronic management of the agitated and aggressive patient involves psychotherapy and pharmacotherapy.

Typology and diagnosis of aggression in the psychiatric patient

- Negative emotions are experienced by most patients with psychiatric diagnoses.
- Negative emotions can be expressed as anger and agitation, which could lead to aggressive and violent behaviors, endangering others.
- Aggression is defined as hostile, injurious, or destructive behavior. It is subtyped as reactive or impulsive vs planned or instrumental.
- Agitation, aggression, and violent behaviors can be found across psychiatric disorders but are core features of some disorders:
  - **Personality disorders** (see Chapter 17) in particular, **antisocial personality disorder (ASPD)** and **borderline personality disorder (BPD)**.
  - **Disruptive, impulse control, and conduct disorders** (Chapter 29). These include oppositional defiant, conduct, and disruptive behavior disorders and pyromania in childhood or adolescence (see Chapter 30) and **intermittent explosive disorder (IED)** and ASPD in adulthood.
- Importantly, anger and aggression in the context of **other psychiatric disorders** can be present and can exacerbate severity and complicate treatment delivery.
  - For example, in psychotic disorders, behavioral dyscontrol is associated with the patient's conviction that they have no control over their own behavior due to external threat and external control of mind and body. Trait anger can also interact with symptoms of psychosis and is associated with increased rates of violent behavior.

Mount Sinai Expert Guides: Psychiatry, First Edition. Edited by Asher B. Simon, Antonia S. New, and Wayne K. Goodman.
© 2017 John Wiley & Sons, Ltd. Published 2017 by John Wiley & Sons, Ltd.
Companion website: www.mountsinaiexpertguides.com/psychiatry

- Other examples include delirium and acute intoxication and withdrawal that are associated with increased risk for violent behavior by the agitated patient.

Primary prevention and education to reduce aggression and violence

- Anger and aggression are partially heritable and appear to be developmental with prenatal risk factors and early indications emerging during the preschool and school years. Therefore, prevention can start with proper education during prenatal care.
  - For example, animal and human studies show that smoking during pregnancy increases the risk of conduct problems in a dose-related manner, particularly in male offspring. The suggested mechanism for this is through tobacco smoke's actions as a monoamine oxidase inhibitor at critical points during prenatal development.
  - Since the aggressive phenotype emerges in early childhood and during school years, interventions to minimize aggression target bullying behaviors. Given the high prevalence of bullying in schools and its strong relationship to externalizing psychopathologies such as conduct disorders and **attention deficit hyperactivity disorder (ADHD)**, many bullying prevention programs have been developed and tested. Meta-analyses of these studies reveal that school-based anti-bullying programs decrease bullying by 20–23% and decrease victimization by 17–20%, resulting in a relatively small odds ratio of ~1.36.
- The most effective elements associated with a decrease in bullying included parent training/meetings, supervision and disciplinary methods, classroom management, teacher training, classroom rules, a whole-school anti-bullying policy, school conferences, information for parents, and cooperative group work. An extensive number of elements and a long duration and intensity of the program for teachers and children were most significantly associated with a decrease in bullying.

Acute management of immediate threat in clinical settings

- Agitation and aggression are commonly encountered in the acute hospital setting. There are numerous de-escalation techniques with which staff should become familiar. The American Association for Emergency Psychiatry published guidelines for Best Practices in Evaluation and Treatment of Agitation, which include:
  - **Verbal de-escalation:** staff should make attempts to collaborate with the patient, rather than yelling back, issuing threats, or resorting to coercion.
  - **Improving patient's comfort and sense of safety.**
  - **Psychopharmacological management:** medications may be required, but as far as possible, patients should be involved in the discussion of type and route. There is no single medication that is preferred in all cases of agitation; rather, there are three general classes that have been studied: first- and second-generation antipsychotics and benzodiazepines (see Table 42.2).
  - **Seclusion and restraint:** rarely, when verbal de-escalation and medication are not yet effective and the patient is so agitated that he or she is an imminent and serious danger to him/herself or others, seclusion or restraint may be required. Standard physical restraint for violent patients involves four-point restraint. The clinician should be familiar with hospital and regulatory guidelines regarding its limited use.
  - **Environmental controls:** ample physical space and adequate staffing. (1) Controls to prevent the availability of weapon use: do not leave any instruments or weapons in the area near the potentially violent patient. (2) Doors should be locked. (3) Surveillance as well

as seclusion should be considered to ensure safety. All staff, including security personnel, should have adequate training and be knowledgeable on response options.
- The essential first step in the management of the agitated patient is to *assess for and treat any life-threatening causes of agitation*. Depending on the severity of agitation, this may need to co-occur with other management strategies noted above. Oftentimes, treatment of underlying medical and psychiatric disorders will be sufficient to treat agitation, but there are times when this alone is not adequate or when the etiology is unknown.

Chronic treatment of the agitated and aggressive patient

The management of aggression in a non-acute setting is most effectively accomplished with targeted psychotherapy; however, there are some medications that seem to have a positive influence in decreasing impulsive aggression.

Psychotherapy
- Studies of aggression per se have shown a high degree of efficacy for **cognitive behavioral therapy (CBT).**
  - CBT reduces the use of negative anger strategies in problem solving and does so at least as effectively in those with Cluster B personality disorders, including APD and BPD, as in those without a Cluster B personality disorder.
  - In male perpetrators of domestic violence who were willing to seek treatment, a 4-month CBT program aimed at decreasing partner violence was much more successful in reducing such violence than control perpetrators on a wait list who were also willing to participate in treatment.
  - In patients specifically diagnosed with IED, 12 weeks of CBT was better than wait list control in improving aggressive acts, anger, and depressed mood, and those improvements persisted 3 months after treatment completion.
- Many other evidence-based psychotherapies for BPD that target emotion regulation reduce impulsive aggression in individuals with BPD (see Chapter 17). These include:
  - **Dialectical behavioral therapy (DBT):** while not studied for outpatient impulsive aggression per se, emotional skills training has been shown to be effective in reducing aggression. Specifically, a corrections-modified DBT program (a 16-week DBT-CM) reduced aggressive behavior in a correctional setting.
  - **Transference focused psychotherapy (TFP).**
  - **Mentalization based therapy (MBT).**
- Overall, diverse approaches to the management of aggression have shown some efficacy, but there have been no head-to-head trials to compare efficacy of CBT to therapies employing emotion regulation skills or social skills training. What the studies share is that short-term (normally ~8 sessions) skills-based therapy targeting anger and aggression demonstrates positive results in reducing anger and aggression.

Psychopharmacology
- Most of the data on the pharmacologic management of impulsive aggression have been gathered in individuals with personality disorders (Chapter 17). Table 36.1 lists medications with demonstrated efficacy in reducing impulsive aggression over an 8- to 12-week period of treatment.
  - The **serotonin-selective reuptake inhibitors (SSRIs),** and particularly **fluoxetine**, have been shown to decrease aggression in men with personality disorders and IED.

- **Atypical antipsychotics** have been shown to decrease impulsive aggression in personality disorder patients and in those with schizophrenia.
- Notably, topiramate is not included in Table 36.1 as it has been shown to decrease aggression in some studies but to increase aggression in others. This mixed effect cuts across diagnoses and even in the studies in which aggression is reduced, the effect size is small.
- Lithium is also not included in Table 36.1 as its efficacy has been demonstrated predominantly in children with aggression, in adults with bipolar disorder, and in adults in an inpatient setting. In those studies, serum levels of 1.0–1.2 mEq/L appeared to be effective.
- The pharmacology of aggression prophylaxis is beyond the scope of this review, but meta-analyses have shown that **stimulants** diminish aggressive behavior in children with ADHD. Pharmacological treatments for agitation in the context of trauma- and stressor-related disorders can be found in Chapter 13.

Table 36.1 Psychopharmacologic agents for management of impulsive aggression.

Drug (dose)	Diagnostic group			
	Personality disorders	Psychotic disorders	ADHD/disruptive behavior	Bipolar disorder
Olanzapine	5 mg/day po	5–10 mg/day		5–10 mg/day
Aripiprazole	5–15 mg/day po	15–30 mg/day po		30 mg/day po
Clozapine		200–800 mg/day*		
Quietiapine	400 mg/day po			400–800 mg/day po
Risperidone			1–2 mg /day	
Depakote	500–750 mg/day			
Lamotrigine	50–200 mg/day			

* More than olanzapine and haloperidol.

Reading list

Brennan PA, Grekin ER, Mednick SA. Maternal smoking during pregnancy and adult male criminal outcomes. Arch Gen Psychiatry 1999;56(3):215–9.

Coccaro E. Treating intermittent explosive disorder. Harvard Mental Health Letter, 2011. Available at http://www.health.harvard.edu/newsletter_article/treating-intermittent-explosive-disorder

Glancy G. Saini MA. An evidenced-based review of psychological treatments of anger and aggression. Brief Treatment and Crisis Intervention 2005;5(2):229–48.

Holloman GH, Zeller SL. Overview of Project BETA: Best practices in Evaluation and Treatment of Agitation. West J Emerg Med 2012;13(1):1–2.

Knox DK, Holloman GH. Use and Avoidance of Seclusion and Restraint: Consensus Statement of the American Association for Emergency Psychiatry Project BETA Seclusion and Restraint Workgroup. West J Emerg Med 2012;13(1):35–40.

Reagu S, Jones R, Kumari V, Taylor PJ. Angry affect and violence in the context of psychotic illness: A systematic review and meta-analysis of the literature. Schizophr Res 2013;146:46–52.

Richmond JS, Berlin JS, Fishkind AB, et al. Verbal De-escalation of the Agitated Patient: Consensus Statement of the American Association for Emergency Psychiatry Project BETA De-escalation Workgroup. West J Emerg Med 2012;13(1):17–25.

Siever L. Neurobiology of aggression and violence. Am J Psychiatry 2008;165:429–42.

Ttofi MM, Farrington DP. Effectiveness of school based programs to reduce bullying: a systematic and meta-analytic review. J Exp Criminol 2011;7:27–56.

Wilson MP, Pepper D, Currier GW, Holloman GH, Feifel D. The Psychopharmacology of Agitation: Consensus Statement of the American Association for Emergency Psychiatry Project BETA Psychopharmacology Workgroup. West J Emerg Med 2012;13(1):26–34.

Additional material for this chapter can be found online at:
www.mountsinaiexpertguides.com/psychiatry

This includes a case study, ICD codes, and multiple choice questions.

CHAPTER 37

Approach to the Suicidal Patient

Marianne Goodman[1] and Violeta Nistor[2]
[1] Icahn School of Medicine at Mount Sinai, New York, NY, USA
[2] Western Carolina Psychiatric Associates, Greenwood, SC, USA

OVERALL BOTTOM LINE

- Suicide was the tenth leading cause of death in the USA for all ages in 2010 and continues to remain a major health problem.
- Suicide risk assessment is the most important tool for the treatment and management of the suicidal patient.
- This chapter reviews the spectrum of suicide ideation, suicide completion, and suicide attempt.
- Management of suicidal patients includes a wide range of interventions addressing suicidal behavior, personality disorders and other major mental illness, psychosocial issues, and interpersonal stressors,
- The least restrictive setting should be used for the treatment of suicidal patients and hospitalization should be selected for patients presenting a threat to self or others.

Introduction

- There were 38,364 suicides in 2010 in the USA, an average of 105 each day or one suicide every 14 minutes.
- It is estimated that there are 25 suicide attempts for every completed suicide.
- Although only a small number of attempts result in death, each attempt increases the risk of death.
- Suicide is one of the most common reasons for psychiatric emergency department visits.

Assessing suicide risk

- Suicide completion leads to long-term and devastating effects for both the family and the treating psychiatrist.
- Suicide risk assessment is the most important tool for the treatment and management of the suicidal patient and it is now a *core competency* element for psychiatrists in training.
- Psychiatrists do not have a reliable tool to predict suicide in individual patients. The current best available tool is a *systematic suicide risk assessment*, which can help organize risks and protective factors that may help in the treatment and safety of the patient.

Mount Sinai Expert Guides: Psychiatry, First Edition. Edited by Asher B. Simon, Antonia S. New, and Wayne K. Goodman.
© 2017 John Wiley & Sons, Ltd. Published 2017 by John Wiley & Sons, Ltd.
Companion website: www.mountsinaiexpertguides.com/psychiatry

Risk factors

Suicidal behavior is multi-axial and numerous risk factors have been described, including those listed in the American Psychiatric Association (APA) Guidelines for the Assessment and Treatment of Patients with Suicidal Behavior:

- *The most powerful risk factor for predicting suicide-related behavior and completed suicide is the history of suicide attempts.*
- Psychiatric diagnoses, such as major depressive disorder, bipolar disorder (primarily in depressive or mixed episodes), schizophrenia, anorexia nervosa, alcohol use disorder, Cluster B personality disorders (particularly borderline personality disorder), comorbidity of axis I and/or axis II disorders.
- Demographics such as male gender, widowed, divorced, or single marital status, particularly for men, elderly age group (age group with greatest proportionate risk for suicide), adolescent and young adult age groups (age groups with highest numbers of suicides), white race, gay, lesbian, or bisexual orientation.
- Traumatic events such as sexual or physical abuse, interpersonal transitions, such as recent lack of social support (including living alone), unemployment, drop in social status, poor relationships with family, recent stressful life event, and previous suicidal behavior.
- Impulsive aggression, substance dependence, and comorbid antisocial personality disorder.
- Disruption in the continuity of care, especially after discharge, in the mental health system.

Protective factors

- Regular contact and care for patients, including those resisting treatment, was beneficial.
  - For example, patients who refused to continue treatment after evaluation but who received a follow-up letter at least four times a year had a considerably lower risk of suicide than patients who did not receive the letters.
  - Other randomized clinical trials established the positive influence of interventions that provide a concerned supportive network through letters, brief interviews, or phone contacts in reducing suicide-related behaviors.
- Another protective factor is the supportive relationship between patient and clinician. Establishing a positive therapeutic alliance leads to a greater tendency to work on improving the quality of communication through individual, couples, and family therapy.
  - Collaborative Assessment and Management of Suicidality (CAMS), a suicide-specific clinical intervention, emphasizes the importance of establishing and maintaining a therapeutic alliance for a better understanding of the suicidal ideation.
  - Trials of CAMS showed less suicidal behavior in both inpatient and outpatient settings.

Suicide attempters vs completion

Definitions:

- Suicide completions are attempts that end in death.
- Suicide attempts are non-lethal behavioral actions with some intent to die.
- Suicidal ideation comprises thoughts, urges, and beliefs about suicide, but does not include a behavioral component.
- Most suicide completions occur *after* the first attempt.
  - A Finnish study of attempters concluded that 38% of females and 62% of males died in the first attempt.
  - Another 39% of females and 19% of males had a non-lethal attempt in the last year prior to the death, illustrating the crucial role of previous attempts for suicide completion, especially in females. For males, suicide completions are often first attempts whereas for females, completion follows a path of multiple and successive attempts and unsuccessful treatments.

Completions

- The most common method of suicide involves guns therefore it is essential to ask patients about firearms.
- The time frame for heightened risk for completions in adults is between 2 and 3 am. Insomnia and nightmares are significant risk factors and should be assessed in at-risk individuals.
- Suicide deaths in youth increased with lower antidepressant prescribing as a result of black box warnings.
- Mood disorders are the mental disorders most frequently associated with suicide completion.
- Individuals with borderline personality disorder (BPD) are at heightened risk for suicide completion.

Attempts

- In adolescents, the ratio of attempts to completions is 100:1. In the elderly, this ratio drops to 4:1.
- A recent study from the Netherlands reported a 2.7% lifetime prevalence rate of suicide attempts.
- One-third of individuals who think about suicide proceed to an attempt; 60% transition within the first year after initial onset of suicidal ideation.
- Females attempt suicide more frequently than males. Males have higher rates of completion.

Management of the suicidal patient

- Suicide prevention has greatly expanded with psychotherapeutic interventions and pharmacologic agents targeted to treat risk factors such as depression and impulsivity. It involves a wide range of interventions addressing suicidal behavior, personality disorder, major mental illness, psychosocial issues, and interpersonal stressors.
- Psychiatric management includes: (1) establishing and maintaining a therapeutic alliance; (2) monitoring patient safety; (3) establishing psychiatric diagnosis and level of functioning to arrive at a plan and setting for treatment.

The APA Guidelines on suicidal behavior

Provide specific indications for psychiatric hospitalization for suicide risk and advocate particular agents to address components of suicide risk.

- **Admission is generally indicated:**
  - After a suicide attempt or aborted suicide attempt if:
    - The patient is psychotic.
    - The attempt was violent, near-lethal, or premeditated.
    - Precautions were not taken to avoid rescue or discovery.
    - Persistent plan and/or intent is present.
    - Distress is increased or the patient regrets surviving.
    - The patient is male and older than age 45 years, especially with new onset of psychiatric illness or suicidal thinking.
    - The patient has limited family and/or social support, including lack of stable living situation.
    - Current impulsive behavior, severe agitation, poor judgment, or refusal of help is evident.
    - The patient has change in mental status with a metabolic, toxic, infectious, or other etiology requiring further work-up in a structured setting.
  - In the presence of suicidal ideation with:
    - Specific plan with high lethality and/or:
    - High suicidal intent.

- Psychosis.
- Major psychiatric disorder.
- Past attempts, particularly if medically serious.
- Possibly-contributing medical condition (e.g., acute neurological disorder, cancer, infection).
- Lack of response to or inability to cooperate with partial hospital or outpatient treatment.
- Need for supervised setting for medication trial or ECT.
- Need for skilled observation, clinical tests, or diagnostic assessments that require a structured setting.
- Limited family and/or social support, including lack of stable living situation.
- Lack of an ongoing clinician–patient relationship or lack of access to timely outpatient follow-up.
- Acute presentation is different from a chronic one.
- Poor compliance with outpatient care.

- Hospitalization may be necessary in the absence of suicide attempts or reported suicidal ideation/plan/intent if evidence from the psychiatric evaluation and/or history from others suggests a high level of suicide risk and a recent acute increase in risk.
- For BPD patients, in addition to having unproven effect, hospitalization can result in negative consequences, including behavioral regression and reinforcing behaviors that clinicians are trying to limit, prompting one group to advocate that individuals with BPD should never be hospitalized.
- The most important decision during the evaluation of a suicidal patient is the selection of the right setting for the management of those patients.
- Suicidal patients should be treated in the least confining environment that will still provide safety for the patient.
  - Hospitals keep patients safe and are appropriate for treatment of acute symptom deterioration in major psychiatric diagnosis, diagnostic clarification, and simplification of medications.
  - There is minimal empirical evidence pertaining to the efficacy of hospitalization for chronic suicidality.
  - Alternative possibilities include partial hospitalization, intensive outpatient programs, and ambulatory care.

No harm contracts

- Although widely used, the APA guidelines advocate for the proper use of the therapeutic alliance to attain safety with skilled clinicians and caution about their use as a substitute for an accurate suicide risk assessment.
- The APA emphasizes that hospitalization or discharge of a patient should never be based on a patient's willingness or reluctance to enter this contract.
- The contract is not recommended for new patients, and such contracts should be made in an established therapeutic alliance with regular outpatient follow-up and proper documentation.
- Guidelines on the use of contracts derive from expert opinion as there are few empirical studies guiding their use.
- Suicide Safety Plans have replaced no harm contracts and are the recommended intervention. Safety Plans are written documents, constructed with the clinician, that help identify warning signs, coping strategies, people to call when in distress, numbers of clinicians, and hot lines and strategies to keep the patient's surroundings safe of lethal ways to harm oneself (Stanley and Brown, 2011).

Medico-legal issues

* During one's career, there is a 50% risk of losing a patient to suicide.
* Risk management methods for working with this challenging group include assessing the patient's competence, outreach to the family, and having the proper documentation and consultation.

Reading list

Brown MZ, Comtois KA, Linehan MM. Reasons for suicide attempts and nonsuicidal self-injury in women with borderline personality disorder. J Abnorm Psychol 2002;111:198–202.

Burgess P, Pirkis J, Morton J, et al. Lessons from a comprehensive clinical audit of users of psychiatric services who committed suicide. Psychiatr Serv 2000;51(12):1555–60.

Goodman M, Roiff T, Oakes AH, Paris J. Suicidal risk and management in borderline personality disorder. Curr Psychiatry Rep 2012;14(1):79–85.

Gutheil TG. Suicide, suicide litigation, and borderline personality disorder. J Pers Disord 2004;18:248–56.

Isometsa ET, Lonnqvist JK. Suicide attempts preceding completed suicide. Br J Psychiatry 1998;173:531–5.

Jobes DA. Suicidal patients, the therapeutic alliance, and the collaborative assessment and management of suicidality. In: Michel K, Jobes DA (eds). Building a therapeutic alliance with the suicidal patient. Washington DC: American Psychological Association, 2011.

Paris J. Is hospitalization useful for suicidal patients with borderline personality disorder? J Pers Disord 2004;18:240–7.

Stanley B, Brown GK. Safety Planning Intervention: A Brief Intervention to Mitigate Suicide Risk. Cogn Behav Pract 2012;19(2):256–64.

Suggested websites

Centers for Disease Control and Prevention: Suicide facts at a glance, 2010. http://www.cdc.gov/violenceprevention/pdf/suicide-datasheet-a.PDF 2015 Suicide Fact Sheet from CDC

American Psychiatric Association: Practice Guideline for the Assessment and Treatment of Patients with Suicidal Behaviors. Am J Psychiatry 2003, 160(Nov suppl.) https://www.psychiatry.org/residents-medical-students/residents/coping-with-patient-suicide

Helping Residents Cope with a Patient Suicide. https://www.psychiatry.org/residents-medical-students/residents/coping-with-patient-suicide

---

Additional material for this chapter can be found online at:
www.mountsinaiexpertguides.com/psychiatry

This includes advice for patients, a case study, and multiple choice questions.

CHAPTER 38

Approach to the Non-Adherent Patient

Nathaniel Mendelsohn[1] and Roy Bachar[2,3]

[1] New York University School of Medicine, New York, NY, USA
[2] Hackensack University Medical Center, at the Debra Simon Center for Integrative Behavioral Health and Wellness, Maywood, NJ, USA
[3] Mount Sinai Hospital, New York, NY, USA

OVERALL BOTTOM LINE

- Poor treatment adherence among patients with psychiatric illnesses is a widespread and serious problem.
- **Determining adherence:** the more flexible and less authoritative/punitive a psychiatrist can be in measuring the extent to which a patient is taking a medication, the greater is the likelihood that best adherence can be assured.
- **Shared decision-making and therapeutic alliance:** the first step in maximizing a patient's adherence to medication is forming a strong therapeutic alliance and including the patient in the decision-making process.
- **Patient education:** informing a patient of possible side effects may decrease the likelihood the patient will stop taking a medication if those side effects occur.
- **Ease of use:** simplifying dosing schedules and decreasing polypharmacy may make compliance less cumbersome for the patient.
- **Make time:** try to carve out a portion of every appointment to assess and address the patient's level of adherence.

Discussion of topic and guidelines

Adherence to medication (and other treatments) is generally understood as the degree to which patients follow the prescriptions and recommendations of their healthcare providers. For some providers, the word "compliance" connotes a sense of the doctor's paternalism and the patient's passivity; for others, the term "concordance" implies the sense of shared decision-making between doctor and patient. Regardless of the terminology, *the psychiatrist or provider should cultivate a means of communication that conveys the importance of following prescriptions without making the patient feel at fault for non-cooperation.* In this chapter the terms "compliance" and "adherence" will be used interchangeably, and all references to medication should be taken to include the entire treatment regimen (e.g., scheduled appointments, therapy, avoiding substances, etc.).

Difficulty maximizing a patient's compliance is not unique to psychiatry (e.g., general practitioners face the constant challenge of helping patients adhere to medications for diabetes and cardiac disease). However, treating someone with a mental illness poses a unique set of problems, as energy, motivation, and cognitive ability are often affected. In addition, the benefits of psychiatric medications can take weeks to months before becoming apparent. The numbers are telling: for patients with major depression who are prescribed antidepressants, 50% will have stopped taking

---

Mount Sinai Expert Guides: Psychiatry, First Edition. Edited by Asher B. Simon, Antonia S. New, and Wayne K. Goodman.
© 2017 John Wiley & Sons, Ltd. Published 2017 by John Wiley & Sons, Ltd.
Companion website: www.mountsinaiexpertguides.com/psychiatry

the medication within 3 months; 33% of those with schizophrenia are poorly compliant and another third do not take medication at all; compliance in patients with bipolar disorder has been measured as low as 35%. The implications of such poor compliance are vast, including a 4-fold increased rate of hospitalization in schizophrenia. The financial impact is staggering, with estimates putting the 2005 US hospitalization costs of antipsychotic non-adherence at $1.479 billion.

Determining and addressing adherence should be a routine part of every encounter. To accurately assess a treatment's effectiveness and make treatment choices, a psychiatrist should have accurate data regarding whether the prescribed treatment is being followed. Methods for measuring compliance can be broadly categorized as either direct or indirect. *Direct methods* include blood levels and directly observing a patient take a medication. *Indirect methods* include patient reports, clinical responses, counting pills, and determining the number of refills filled. No matter the method used, using flexible and non-punitive methods is paramount in assuring the best compliance.

Barriers to adequate compliance are numerous and can include everything from factors related to the patient (e.g., demographics, cognitive impairment, conflict) to problems with the healthcare system and delivery of medications (e.g., cost, inability to see a provider when prescriptions need to be renewed). Obstacles to compliance can be further divided into those hindering the actual capability of the patient to follow the treatment (e.g., comorbid substance abuse, inadequate social support) and those affecting the patient's desire for treatment (e.g., poor insight, stigma, side effects); the latter is often particularly salient in psychiatric patients. Not surprisingly, studies show that patients' poor insight and beliefs about their need for medication correlate with medication adherence. While some patients may openly inform the provider of their doubts concerning the need for medication or the seriousness of their mental illness, others may be more guarded. The provider should make an effort to assess a patient's attitudes and beliefs regarding her or his symptoms and syndromes and the recommended treatments. While simply asking a patient how she or he feels a medication can help may be sufficient in some cases, a more focused – but still collaborative and non-punitive approach – may be necessary for other patients.

Side effects of recommended treatments are thought to hinder a patient's willingness to follow the doctor's advice. However, studies regarding the impact of side effects on medication adherence show mixed results ranging from no correlation to strong agreement between both physician and patient that side effects are the primary cause of non-adherence. Nonetheless, physicians should employ multiple methods to address and minimize the role of side effects, and successful management begins with patient education. Before prescribing a medication, providers should inform patients of potential side effects *as well as encourage them to bring any such side effects to the clinician's attention*. Psychiatrists should be aware of the most common side effects and those most concerning to patients. (Mentioning all the numerous side effects that could occur is neither efficient nor helpful.) Weight gain and excessive sedation have been identified as having the greatest contribution to non-adherence in patients with schizophrenia and bipolar disorder; sexual dysfunction may be equally important, but the correlation with non-adherence is higher in polypharmacy than monotherapy. Providers should address these side effects before starting medications as well as on a regular basis during the course of treatment.

After a psychiatrist has determined the degree to which a patient is compliant and has identified obstacles hindering maximal compliance, she or he is able to make a better intervention, including maximizing patient education and ease of use (simplifying dosing schedules or providing long-acting injectable forms of the medications), decreasing polypharmacy, discussing potential side effects, and preparing the patient for the possibility the medication might not be immediately effective.

Different psychotherapeutic modalities for improving adherence are also available. In cognitive behavioral therapy (CBT), the provider assists the patient in recognizing and challenging her or his automatic thoughts about medications. Successful CBT may result in the patient's building a connection between medication adherence and improved mental health. Motivational interviewing (MI) is a psychotherapy for addiction, but in medication non-adherence it can involve tailoring an approach to the patient's level of motivation to adhere and then rolling with the patient's resistance rather than challenging it. In MI the presence of resistance indicates that the provider is using an intervention inappropriate to the patient's level of motivation. Resistance also suggests the need for a stronger therapeutic alliance between clinician and patient.

A common theme in these and other interventions – and an essential element beginning in the initial encounter – is the importance of fostering a strong therapeutic alliance and making treatment decisions in concert with the patient. If the patient has not taken an active role in the decision-making process, she or he may be less inclined to adhere to the regimen, and the more authoritative the physician appears, the less likely the patient might see him or herself as having contributed. Ultimately the provider is responsible for choosing the most effective and safest treatment, but in doing so she or he should be attentive to the patient's interests and openly address any concerns and opinions. This collaborative approach is key to maximizing adherence.

Reading list

Aronson JK. Compliance, concordance, adherence. Br J Clin Pharmacol 2007;63(4):383–4.

Colom F, Vieta E, Martinez-Aran A, Reinares M, Benabarre A, Gasto C. Clinical factors associated with treatment noncompliance in euthymic bipolar patients. J Clin Psychiatry 2000;61:549–55.

Copeland LA, Zeber JE, Salloum IM, et al. Treatment adherence and illness insight in veterans with bipolar disorder. J Nerv Ment Dis 2008;196:16–21.

Day JC, Bentall RP, Roberts C, et al. Attitudes toward antipsychotic medication. Arch Gen Psychiatry 2005;62:717–24.

Fenton WS, Blyler CR, Heinssen RK. Determinants of medication compliance in schizophrenia: Empirical and clinical findings. Schizophr Bull 1997;23:637–51.

Frank AF, Gunderson JG. The role of the therapeutic alliance in the treatment of schizophrenia. Arch Gen Psychiatry 1990; 47:228–36.

Julius RJ, Novitsky MA Jr, Dubin WR. Medication adherence: a review of the literature and implications for clinical practice. J Psychiatr Pract 2009;15(1):34–44.

McDonald HP, Garg AX, Haynes RB. Interventions to enhance patient adherence to medication prescriptions. JAMA 2002;288:2868–79.

Oehl M, Hummer M, Fleischhacker WW. Adherence with antipsychotic treatment. Acta Psychiatr Scand Suppl 2002;102(Suppl. 407):83–6.

Olfson M, Marcus SC, Wilk J, et al. Awareness of illness and nonadherence to antipsychotic medications among persons with schizophrenia. Psychiatr Serv 2006;57:205–11.

Osterberg L, Blaschke T. Adherence to medication. N Engl J Med 2005;353(5):487–97.

Thompson L, McCabe R. The effect of clinician-patient alliance and communication on treatment adherence in mental health care: a systematic review. BMC Psychiatry 2012;12:87.

Velligan DI, Weiden PJ, Sajatovic M, et al. The expert consensus guideline series: adherence problems in patients with serious and persistent mental illness. J Clin Psychiatry 2009;70 Suppl 4:1–46.

Vergouwen AC, van Hout HP, Bakker A. Methods to improve patient compliance in the use of antidepressants. Ned Tijdschr Geneeskd 2002;146:204–7.

Additional material for this chapter can be found online at:
www.mountsinaiexpertguides.com/psychiatry

This includes advice for patients, a case study, and multiple choice questions.

CHAPTER 39

Psychiatric Ethics

Alison Welch and Jacob M. Appel
Icahn School of Medicine at Mount Sinai, New York, NY, USA

OVERALL BOTTOM LINE
- Psychiatric ethics is a broad field that encompasses psychiatrists' duties to patients, third parties, and communities.
- Core values in psychiatric ethics include autonomy, non-malfeasance, beneficence, justice, and respect for persons.
- Vast changes in the healthcare system and in the profession have led to significant shifts in ethical norms related to confidentiality and boundary violations.
- The Ethics Committee of the American Psychiatric Association issues guidelines on challenging ethical subjects.

Discussion of topic and guidelines
History

The history of psychiatric ethics is reflective of the evolution of medical ethics. As early as the fifth century BC, the Hippocratic Oath outlined physician duties; another millennium elapsed before the *Formula Comitis Archiatrorum* first codified ethical healthcare practices. The English physician Thomas Percival (1740–1804) coined the term "medical ethics" in his *Medical Ethics, or a Code of Institutes and Precepts, Adapted to the Professional Conduct of Physicians and Surgeons* (1803) and established the standards of ethical care that heavily influenced the American Medical Association's first official code of ethics in 1847.

Public awareness of abuses in the healthcare system – most notably revelations regarding the Tuskegee syphilis experiment – led to demands for increased protection of the rights of patients during the 1960s and 1970s. In psychiatry, Geraldo Rivera's 1972 investigation of deplorable conditions for the mentally disabled at the Willowbrook State School on Staten Island, as well as patient Kenneth Donaldson's Supreme Court challenge to 15 years of confinement without treatment in the Florida State Hospital at Chattahoochie (1975), drew attention to the ethical shortcomings in state institutions. Increasingly, psychiatrists found their profession challenged both by young legal veterans of the Civil Rights movement (who saw the mentally ill as a vulnerable population to be protected) and by "anti-psychiatrists" such as Thomas Szasz and Ronald Laing. Deinstitutionalization in the subsequent decades, often driven by a concern for patient rights, generated additional ethical challenges in balancing the wishes and welfare of the chronically mentally ill.

To assist practitioners, the American Psychiatric Association (APA) published *The Principles of Medical Ethics with Annotations Especially Applicable to Psychiatry* in 1973.

Mount Sinai Expert Guides: Psychiatry, First Edition. Edited by Asher B. Simon, Antonia S. New, and Wayne K. Goodman.
© 2017 John Wiley & Sons, Ltd. Published 2017 by John Wiley & Sons, Ltd.
Companion website: www.mountsinaiexpertguides.com/psychiatry

Values

Beauchamp and Childress laid out "Four Principles" of biomedical ethics in their seminal text-book, first published in 1979 (see Reading list): *autonomy*, *beneficence*, *non-malfeasance,* and *justice*. An additional principle, *respect for persons*, was outlined in a Congressional response to abuses in medical research, The Belmont Report (1979). These five values govern contemporary psychiatric ethics.

- **Autonomy** refers to a competent patient's right to make informed decisions regarding his or her care. Reasonable disclosure by the physician of appropriate clinical information is a necessary prerequisite for patients to exercise autonomy, and one that has been recognized by the legal system in the case of *Canterbury v. Spence* (1972). Psychiatric advance directives (PADs), so-called "Ulysses contracts," through which patients stipulate future forms of care they will accept or refuse, reflect an effort to increase autonomy. PADs are enforceable in a minority of states.
- **Beneficence** (to "do good") reflects the value of serving the patient's interests, even when such interests come into conflict with the patient's autonomous wishes or the needs of third parties. Involuntarily hospitalizing suicidal patients is a paradigmatic example of this type of tradeoff favoring beneficence.
- **Non-malfeasance** (to "do no harm") serves as a reminder that psychiatrists have fiduciary duties to their patients and cannot undermine patient welfare for their own benefit. Breaches of non-malfeasance include exploiting the inequality of power between provider and patient for financial gain or sexual gratification. *Beneficence* and *non-malfeasance* discussions arise when patient autonomy conflicts with the welfare of third parties, as in *Tarasoff warnings* reflecting the duty to warn and protect potential victims of violence.
- **Justice** ensures that patients receive both an equitable share of care and have an equal burden of risk without regard to their economic circumstances. Due to the limited number of medical licenses in the US, physicians have an ethical (although not legal) duty to provide care to the indigent and those covered by Medicare or Medicaid. APA guidelines state that "a physician shall support access to medical care for all people." Just practice ensures that patients are not abandoned and prohibits treating patients prejudicially on the basis of such criteria as race, religion, gender, or sexual orientation. Historical bias against gay therapists in some psychoana-lytic training programs reflects a particularly pernicious transgression of justice not widely acknowledged by the profession.
- **Respect for persons** includes not only respect for patient autonomy, but also pays particular attention to the needs of vulnerable populations such as children, prisoners, and the cognitively impaired. Legal safeguards have been imposed in many states to protect such individuals from exploitation in care and research.

Duties to patients

Historically, the ethical duty of psychiatrists was principally bound to the individual patient. No provider is ever obligated to treat a particular patient, except under emergent circumstances; however, once a psychiatrist does engage in caring for a patient, she or he must follow certain professional standards and ensure a safe transfer of patient care. These duties include the following:

Respect for boundaries/avoiding conflicts of interest

In order to serve the needs of patients and to avoid mismanaging transference, psychiatrists must avoid social and professional interactions with patients that jeopardize the physician–patient rela-tionship. Sexual relations between psychiatrists and patients (including former patients) are unethical and stand so far beyond the bounds of care that they are often not covered by malpractice insurance. Consent is never a defense for this boundary violation. The taboo surrounding this subject was addressed in the film *Betrayal* (1978), which drew public attention to the case of *Roy v. Hartogs* (1976) upon which it was based. Romantic relationships with "key third parties," such as spouses and parents of current patients, are also impermissible. Psychiatrists should also avoid economic endeavors, such as inviting a patient to invest in a business, hiring a patient for office work, or accepting "stock tips" from patients. An undisclosed duty to a third party should never impact patient care.

Confidentiality

The foundation for honest communication between patient and therapist is the knowledge that information divulged will not be shared gratuitously with third parties. This principle is legally codified in the Health Insurance Portability and Accountability Act of 1996. Psychotherapy notes are protected even from subpoena by the patient–therapist privilege established in *Jaffe v. Redmond* (1996). Only a significant threat to a third party or to the public can justify a breach in confidentiality. Patients should be warned in advance of such competing obligations. Even when breach of confidentiality is ethically permitted, the psychiatrist must weigh what harm is to be avoided against the damage to the physician–patient relationship, as a decline in patient confidence also raises the risk of future harms through the patient's failing to disclose injurious intent. Of note, psychiatric confidentiality may transcend the death of the patient.

Practice within area of competence

APA guidelines state that "a psychiatrist who regularly practices outside his/her area of professional competence should be considered unethical." Such conduct might range from performing gynecological exams to supervising Chinese acupuncture. Falsely representing one's skills or training – such as claiming to be a "certified psychoanalyst" without analytic training – is unethical.

Unexamined patients

The colloquially-named "Goldwater rule" prevents psychiatrists from offering opinions about the mental health of patients they have not personally evaluated. This rule applies to media commentary regarding public figures and was enacted as a response to unfounded criticism of the mental health of presidential candidate Barry Goldwater in 1964.

Conversion therapy

APA guidelines now expressly prohibit "reparative or conversion therapy" designed to alter a patient's sexual orientation.

Involvement in torture and executions

The ongoing debate over capital punishment and the alleged use of torture at Guantanamo Bay has renewed concerns over the role of mental health professionals in these areas. The APA's position is that psychiatrists cannot take part in executions or torture under any circumstances; this presumably includes the force-feeding of competent prisoners, which has been deemed torture by both the AMA and World Medical Association (WMA) and yet continues in American prisons.

Duties to third parties and society

Psychiatrists are increasingly called to fulfill duties to third parties or to the public at large. While internal medicine providers have long confronted these dual (and often conflicting) obligations in matters such as public health and quarantine, only recently has the mental health profession experienced considerable pressures to serve the interests of third parties. Two specific events led to this change. The first was the publication of pediatrician Henry Kempe's article, *The Battered Child Syndrome* (1962), which led to the enactment of state statutes requiring physicians, including psychiatrists, to report child abuse. The second was the California Supreme Court's decision in *Tarasoff v. Regents* (1976) that established a "duty to protect" third parties from dangerous patients, entailing breaching confidentiality to warn third parties directly. Although all states mandate the reporting of child abuse, they vary widely on which other hazards *may* or *must* be reported to the authorities; these may include elder abuse, domestic violence, and impaired driving. Passed in 2013, New York State's SAFE Act requires psychiatrists to report to the state patients deemed too dangerous to possess firearms. Recently, some states have enacted *Tarasoff*-limiting statutes that specifically shield psychiatrists from duties to warn or protect third parties.

Hospital ethics
The last three decades have seen a formal structure arise for addressing ethical issues within hospital settings. These include federally-mandated institutional review boards (IRBs) to supervise research as well as ethics committees to address clinical cases. Many hospitals also have an ethics consult service to offer expert opinions on ethical matters. Psychiatrists are often leaders in this infrastructure, and in its absence may be called upon for their ethical insights. The APA guidelines echo the advice of Karl Menninger regarding how to handle difficult ethical challenges in clinical settings: "When in doubt, be human."

Reading list
American Psychiatric Association. The Principles of Medical Ethics with Annotations Especially Applicable to Psychiatry 2013 Edition. Arlington, VA: American Psychiatric Association, 2013.
Beauchamp T, Childress J. Principles of Biomedical Ethics, 6th edn. New York: Oxford University Press, 2008.
Bloch S, Green S. Psychiatric Ethics. Oxford: Oxford University Press, 2009.
Bloch S, Pargiter R. A history of psychiatric ethics. Psychiatr Clin North Am 2002;25(3):509–24.
Brendel DH. Introduction: the diversification of psychiatric ethics. Harv Rev Psychiatry 2008;16(6):319–21.
Gabbard GO, Lester EP. Boundaries and Boundary Violations in Psychoanalysis. New York: Basic Books, 2002.
Horn P. Psychiatric ethics consultation in the light of DSM-5. HEC Forum 2008;20(4):315–24.

Suggested websites
American Academy of Psychiatry and the Law, Ethics Guidelines.http://www.aapl.org/ethics.htm
Appel, Jacob M. What is bioethics? http://bigthink.com/videos/big-think-interview-with-jacob-appel-2
World Psychiatric Association's "Madrid Declaration on Ethical Standards for Psychiatric Practice." http://www.wpanet.org/detail.php?section_id=5&content_id=48

Additional material for this chapter can be found online at:
www.mountsinaiexpertguides.com/psychiatry

This includes advice for patients, a case study,
and multiple choice questions.

CHAPTER 40

Psychiatric Illness during Pregnancy and the Postpartum Period

Michael E. Silverman and Betsy O'Brien
Icahn Medical School at Mount Sinai, New York, NY, USA

OVERALL BOTTOM LINE
- Psychiatric illness during pregnancy and the postpartum period represents the most common complication associated with childbirth.
- Women with a prior history of psychiatric illness are at greatest risk and should be continually monitored from the early stages of pregnancy.
- Numerous studies demonstrate the ease, acceptability, and utility of screening.
- High-quality evidence demonstrates that effective treatments are available.
- The inability to cope effectively with the demands of the early maternal period may constitute a serious threat to the infant's wellbeing.

Discussion of topic and guidelines

- Psychiatric disturbance in the perinatal period ranges from transient "baby blues," a common response to the physiological and psychological events surrounding pregnancy and infant care, to acute anxiety, depressive, and psychotic episodes.
- Many of the somatic symptoms (such as sleep disorders, appetite changes, and fatigue) are common among healthy individuals during this period and can be misinterpreted as indicators of a more severe clinical disorder.
- While the vast majority of perinatal mood symptoms are short-lived and self-remitting, some women will experience a clinically significant mood disorder that requires medical intervention.

Impact of peripartum depression

- Depression is the most prevalent psychiatric illness in the perinatal period.
- Postpartum depression affects 11–19% of all new mothers and is the leading cause of non-obstetric hospitalization among women of childbearing age.
- Perinatal depression negatively impacts maternal behavior and may impair the child's cognitive and emotional development.
- Despite the fact that pregnant and postpartum women often receive regular medical care (and therefore could be easily screened and treated) many cases go unrecognized.

Mount Sinai Expert Guides: Psychiatry, First Edition. Edited by Asher B. Simon, Antonia S. New, and Wayne K. Goodman.
© 2017 John Wiley & Sons, Ltd. Published 2017 by John Wiley & Sons, Ltd.
Companion website: www.mountsinaiexpertguides.com/psychiatry

Impact on the infant of peripartum depression

- Perinatal mood disorders constitute a serious threat to the infant's wellbeing, as the period immediately surrounding the birth of a child is a critical window for many developmental events.
- Perinatal depression results in common morbidities among psychiatric illnesses including marked functional impairment, distress, and increased risk of suicide.
- Early maternal psychiatric illness is associated with diminished enrichment behavior, a shortened duration of breastfeeding, and renewal of maternal smoking, factors known to adversely affect physical growth and neurobehavioral development of the infant.
- Maternal psychiatric illness is linked to increased risk of conduct disorders and psychiatric disturbances among children – diagnoses that may persist into adulthood.

Postpartum "baby" blues

Postpartum blues, often referred to as "the baby blues," is a transient, mild, down-regulation of mood that often presents with sadness, mood lability, anxiety, irritability, and sleep disturbance. Because of its prevalence and self-remitting nature, postpartum blues is not considered a clinically relevant mood disorder.

Incidence

- Up to 85% of women report at least one depressive mood symptom in the perinatal period.

Course

Onset typically occurs within the first few days postpartum. A "peaking phenomenon" has been established that occurs within the first postpartum week and subsides without intervention around 14 days postpartum.

Etiology

- The etiology of the postpartum blues remains poorly understood.
- Because the hormonal changes that occur in the perinatal period are unprecedented across the female lifecycle, a biological basis is generally assumed.
- Treatment for postpartum blues is not generally indicated as it resolves without intervention. However, sleep, stress reduction, and infant care support can assist in reducing symptoms.
- Women with postpartum blues are at a 4-fold risk of experiencing a more significant perinatal depression.

Peripartum/postpartum depression

The DSM-5 defines peripartum depression with the same diagnostic criteria as major depression: the presence of five of the symptoms listed in Table 10.1 over a 2-week period.

Incidence

- Peripartum depression occurs in 11–19% of all postpartum women.

Course

- Onset occurs within the first 4 weeks following delivery.
- Peak prevalence for depression following delivery generally occurs between 0 and 3 months, but depression may extend throughout the first postpartum year.

BOX 40.1 FACTORS ASSOCIATED WITH PERINATAL DEPRESSION
- Prior history of depression
- Significant (stressful) life events
- Newborn illness/abnormality/hospitalization
- History of physical or sexual abuse
- Difficult pregnancy
- Poor social support/marital instability
- Anxiety during pregnancy
- Low socioeconomic status

Etiology

- Perinatal depression is likely the culmination of a number of influences. While the stress of motherhood poses a challenge for most new mothers, pathogenic antecedents of perinatal depression likely precede pregnancy and extend through delivery.
- Factors associated with perinatal depression are listed in Box 40.1, and are shown to have a cumulative effect.
- The importance of detecting peripartum depression is highlighted by data showing that effective treatments exist and result in improved quality of life.
- **The Edinburgh Postnatal Depression Scale** (http://psychology-tools.com/epds/), the most widely validated depression symptom inventory, is a 10-item self-report instrument designed to assess symptoms associated with depression and anxiety using a scale of 0–30.
  - It does not provide a diagnosis of depression and should not replace clinical judgment.
  - However, it is an effective screening tool and considered a reliable and valid measure for differentiating between women with and without perinatal depression.

Treatment

- According to the American College of Obstetrics and Gynecology, the goal of treatment is symptom remission. Treatment should be based upon psychoeducation, inclusion of support structures, psychotherapy and, when appropriate, psychopharmacology.
  - For mild postpartum depression or anxiety, psychotherapy alone is often the first option. As a range of psychotherapeutic interventions are effective, the type of therapist and therapy indicated should be determined by the underlying psychosocial factors active in the mother's life.
  - For those with prior depression treatment or who present with more severe depressive and anxiety symptoms and/or suicidal ideation, serotonin-selective reuptake inhibitors (SSRIs) are generally recommended as first-line treatment, especially when breastfeeding is desired.
  - Because of a lack of well-constructed randomized trials on psychopharmacotherapy during pregnancy and lactation, psychopharmacology in the perinatal period is more complicated than in the general population.
  - Because medications may cross the placenta, and some exposure is presumed inevitable *in utero*, psychopharmacotherapy should be initiated with a single agent and at the lowest possible dose.
  - Providers should review psychopharmacologic history, risks, benefits, and side-effect profile, emphasizing the risks of untreated depression on infant development while simultaneously maintaining awareness that diminished decision-making capacity is a symptom of perinatal depression.
  - Medication dosages should consider postpartum metabolic changes.

- The impact of untreated depression during the perinatal and neonatal period includes adverse outcomes for both mother and child.
  - Perinatal depression is associated with fetal distress, preterm delivery, low birth weight, and other delivery complications.
  - Postpartum depression and anxiety adversely affect physical and cognitive development in the child and in the most severe cases contribute to maternal suicide and maternal filicide.

Postpartum psychosis and postpartum mania/hypomania

Psychotic illness in the postpartum period is a rare, but severe condition. It is defined as the development of psychotic symptoms such as hallucinations (visual and/or auditory), paranoia, and/or delusions that generally focus on the infant.

Incidence

- Approximately 1 in 1000.
- A family history of bipolar disease increases incidence to 1 in 300, a family history of postpartum psychosis to 1 in 4, and a personal history of postpartum psychosis increases this further to 1 in 2.
- Postpartum psychotic episodes most frequently follow primiparous delivery.

Course

- Postnatal psychosis occurs rapidly, as early as the first 48–72 hours, with the majority of episodes within the first 2 weeks postpartum.
- If the psychosis is associated with a major depressive episode, it can manifest as late as several months postpartum.
- Initial symptom presentation includes restlessness and irritability, fluctuant mood (elated–depressed), and insomnia.
- Course durations are similar to bipolar disorder and based on presenting phenomenology with manic/depressed symptomatology generally extending longer than manic/psychotic.

Etiology

- Postpartum psychosis is generally believed to be a manifestation of underlying bipolar diathesis with the first episode conceptualized as the incipient clinical presentation.

Treatment

- Psychosis in the postpartum period is a psychiatric emergency and requires immediate treatment.
  - A mother with postpartum psychosis should not be left alone with her child(ren).
  - Hospitalization may be required for the safety and stabilization of severely ill patients with symptoms that include suicidal or homicidal behavior, aggression, delusions, and/or exhibition of poor judgment.
  - If not hospitalized, treatment includes close monitoring in an outpatient setting by a psychiatrist. Psychotropic medication is usually necessary, with treatment predicated on medical history and breastfeeding intent.
  - Because psychotropic medications are commonly secreted in breast milk and breastfeeding often results in sleep disturbance (a known trigger for psychotic relapse), formula feeding is recommended.
  - If the patient was not taking medications during the intrapartum period, but had been effectively maintained on psychotropic medications prior to pregnancy, those medications are generally preferred.

- For mothers experiencing a first episode of psychosis during the postpartum period, the mood stabilizer or antipsychotic medication chosen is predicated on standards of care of treatment for bipolar disorder.
- Long-term systematic data for most drugs remain unavailable and therefore firm evidence-based conclusions cannot be reached.
  - If the patient is breastfeeding and presents with postpartum psychosis, mania, or hypomania, a medication such as olanzapine and quetiapine can be considered, with chlorpromazine and haloperidol as secondary options.
  - Lithium and lamotrigine are not compatible with lactation and have been associated with adverse infant events.
  - Medication dosages must consider postpartum metabolic changes.

The impact of untreated postpartum psychosis includes infanticide and suicide. More than half the women who experience a postpartum psychosis will have another episode unrelated to childbirth.

Postpartum obsessive-compulsive disorders (ppOCD)

Obsessive-compulsive disorders (OCD) in the perinatal period are characterized by recurrent, intrusive thoughts and compulsive rituals.

- Unwanted thoughts generally involve disturbing themes of contamination, illness, harm, sexual assault, accident, or loss.
- Compulsive rituals may include washing and/or checking or covert symptoms such as counting and/or ruminating.
- ppOCD obsessions most frequently include fears of intentional harm (e.g., stabbing, beating, choking, molesting), are ego-dystonic in nature, and are associated with depression as opposed to psychosis.
- Such thoughts are rarely disclosed to practitioners, are associated with feelings of guilt and shame, and are believed to contribute to depression.

Incidence

- There is an increased risk of OCD in the perinatal period, beyond that of the general population, with an estimated prevalence in women of approximately 3–4%.
- Research has demonstrated unwanted intrusive thoughts in as many as 70% of all postpartum mothers.

Course

- Symptoms can occur early in pregnancy or any time thereafter.
- Postpartum symptoms are generally observed by week 6 postpartum.
- A preexisting OCD diagnosis is associated with greater severity in the peripartum period.

Etiology

- **The etiology** of ppOCD is unknown.
- Behaviorally, perinatal OCD is generally believed to reflect the mother's current concerns and interests.
- The cognitive model of OCD characterizes the discomfort associated with intrusive thoughts as secondary to the overvaluation of significance of minor concerns.
- It is unclear whether symptoms represent discrete onset or an exacerbation of underlying or previously prodromal behaviors.
- A pre-pregnancy history of OCD is strongly correlated to perinatal OCD.
- Because ppOCD obsessions generally create unexpressed shame, coexisting depression is frequently observed.

Treatment

- Cognitive behavioral therapy is effective in ppOCD although comorbid depression adversely affects treatment outcomes.
- The gold standard pharmacologic treatment for OCD is SSRIs; however their efficacy is unknown in the perinatal population.
- If the patient is refractory to SSRI treatment, augmentation with atypical antipsychotic medication is recommended.
- Because there are limited data on atypical medications and lactation, the risks, benefits, and side effects of these medications should be thoroughly reviewed.
- Mothers often hide symptoms for a considerable amount of time before seeking treatment.
- Maternal anxiety adversely affects the woman and her interactions with her infant as well as her family.
- If left untreated, ppOCD often has a chronic course.

Reading list

Abramowitz JS, Schwartz SA, Moore KM, Luenzmann KR. Obsessive-compulsive symptoms in pregnancy and the puerperium: A review of the literature. J Anxiety Disord 2003;17:461–78.

American College of Obstetrics and Gynecologists. Clinical management guidelines for obstetrician-gynecologists number 92, April 2008. Use of psychiatric medications during pregnancy and lactation. ACOG Committee on Practice Bulletins – Obstetrics. Obstet Gynecol 2008;111(4):1001.

Di Florio A, Forty L, Gordon-Smith K, et al. Perinatal episodes across the mood disorder spectrum. JAMA Psychiatry 2013;70(2):168–75.

Gaynes BN, Gavin N, Meltzer-Brody S, et al. Perinatal Depression: Prevalence, Screening Accuracy, and Screening Outcomes. Rockville, MD: Agency for Healthcare Research and Quality; 2005. Evidence Report/ Technology Assessment 119. AHRQ Publication 05-E006-2.

Klinger G, Stahl B, Fusar-Poli P, Merlob P. Antipsychotic drugs and breastfeeding. Pediatr Endocrinol Rev 2013;10(3):308–17.

Nonacs R, Cohen LS. Depression during pregnancy: diagnosis and treatment options. J Clin Psychiatry 2002;63 Suppl 7:24–30.

O'Hara, MW. Postpartum depression: What we know. J Clin Psychol 2009;65:1258–69.

Pilowsky DJ, Wickramaratne PJ, Rush AJ, et al. Children of currently depressed mothers: a STAR*D ancillary study. J Clin Psychiatry 2006;67(1):126–36.

Wisner KL, Parry BL, Piontek CM. Postpartum depression. N Engl J Med 2002;347(3):194–9.

Yonkers KA, Wisner KL, Stowe Z, et al. Management of bipolar disorder during pregnancy and the postpartum period. Am J Psychiatry 2004;161(4):608–20.

Suggested websites

Edinburgh Postnatal Depression Scale. https://psychology-tools.com/epds/

MedEd Postpartum Depression. http://www.mededppd.org/

MedlinePlus – Postpartum Depression. http://www.nlm.nih.gov/medlineplus/postpartumdepression.html

Postpartum Support International. http://www.postpartum.net/

Additional material for this chapter can be found online at:
www.mountsinaiexpertguides.com/psychiatry

This includes advice for patients, a link to case studies, ICD codes, and multiple choice questions.

CHAPTER 41

Resilience

Adriana Feder[1], Mariana Schmajuk[2], Dennis S. Charney[1], and Steven M. Southwick[1,3]

[1] Icahn School of Medicine at Mount Sinai, New York, NY, USA
[2] Columbia University Medical Center/New York-Presbyterian Hospital, New York, NY, USA
[3] Yale University School of Medicine, New Haven, CT, USA

OVERALL BOTTOM LINE

- Resilience refers to the ability to successfully adapt, maintain, or regain mental health when faced with stress, trauma, or chronic forms of adversity.
- Common to resilient individuals are active coping, having a positive attitude, maintaining flexible thinking, and possessing the ability to form supportive social networks, among other psychosocial characteristics summarized below.
- Neurobiological correlates of resilience help practitioners understand how individuals regulate responses to stress.
- Healthcare providers can promote resilience with brief therapeutic interventions to foster patients' own natural strengths and help them incorporate new coping strategies into their everyday lives.

Discussion of topic and guidelines

We must never forget that we may also find meaning in life even when confronted with a hopeless situation, when facing a fate that cannot be changed. For what then matters is to bear witness to the uniquely human potential at its best, which is to transform a personal tragedy into a triumph, to turn one's predicament in a human achievement. When we are no longer able to change a situation – just think of an incurable disease such as an inoperable cancer: we are challenged to change ourselves.
FranklVE *Man's Search for Meaning*. Boston, MA: Beacon Press, 2006, p. 116.

Introduction

Resilience refers to a person's ability to successfully adapt, maintain, or regain mental health in the face of acute stress, trauma, or more chronic forms adversity, including physical illness. Resilient individuals are those who have been tested by such adversity and continue to demonstrate adaptive psychological and physiological stress responses. In delivering the forms of psychosocial care enumerated below, healthcare providers may strengthen patients' abilities to bounce back from hardship as well as provide prophylactic and ongoing benefits to patients' wellbeing. Studies have linked a range of psychosocial characteristics to higher resilience in the face of stress, and practitioners may use knowledge of these attitudes and characteristics to help promote and facilitate healthy coping in patients during day-to-day clinical practice.

Mount Sinai Expert Guides: Psychiatry, First Edition. Edited by Asher B. Simon, Antonia S. New, and Wayne K. Goodman.
© 2017 John Wiley & Sons, Ltd. Published 2017 by John Wiley & Sons, Ltd.
Companion website: www.mountsinaiexpertguides.com/psychiatry

For each strategy described in detail below, we include neurobiological correlates as well as concrete interventions that providers should consider.

A prescription for resilience: strategies to facilitate resilience

Active coping and facing one's fears: seeking solutions and managing emotions

Certain forms of coping (e.g., behavioral or psychological techniques) to reduce or overcome stress have been linked to resilience and are becoming increasingly recognized as potential entry points for intervention. In particular, active coping must be distinguished from avoidant coping. Individuals who use avoidant coping (e.g., emotional/behavioral withdrawal, giving up attempts to cope, or drinking alcohol instead of dealing directly with stressors) have increased risk of psychological distress and depression. On the other hand, active coping is associated with adaptability and resilience. For example, planning and problem-solving, often with help from family, friends, or providers, direct patients to focus on and manage more controllable aspects of a stressor.

Neurobiological correlate: active as opposed to avoidant coping is thought to be associated with more transient activation of the hypothalamic-pituitary-adrenal (HPA) axis in response to stress.

Provider intervention:

- Help patients to recognize and use their personal strengths to improve their sense of control. With more confidence, patients are able to reduce the perception of being threatened by illness and are able to engage in finding solutions to help manage stress.
- Foster active problem-oriented coping, which may improve motivation, compliance, and perseverance to overcome medical issues.

Positive emotions

Positive affect and the expectation of a good outcome (optimism) have been found to be protective in the face of stress and are associated with improved recovery times and better physical health. Humor is also known to alleviate tension, protect against stress, and attract social support.

Neurobiological correlate: positive emotions activate dopaminergic reward systems. During times of stress, optimism and the ability to experience positive emotions alongside negative ones are associated with decreased autonomic arousal and might contribute to healthier cognitions.

Provider intervention:

- While optimism may be genetically influenced, it can also be learned.
- Help patients maintain hope, and encourage them to engage in pleasurable activities and seek social support.
- Maximize patients' abilities to experience positive emotions. Assess for depression and consider need for antidepressant medication.
- A referral for psychotherapy might be helpful and necessary to help a patient gain perspective.

Flexible thinking

Resilience is associated with the ability to find the silver lining in difficult situations, and resilient individuals find it easier to reinterpret and reframe negative events in a better light. This positive reframing may reduce emotional responses and lessen stress. Helping patients find more adaptive ways of perceiving challenging situations can facilitate resilience, and when individuals feel that they have the capacity and necessary support to tackle a problem, they are more likely to appraise the problem as a challenge than as a threat.

Neurobiological correlate: processes that underlie cognitive reappraisal include memory reconsolidation, and cognitive control of emotion.

Provider intervention:

• Work together with patients to break down a problem into smaller parts so as to enable them to realize that they have the skills and support needed to tackle it.

• Help patients view their losses in less extreme terms and find activities that they can still enjoy despite new limitations. While some patients react to illness by feeling that all is lost if they cannot maintain their previous level of activity, flexible thinking includes accepting new limitations brought about by illness, while simultaneously focusing on aspects of illness or stress that can be controlled.

• Help patients view the positive side of challenging situations, e.g., the discovery of the patient's own natural strength and ability to cope with hardship, or the deepening of an interpersonal relationship which began by seeking support from others to cope with a progressive illness.

Establishing a nurturing social network

Low levels of social support are associated with depression and higher medical morbidity. Higher levels of social support have been linked to active problem-solving, improved self-esteem and optimism, and better mental and physical health outcomes despite stressors. The ability to utilize social support, work in groups, and engage in altruistic behaviors activates brain reward circuitry. In turn, this helps reduce fear responses and improves resilience. Dampened neuroendocrine and cardiovascular responses to stress might prevent or lower levels of depression. Social support also reduces functional impairment and can improve treatment adherence.

Neurobiological correlate: social cooperation is associated with activation of reward circuitry in the brain. Oxytocin is involved in enhancing the rewarding value of social interactions and reducing stress responses.

Provider intervention:

• Help patients find supportive networks.

• Encourage patients to find role models who may relate to their experiences. Resilient role models can reinforce positive changes and behaviors. For example, introducing a patient to another patient who has successfully adapted to a medical condition can facilitate a patient's own adaptation to illness.

Having a moral compass

The existence of an internal belief system that provides a sense of purpose is common among resilient individuals. Having core belief systems can offer patients structure and help them maintain a positive outlook. For many, spirituality may facilitate recovery, the ability to find meaning when faced with trauma or stress, and psychological growth in the face of challenging situations.

Neurobiological correlate: research findings suggest that the serotonin system might be implicated in spiritual experiences. Brain imaging studies are starting to identify the neural correlates of human morality.

Provider intervention:

• Explore patients' belief systems to help them regain a sense of purpose that might have been shaken by illness.

• A referral for psychotherapy might be helpful.

• Religious individuals who might have stopped practicing or attending services can be encouraged to resume.

• Encourage altruistic behavior.

Attending to physical wellbeing

The quality of the diet, amount of exercise, capacity to relax, and quantity and quality of sleep are important in determining how the body and brain respond to stress.

Table 41.1 Neurochemical responses to acute stress.

Neurochemical	Acute effects	Associated with	
		Resilience	Vulnerability
Corticotropin-releasing hormone (CRH)	Activates fear behaviors, inhibits neurovegetative functions	Reduced CRH release	Chronically increased CRH may predispose to PTSD and depression
Cortisol	Mobilizes energy and focuses attention	Rapid termination of acute release via negative feedback	Dysregulated cortisol release and feedback mechanisms
Dehydroepiandrosterone (DHEA)	Counteracts high cortisol, positive effects on mood	High DHEA/cortisol ratios protect against PTSD and depression	Low DHEA response may predispose to PTSD and depression
Locus coeruleus–norepinephrine (LC-NE) system	Increases arousal, attention, and fear memory formation	Reduced responsiveness of LC-NE system	Unconstrained response of LC-NE system
Neuropeptide Y (NPY)	Anxiolytic, improves performance during stressful situations	Adaptive increase in amygdalar NPY	Low NPY is associated with PTSD
Serotonin (5-HT)	Mixed effects, modulatory	High postsynaptic 5-HT$_{1A}$ receptor activity may facilitate recovery from stress	Low postsynaptic 5HT$_{1A}$ receptor activity may predispose to anxiety and depression
Dopamine	Important in reward responses and conversely in anhedonic/helpless behaviors	Optimal dopamine system function preserves reward responses and fear extinction	Excessive mesocortical dopamine release
Brain-derived neurotrophic factor (BDNF)	Supports neuronal growth, involved in fear conditioning and extinction	High BDNF level in hippocampus	Stress can induce decrease in hippocampal BDNF expression
Endocannabinoids (eCBs)	Regulate HPA axis activity	Optimal eCB signaling regulates stress hormone response	Insufficient eCB action at CB1 receptor might increase anxiety
Glutamate	Excitatory synaptic signaling	Increased AMPA receptor activation might promote antidepressant and antianxiety effects	Glutamate system dysregulation has been observed in chronic stress

Neurobiological correlate: exercise has been shown to be associated with resilience by promoting neurogenesis.

Prescriber intervention:

- Provide education about sleep hygiene.
- Prescribe exercise regimens or relaxation practice to encourage patients to seek exercise classes to promote social involvement.

- Teach patients about the benefits of nutrition.
- Provide positive feedback for patients' successes in each of the above.

Biological model of resilience

Complex systems of hormones, neurotransmitters, and neuropeptides help regulate the neuro-biological response to stress, and interactions between these factors underlie individual variability in stress resilience (Table 41.1). Key systems include the HPA axis, the noradrenergic, serotonergic, and dopaminergic systems, and neuropeptide Y (NPY), among others.

Summary

All people experience stress, illness, and loss. Although most individuals are resilient to the worst outcomes, clinicians can help all patients successfully adapt to adversity and potentially prevent resultant depression, uncontrollable anxiety, or maladaptive consequences. Understanding the psychological features and neurobiology of resilience can enable practitioners to employ interventions that maximize successful coping in patients and their families. Along a variety of axes, clinicians can improve resilience by helping patients:

1. engage in more adaptive forms of coping;
2. gradually accept losses while maintaining a positive outlook and focusing on controllable aspects of the situation;
3. pursue pleasurable activities;
4. seek the company, support, and assistance of others;
5. find role models who have learned to cope successfully;
6. grow stronger by gradually facing fears;
7. find meaning and purpose in life;
8. attend to their physical wellbeing.

When necessary, clinicians can initiate a referral for psychotherapy, treat with antidepressant medication, or pursue a psychiatric consultation. As our understanding of resilience continues to grow, so will the range of interventions available to us in general clinical practice.

Reading list

Cotman CW, Berchtold NC. Exercise: A behavioral intervention to enhance brain health and plasticity. Trends Neurosci 2002;25:295–301.

Davidson RJ, McEwen BS. Social influences on neuroplasticity: stress and interventions to promote well-being. Nat Neurosci 2012;15:689–95.

Feder A, Haglund M, Wu G,Southwick SM, Charney DS. The neurobiology of resilience. In: Charney DS, Buxbaum JD, Sklar P, Nestler EJ (eds). Neurobiology of Mental Illness, 4th edn. New York: Oxford University Press, 2013.

Feder A, Nestler EJ, Charney DS. Psychobiology and molecular genetics of resilience. Nat Rev Neurosci 2009;10:446–57.

Fredrickson BL. The broaden-and-build theory of positive emotions. Philos Trans R Soc Lond B Biol Sci 2004;359:1367–78.

Mobbs D, Greicius MD, Adbel-Azim E, Menon V, Reiss AL. Humor modulates the mesolimbic reward centers. Neuron 2003;40:1041–8.

Southwick SM, Charney DS. Resilience: the Science of Mastering Life's Greatest Challenges. Cambridge, UK: Cambridge University Press, 2012.

Southwick SM, Charney DS. The science of resilience: implications for the prevention and treatment of depression. Science 2012;338:79–82.

Southwick SM, Bonanno GA, Masten AS, Panter-Brick C, Yehuda R. Resilience definitions, theory, and challenges: interdisciplinary perspectives. Eur J Psychotraumatol 2014;5:10.3402/ejpt.v5.25338.

Thompson RW, Arnkoff DB, Glass CR. Conceptualizing mindfulness and acceptance as components of psychological resilience to trauma. Trauma Violence Abuse 2011;12:220–35.

Wu G, Feder A, Cohen H, et al. Understanding resilience. Front Behav Neurosci 2003;7:10.

Suggested websites

American Psychological Association, "The Road to Resilience." http://www.apa.org/helpcenter/road-resilience.aspx

"Resilience: Build skills to endure hardship." http://www.mayoclinic.org/tests-procedures/resilience-training/in-depth/resilience/art-20046311

"The Resilience Prescription." https://icahn.mssm.edu/static_files/MSMC/Files/Patient%20Care/Occupational%20Health/ResiliencePrescriptionPromotion-082112.pdf

University of Pennsylvania, "Authentic Happiness." https://www.authentichappiness.sas.upenn.edu/

Dr. Charney: "Resilience Lessons from our Veterans." https://www.youtube.com/watch?v=XoN1pv2JKpc

Dr. Southwick: "How to Become More Resilient", focus on social relationships. https://www.youtube.com/watch?v=DJYC6Ymp8JQ

Dr. Southwick: "The Science of Resilience: Implications for Prevention and Treatment of Depression in College Students", on ways to enhance resilience in students, also applicable to many life situations. https://www.youtube.com/watch?v=2dVZMGMMr90

Additional material for this chapter can be found online at:
www.mountsinaiexpertguides.com/psychiatry

This includes advice for patients, a case study,
and multiple choice questions.

CHAPTER 42

Emergency Psychiatry

Amy L. Johnson[1], Naomi Schmelzer[2], Maria Linden[3], and Claudine Egol[4]

[1] Weill Cornell Medical College, New York, NY, USA
[2] Brigham and Women's Hospital, Boston, MA, USA
[3] Icahn School of Medicine at Mount Sinai, New York, NY, USA
[4] Northport Veterans Affairs Medical Center, Northport, NY, USA

OVERALL BOTTOM LINE
- A psychiatric emergency is an acute disturbance of thought, behavior, or social relationship that requires an immediate intervention as defined by the patient, the family, or the community.
- The proper management of agitation in a psychiatric emergency includes assessing and treating the underlying etiology, collaborating with the patient, using verbal de-escalation and other non-pharmacological interventions, and *pro re nata* (prn) medications. Seclusion and restraint should be used infrequently and only as a last resort.
- One of the most important and frequent tasks in emergency psychiatry is assessing risk of suicide and violence and the related need for psychiatric hospitalization.
- Emergency psychiatrists must be familiar with a multitude of legal, ethical, and regulatory issues.

Discussion of topic and guidelines
Introduction
Emergency psychiatry is a relatively new subspecialty, developing over the last 25 years. While just a few decades ago it consisted solely of psychiatric consultants in large urban medical emergency departments, it is now comprised of numerous practitioners, dedicated psychiatric emergency services, and its own association (the American Association for Emergency Psychiatry). According to the American Psychiatric Association's (APA) Task Force on Psychiatric Emergency Services, a psychiatric emergency is "an acute disturbance of thought, behavior, or social relationship that requires an immediate intervention as defined by the patient, the family, or the community." This could represent a plethora of possibilities, including an acutely suicidal patient, a patient intoxicated with synthetic marijuana, an adolescent with disruptive behavior at school, a homeless patient with schizophrenia, or an elderly patient with paranoia related to dementia. Many factors, including the ongoing shift of mental health services to outpatient settings and the growth of managed care, are leading more patients than ever to present to psychiatric emergency services. From the multitude of emergency psychiatry topics, we have chosen to focus on the following:
1. non-psychiatric medical evaluation;
2. acute intoxication;
3. agitation;
4. suicide and violence risk assessments;
5. legal issues.

Mount Sinai Expert Guides: Psychiatry, First Edition. Edited by Asher B. Simon, Antonia S. New, and Wayne K. Goodman.
© 2017 John Wiley & Sons, Ltd. Published 2017 by John Wiley & Sons, Ltd.
Companion website: www.mountsinaiexpertguides.com/psychiatry

Non-psychiatric medical evaluation

In the emergency room, a psychiatric symptom may reflect a primary psychiatric disorder (in which coexisting medical conditions are either stable or do not exist), a primary medical illness, or worsening of an established psychiatric disorder due to unstable coexisting medical illness. The initial management goal is prompt identification and stabilization of immediately life-threatening conditions. Next, a medical screening should evaluate whether the presenting psychiatric complaint is a manifestation of underlying medical illness or related to a primary psychiatric process.

The extent of medical screening remains a controversial topic and lacks clinical consensus, with emergency medicine and psychiatric specialists sometimes disagreeing about the appropriateness of clinical tests in the emergency setting. Numerous studies suggest that a thorough medical history and physical examination, including review of systems and cognitive testing, are high yield for detecting active medical conditions in patients presenting solely with psychiatric complaints, and that these findings rather than routine screening labs should be used to further focus clinical testing. On the other hand, screening may uncover medical illnesses that are incidental to the presenting complaint but require urgent care or ongoing management once a patient is transferred to psychiatry. Psychiatrists are often cautious about admitting patients to inpatient wards if contributing or comorbid medical illness cannot be safely or effectively managed.

Although several studies have shown that routine labs are low yield for clinically significant findings, several high-risk patient groups require comprehensive testing:
- the elderly;
- new-onset psychiatric symptoms;
- atypical complaints in an existing psychiatric patient;
- developmental disabilities;
- substance abuse disorders;
- pre-existing medical conditions.

Nearly all psychiatric symptoms can be seen in primary medical illness, making for a broad and diverse differential diagnosis:
- CNS disorders;
- metabolic or electrolyte abnormalities;
- cardiopulmonary disease;
- medication effects;
- substance intoxication or withdrawal;
- endocrine disorders;
- infection;
- rheumatologic conditions.

Commonly ordered laboratory tests:
- CBC;
- metabolic panels;
- urinalysis;
- urine toxicology;
- blood alcohol level.

Other ancillary tests to consider:
- CPK;
- prothrombin time;
- EKG;
- cardiac enzymes;
- liver function tests;
- TSH;

- head imaging;
- chest x-ray;
- relevant drug levels, particularly if overdose is suspected.

Acute intoxication

Acute intoxication, which may have both medical and psychiatric manifestations, is a common presentation in the emergency department. An initial step in a careful assessment is to obtain a detailed history from both the patient and any collateral sources (as intoxicated patients are often unable to provide a reliable history). The next step is to perform physical and mental status examinations, looking for evidence of autonomic instability, trauma, and treatable medical and psychiatric conditions. Objective findings can yield important clues regarding the specific substance ingested (see Table 42.1). In addition, lab tests such as CBC and metabolic panels, as well as imaging studies, should be considered as they may contribute to clinical decision-making.

Agitation

Agitation is common and is a significant cause of both patient and staff injury. The AAEP developed Project BETA (Best Practices in Evaluation and Treatment of Agitation) guidelines in 2012.

An acutely agitated patient may be unwilling or unable to cooperate with a formal psychiatric assessment, necessitating the postponement of a full evaluation until the patient is calmer. However, a brief initial evaluation (including focused mental status exam and history obtained from available collateral sources such as family, friends, emergency responders or police, and medical records) should be aimed at determining the most likely etiology for agitation. Preliminary interventions to calm the patient should be initiated simultaneously or shortly afterwards.

Umbrella diagnostic categories in the differential for acute agitation are:

- delirium;
- chronic cognitive impairments (e.g., traumatic brain injury, developmental disability, dementia);
- intoxication or withdrawal;
- primary psychosis;
- other miscellaneous causes (e.g., depression, anxiety, poor behavioral control or intense anger often seen in persons with personality disorders).

The overall approach to managing a patient with agitation is to use collaboration rather than coercion to achieve calm and maintain safety. Addressing any underlying medical cause of agitation in a timely manner should be the first step and may be sufficient. Next, non-pharmacological interventions such as verbal de-escalation and reduction of environmental stimuli should be implemented. If a patient requires medication, efforts should be made to include him or her in the choice and route, and the medication should be used to restore calm rather than induce sleep or serve as chemical restraint (see Table 42.2).

For patients who are immediately dangerous to themselves or others, restraint or seclusion can be used for brief periods of time; however this should be avoided whenever possible. Staff must be familiar with the relevant hospital and regulatory guidelines.

Suicide and violence risk assessments

Because danger to self or others is a frequent presenting symptom in emergency psychiatry, and because it is the most common indication for hospitalization, suicide and violence risk assessments are performed routinely by emergency psychiatrists. The evaluation of suicidal and violent patients requires thorough and careful interviewing of the patient and any available collateral sources (family, friends, other providers).

Table 42.1 Objective signs in acute intoxication.

Objective findings	Cocaine, amphetamines	Antihistamines, tricyclic antidepressants, antiparkinsonian agents	PCP, MDMA, LSD	Opiates	MAOIs, SSRIs, or TCAs in combination with other serotonergic drugs	Benzodiazepines, barbiturates, alcohol, zolpidem
Tachycardia	×	×	×		×	
Bradycardia				×		×
Hypertension	×	×	×		×	
Hypotension				×		×
Hyperthermia	×	×	×		×	
Hypothermia				×		×
Tachypnea	×	×	×		×	
Bradypnea				×		×
Hyperreflexia	×				×	
Hyporeflexia				×		×
Nystagmus			×			
Mydriasis	×	×	×		×	
Miosis				×		×
Psychosis	×	× (delirium)	×			
Tremor	×				×	
Diaphoresis	×				×	

Table 42.2 Selection of pharmacologic agent based on differential diagnosis of acute agitation.

Suspected diagnosis	Medication recommendations
Delirium	If alcohol/benzodiazepine withdrawal, give oral or parenteral benzodiazepines If no alcohol/benzodiazepine withdrawal, avoid benzodiazepines and give antipsychotic (second or first generation)
Intoxication	If due to CNS stimulant, give oral or parenteral benzodiazepines If due to CNS depressant, give oral first-generation antipsychotic (haloperidol)
Psychosis	Give antipsychotic (second or first generation)
Unknown cause	If no psychosis evident, give oral or parenteral benzodiazepines If psychosis evident, give antipsychotic (second or first generation)

When assessing suicide risk, it is important to inquire about history of suicidal ideation and past attempts as well as current thoughts and plans. One must inquire about the chronicity and any recent change in suicidal thoughts, differentiate passive from active ideation, and determine whether specific plans have been formulated. Assessing the degree of lethality and the patient's intent and ability to follow through on plans is of paramount importance. If it is determined that a patient cannot be maintained safely in the outpatient setting, hospitalization is indicated. (Note that danger to self includes not only suicidality but also being unable to meet basic needs such as shelter, food, basic ADLs, and medical care.)

The most reliable predictor of future violence is a history of violence. The clinician must elicit this history as well as assess acute and static risk factors. Acute factors that can be modified with time or treatment include acute intoxication/withdrawal, impulsivity, mania, command auditory hallucinations urging violence, psychotic paranoia, and access to weapons. Static factors include male gender, young age (teens to 20s), antisocial personality disorder, and a history of destruction of property.

Legal issues

Emergency psychiatrists must be familiar with a number of legal, ethical, and regulatory issues, including but not limited to the following:
- requirement to provide emergency care;
- city, state, federal regulations;
- confidentiality;
- capacity and informed consent;
- standards for voluntary and involuntary admission;
- seclusion and restraint regulations;
- managed care issues;
- mandated reporting.

A few of the above warrant specific comment:
- EMTALA (the Emergency Medical Treatment and Labor Act) – also known as COBRA or the Patient Anti-Dumping Law – is a 1986 federal law that requires hospitals to provide an examination and stabilizing treatment when a patient presents to an emergency room, regardless of insurance coverage or ability to pay. The statute is primarily a non-discrimination law whose purpose is to prevent hospitals from rejecting or refusing to treat patients, or transferring them to other hospitals, because of a patient's inability to pay.
- Confidentiality is an extremely important standard, though not absolute. There are multiple psychiatric emergency situations in which the harm in maintaining confidentiality is greater than the harm in disclosing information, such as when emergency treatment is needed or when there is a duty to warn or protect another party.

- Statutes and practices pertaining to both voluntary and involuntary admissions vary by state (see http://www.treatmentadvocacycenter.org), but it is generally true that while the need for treatment was the main trigger for admission in past decades, the main determinant in recent years is the patient's dangerousness to self or others.
- Mandated reporting obligations are state-specific, and may include cases of neglect or abuse to Child and Adult Protective Services, reportable diseases to the Department of Health, and even reporting of potentially dangerous patients to state agencies in order to limit gun access, as with the newly enacted New York State SAFE Act.

Reading list

Glick RL, Berlin JS, Fishkind AB, Zeller SL (eds). Emergency Psychiatry Principles and Practice. Philadelphia, PA: Lippincott Williams & Wilkins, 2008.

Haukka J, Suominen K, Partonen T, Lönnqvist J. Determinants and outcomes of serious attempted suicide: a nationwide study in Finland, 1996–2003. Am J Epidemiol 2008;167(10):1155.

Holloman GH, Zeller SL. Overview of Project BETA: Best Practices in Evaluation and Treatment of Agitation. West J Emerg Med 2012;13(1):1–2.

Riba MB, Ravindranath D (eds). Clinical Manual of Emergency Psychiatry. Arlington, VA: American Psychiatric Press, 2010.

Sederer LI. The Family Guide to Mental Health Care. New York: W. W. Norton & Company, 2013.

Simon RI, Tardiff K. Textbook of Violence Assessment and Management. Arlington, VA: American Psychiatric Press, 2008.

Suggested websites

American Association for Emergency Psychiatry. http://www.emergencypsychiatry.org

New York State Office of Mental Health, Violence Prevention: Risk Factors. http://www.omh.ny.gov/omhweb/sv/risk.htm

---

Additional material for this chapter can be found online at: www.mountsinaiexpertguides.com/psychiatry

This includes advice for patients, a case study, and multiple choice questions.

CHAPTER 43

Forensic Psychiatry

Jacob M. Appel[1], Amir Garakani[1,2], and Michal Kunz[3]
[1] Icahn School of Medicine at Mount Sinai, New York, NY, USA
[2] Yale School of Medicine, New Haven, CT, USA
[3] Kirby Forensic Psychiatric Center, New York, NY, USA

OVERALL BOTTOM LINE
- Forensic psychiatry encompasses all aspects of the psychiatric and the legal professions, both civil and criminal.
- The duties of forensic psychiatrists include writing reports, testifying in court, and performing therapeutic work in the correctional setting.
- Forensic psychiatrists wear "two hats" and owe distinct duties to the patient and to third parties.
- Among the subjects addressed by forensic psychiatry are competence, insanity defenses, psychopathy, malpractice claims, civil commitment, and the handling of sexual offenders.

Discussion of topic and guidelines

What is forensic psychiatry?

- Forensic psychiatry represents the interface of law and mental health. The field encompasses many aspects of the psychiatric and the legal profession, both civil and criminal.
- Completion of a 1-year fellowship after psychiatric residency training is required in order to sit for the board certification exam.

What do forensic psychiatrists do?

- They practice in a wide range of areas, including corrections, hospital and academic medical schools, research, hospital administration, state and local health boards, public and community mental health programs, and private practice.
- They serve as expert witnesses in civil or criminal court or disability hearings.
- As dual agents who wear "two hats," they have distinct obligations to third parties, often at odds with the traditional therapeutic role of psychiatrists.
- Forensic psychiatrists have an obligation to inform the patients they evaluate of their external obligations.

Issues in forensic psychiatry – criminal

Insanity and competence

Forensic psychiatrists are often called upon to offer expert testimony regarding the competence of criminal defendants to stand trial and the criminal responsibility of defendants for their actions.

Mount Sinai Expert Guides: Psychiatry, First Edition. Edited by Asher B. Simon, Antonia S. New, and Wayne K. Goodman.
© 2017 John Wiley & Sons, Ltd. Published 2017 by John Wiley & Sons, Ltd.
Companion website: www.mountsinaiexpertguides.com/psychiatry

- Historically, criminal responsibility required a *mens rea* ("guilty mind") and insanity offered an affirmative defense against guilt.
- Many jurisdictions follow the **M'Naghten Test:**
  - Established during an English murder trial in 1843.
  - Requires a defendant to "not know he was doing what was wrong."
- Alternative approach:
  - The **"irresistible impulse" test**, originating in *Commonwealth v. Rodgers* (1844), requires proof that the crime arose from "an irresistible and incontrollable impulse" in order for the defense to succeed.
- The **Durham Test:**
  - Broader and largely rejected.
  - Advanced by Judge David Bazelon in 1954, it absolves a defendant if "his unlawful act was the product of a mental disease or defect."
- The model penal code of the American Law Institute adopts a combination of the M'Naghten and irresistible impulse standards.
- During the 1980s, many states and the federal government shifted the burden of evidence to the defendant in trials following the public outcry after the acquittal of John Hinckley, who was charged with the attempted assassination of President Ronald Reagan.
- Some states allow a plea of "Guilty but Mentally Ill" that affords both incarceration and treatment.
- An insanity defense is raised in only 1–2% of cases that go to trial and is successful approximately 10% of the time.
- In *Dusky v. United States* (1960), the Supreme Court established a standard for competence to stand trial that includes a defendant having a "rational as well as factual understanding of the proceedings" and "sufficient present ability to consult with his lawyer with a reasonable degree of rational understanding."
- Courts have also established standards for determining competence to be executed, but psychiatric participation in this process is ethically controversial.
- APA guidelines state that "a psychiatrist should not be a participant in a legally authorized execution" because "the [ethical] physician–psychiatrist is a healer, not a killer, no matter how well purposed the killing may be."

Psychopathy
Forensic psychiatrists are often called upon to evaluate and treat "psychopathic" patients.
- Hervey Cleckley's *Mask of Sanity* (1941), the pioneering work in the field, posited 16 traits that composed the "psychopathic" personality including an inability to love and an absence of remorse.
- His work shaped the DSM-I's definition of "sociopathic personality disturbance," the precursor of the DSMI-III's "antisocial personality disorder," but the criteria for ASPD and psychopathy remain distinct.
- Robert Hare, in his *Psychopathy Checklist, Revised (PCL-R)*, attempted to create specific criteria for the diagnosis.
- A number of environmental factors predispose individuals toward psychopathy, including inadequate parenting styles, but genetic predisposition also likely plays a role.
- 15% of male inmates in US prisons are believed to qualify for a diagnosis of psychopathy, but the number rises to 12–40% among rapists.
- Approximately 1% of the population at large meets PCL-R criteria. Although scales such as the HCR-20 (Historical Clinical Risk) are used to determine the violence potential of patients, violence is notoriously difficult to predict with meaningful accuracy.

Sexual offenders

The diagnosis, treatment, and commitment of sexual offenders are the subject of both serious forensic inquiry and public passions.

- Starting in the 1930s, states enacted "sexual psychopath" statutes that permitted the civil commitment of individuals who allegedly fell into this often poorly-defined class, but many were repealed during the civil rights revolutions of the 1960s and 1970s.
- Outcry over the murders of Megan Kanka in New Jersey and Polly Klass in California led to a renewed interest in such measures, including the passage of sexually violent predator legislation, in the 1990s.
- The Supreme Court upheld the indefinite civil commitment of some sexual offenders in *Kansas v. Hendricks* (1997).
- Sex offender registration has become widespread. Complex treatment programs that utilize psychosocial as well as biological (hormonal) methods have been developed.
- While indefinite civil commitment reduces recidivism by those confined, it is unclear whether sex offender registration has any impact on reducing recidivism or sexual violence.

Correctional psychiatry

- In *Bowring v. Godwin* (1977) and *Ruiz v. Estelle* (1980), federal courts established a right for prison inmates to obtain psychiatric care and laid out basic parameters for its provision.
- The prevalence of serious mental illness among inmates may be as high as 14.5% among males and 31% among females.
- A large number of specialists in correctional psychiatry is therefore necessary to meet prisoners' needs.
- These providers confront the problem of "dual loyalty" as they must meet the therapeutic needs of patients while also serving the interests of correctional facilities.
- Forensic psychiatrists may also be called upon to distinguish genuine psychiatric illness from malingering.

Issues in forensic psychiatry – civil

Malpractice

- Forensic psychiatrists are often called upon for their expertise and testimony in cases of alleged malpractice.
- Malpractice requires four components:
  - a duty to a patient;
  - a breach of that duty;
  - proximate cause;
  - damages.
- The standard of care expected of providers is generally *descriptive* (based upon what other reasonable providers do), but may occasionally prove *prescriptive* if the customary practice is seriously deficient.
- Experts are generally called upon to testify as to whether the acts in question violated professional standards.
- The "respected minority" doctrine may provide a malpractice defense even when the treatment afforded does not conform to majority norms.
- Although lawsuits against psychiatrists have risen since the 1970s, the field faces less litigation than many other specialties.

- Among the most frequent bases for claims are:
  - incorrect treatment;
  - attempted or completed suicide;
  - incorrect diagnosis.
- Successful suits for wrongful hospitalization are rare.
- Some intentional torts, including sexual misconduct, may not be covered by malpractice insurance.
- Malpractice claims can also influence the standard of care. The case of *Osheroff vs. Chestnut Lodge* (1982), although settled out of court, played an instrumental role in the field's shift from favoring psychotherapy alone to privileging pharmacotherapy.

Third-party duties

- Although many medical specialties have grappled with physicians' duties toward third parties, such as in matters of public health, psychiatry proved largely immune to these concerns until the 1970s.
- This changed as a result of a California Supreme Court decision in *Tarasoff v. Regents of the University of California* (1976) that established an affirmative duty of psychiatrists to breach confidentiality "to protect" specific third parties from potential violence.
- In the wake of *Tarasoff*, many jurisdictions imposed upon mental health professionals either a "duty to warn" and/or a "duty to protect" third parties.
- More recently, so-called *Tarasoff*-limiting statutes have shielded psychiatrists from such duties.
- Approaches vary widely among states.
- Concern over gun violence has led several states, starting with New York's SAFE act, to require psychiatrists to report patients who are potentially unfit to own firearms.

Civil commitment

Few areas in forensic psychiatry have generated more debate, or criticism from "mental health liberation" attorneys like Bruce Ennis and dissident psychiatrists like Thomas Szasz, than the practice of involuntarily committing patients to psychiatric hospitals.

- In the landmark case of *O'Connor v. Donaldson* (1975), the Supreme Court wrote that "State cannot constitutionally confine, without more, a non-dangerous individual who is capable of surviving safely in freedom," marking an evolving shift from patient welfare to dangerousness as the standard for forcible commitment.
- In the case of *Zinermon v. Burch* (1991), the Supreme Court held that a patient lacking the capacity to consent to voluntary admission must be afforded the procedural rights due involuntarily-committed patients.
- A series of cases, most notably *Rogers v. Okin* (1979), require judicial approval for involuntary, non-emergent treatment in most jurisdictions.
- Starting with "Kendra's Law" (1999) in New York State, some jurisdictions permit assisted outpatient treatment (AOT), a form of involuntary outpatient commitment to care for historically dangerous patients.
  - AOT allows either a provider or certain specified relatives and caregivers to petition the court on the grounds that the patient cannot live safely in the community without judicially-mandated medication.
  - If a judge agrees, an AOT order allows authorities to bring a non-compliant individual to the hospital for potential involuntary hospitalization.
- In the widely-followed opinion of *Wyatt v. Stickney* (1971), Federal Judge Frank Johnson established minimum standards for care within state institutions.

Civil competence

Forensic psychiatrists may be called upon to assess the capacity of individuals to engage in various legal and civil functions, such as writing a will ("testamentary capacity") and signing a contract.

Psychiatric disability determination and personal injury litigation

Assessment of disability is the most common evaluation performed by forensic psychiatrists.

- A determination of disability is required for a patient to receive compensatory benefits from Social Security Disability Benefits (SSD) to worker's compensation.
- The role of the psychiatrist is complicated by the differing definitions of disability used by the Social Security Administration and various private insurance plans, as well as by the waxing and waning nature of some disabilities and a competing concern for malingering.

Forensic psychiatry and parent–child relationship

The rise of divorce has led to an increased role for psychiatric experts in testifying at child custody proceedings.

- Most jurisdictions now determine custody based on a standard related to the best interests of the child, which entails determinations of parental fitness and may include the child's personal preferences.
- In making such determinations, judges often rely heavily on the guidance of forensic psychiatrists.

Reading list

American Psychological Association. Specialty Guidelines for Forensic Psychiatry. Available at http://www.apa.org/practice/guidelines/forensic-psychology.aspx

Appelbaum PS, Gutheil TG. Clinical Handbook of Psychiatry and the Law, 4th edn. Philadelphia, PA: Lippincott Williams & Wilkins, 2006.

Bonnie RC, Jeffries JC Jr., Low PW. A Case Study in the Insanity Defense – The Trial of John W. Hinckley, Jr, 3rd edn. St Paul, MN: Foundation Press, 2008.

Rosner R. Principles and Practice of Forensic Psychiatry. Boca Raton, FL: CRC Press, 2003.

Slovenko R. Psychiatry in Law, Law in Psychiatry. New York: Routledge, 2009.

Suggested websites

American Academy of Psychiatry and the Law. http://www.aapl.org/

Additional material for this chapter can be found online at:
www.mountsinaiexpertguides.com/psychiatry

This includes advice for patients, a case study, and multiple choice questions.

CHAPTER 44

Global and Disaster Psychiatry

Diana Samuel[1], Jan Schuetz-Mueller[2], and Craig L. Katz[2]
[1] Columbia University Medical Center/New York-Presbyterian Hospital, New York, NY, USA
[2] Icahn School of Medicine at Mount Sinai, New York, NY, USA

OVERALL BOTTOM LINE

- Global mental health is an area of study, research, and practice that emphasizes improving mental health and achieving mental health access for everyone.
- Vast unmet mental health needs throughout low- and middle-income countries have significant impact on worldwide morbidity.
- In these countries, available mental health resources (human and otherwise) are often profoundly insufficient.
- Western psychiatric practice may be practically adapted to reduce the disparity between the need and provision of services; this should be accomplished with cultural sensitivity.

Discussion of topic and guidelines

Global mental health reflects an ambitious agenda that strives to apply all that psychiatry has to offer to all people, in all places. As such it is less of a field than an outlook, and for the Western practitioner reading this Western book, it provides a framework looking outward from a relatively local psychiatric practice. Ultimately, global mental health guides us on how to apply each and every chapter in this book to any community's children, adults, and elderly.

Although the imperative of equitable access to care knows no boundaries, global mental health traditionally focuses on low resource settings and particularly low- and middle-income countries. In this chapter we address international psychiatric practice in such areas as well as that in disaster-stricken communities; we will not explicitly address rural or community psychiatry, even if they surely inhere in the portfolio of global mental health. We have two overarching objectives for all health practitioners in resource-poor global settings: (1) to convince you why it is important to include mental health in your global health practice, and (2) to help you figure out how to do so.

We have organized this chapter according to a model we call the *wheel of global mental health* (Figure 44.1), incorporating mutually interdependent elements to be considered when embarking on practicing mental health care in resource-poor settings; a shift in one area dynamically affects the status of the others. The language that is used to define the roles of the parties involved should be carefully noted: to move beyond the idea that one party is *receiving* help and another *providing* it, we have chosen the terms *collaborator* and *host*.

Mount Sinai Expert Guides: Psychiatry, First Edition. Edited by Asher B. Simon, Antonia S. New, and Wayne K. Goodman.
© 2017 John Wiley & Sons, Ltd. Published 2017 by John Wiley & Sons, Ltd.
Companion website: www.mountsinaiexpertguides.com/psychiatry

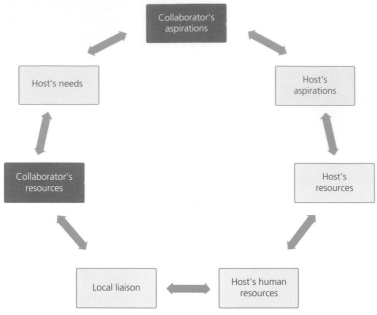

Figure 44.1 The wheel of global mental health.

The host's needs

To describe the host's needs is to describe the worldwide need for psychiatric care. Mental illness is often a major factor – whether florid or hidden, but certainly underdiagnosed and under-treated – among patients in all healthcare settings. Neuropsychiatric disorders make up 4 of the top 10 leading causes of years of life lived with disabilities (YLDs) and comprise nearly one-third of all YLDs. Unipolar depression leads this statistic and is estimated to cause more than 10% of YLDs worldwide. Approximately 800,000 people commit suicide every year, the majority of whom live in low- and middle-income countries (given the stigma of suicide and lack of consistent reporting, this estimate is probably quite low). Psychiatric conditions greatly affect medical morbidity/mortality (e.g., cardiovascular disease, smoking, obesity, etc.), as well as the treatment and spread of communicable diseases prevalent in developing countries (e.g., by interfering with treatment adherence).

The host's human resources

Many factors determine a community's access to mental healthcare: geography, demography, language, culture, history, development, politics, civil movement, stigma, public awareness, conflict, financing of services, etc. There is an estimated shortage of over 1 million mental health workers in low- and middle-income countries; this is likely to become only more pronounced. In 2009, the annual cost to alleviate this shortage was estimated at $4.4 billion. Low-income countries have 0.06 psychiatrists per 100,000 people, while high-income countries have roughly 200 times more (10.5/100,000). As developing countries lack adequate training facilities, the scarcity of child psychiatrists, psychiatric nurses, social workers, and other mental health workers is equally as dramatic, and human resources are further depleted by large-scale migration of mental health workers from low- to higher-income countries. Research has thus focused on finding alternative routes of access to care, and a cost-effective alternative has been found in utilizing primary care services to identify and treat people with mental illness. In this scenario, only a few specialists are required to train and supervise primary care clinicians and ensure provision of adequate care. Whatever the specialty of practitioners working in low- and middle-income countries, they should expect to be *de facto* mental health practitioners.

The host's other resources

In order for human resources to be implemented effectively, other resources must be present: finances, mental health policies, access to healthcare, access to medication, etc. These must include efforts to reduce stigma and improve awareness. Mental health lacks in prioritization and is completely absent from public budgets in almost one-third of all countries. In those that have allocated such funding, the poorest seem to spend the smallest budgetary proportion on mental health. In the minority of countries that have mental health policies, only 40% have been revised since 1990. The mentally ill have no legal protection in 22% of countries. The effects of limited financial resources also become evident in the availability of medications. While the WHO list of essential medications includes a reasonable formulary of psychiatric medications, these are often not available or accessible to patients. A particular medication may be in low supply at any given moment, leading to forced medication switching or discontinuation. Patients are often required to buy medications at higher costs in private pharmacies.

On the upside, certain resources are more readily available in low- and middle-income countries, including informal community resources (e.g., family, friends) and non-governmental organizations (NGOs). Enlisting the help of family while providing psychoeducation can greatly reduce a patient's distress, while creating a more supportive environment and promoting recovery. Given that 88% of countries have at least one NGO with a mental health program, chances are high that a practitioner would be able to connect with such an organization.

Your resources

Sustainability of the healthcare practitioner's role and resources is essential; this includes medication availability. Many countries prohibit non-physicians, and some forbid non-specialists, from prescribing psychotropics, severely limiting access to care. Although guidelines have been created in hopes of providing available treatment to cover a large breadth of psychopathology, the 2011 Interagency Emergency Kit for crises contains only 5 psychotropics (1 from each of the 5 classes). Without a crisis, the availability of even these basic medications is limited.

When determining what services you can deliver or oversee, you must consider local factors: consumer and staff preferences, service traditions, how evidence is interpreted and used, the strengths and weaknesses of the existing services, etc. Although evidence supports having a balance of hospital and community care, low- and middle-income countries with budgeted mental health services usually allot the money toward the former. There is a significant need for more community-based programs to improve service access and quality while promoting independent living. Without the relative luxury of outpatient clinics, your focus may need to be on integrating mental health into primary medical settings. Mental healthcare specialists are often best deployed as consultants to primary care staff.

Your aspirations

One's ideals can encounter a daunting reality in global mental health work, namely human rights violations against this vulnerable population. Protective laws and regulatory mechanisms are often absent, and resource-poor countries have come to rely on international human rights organizations for justice. International NGOs have played a crucial role. For example, the Mental Disability Advocacy Center (MDAC) has successfully formed litigation at international and national levels that has brought about legislative reform. Addressing mental health needs in countries without adequate protections can challenge the ideals of even the most well-meaning healthcare professional from overseas. An unsettling dilemma arises when caring for an acutely psychotic patient when the only psychiatric hospital is plagued by overcrowding and indefinite commitment; meanwhile, attempts at clinically managing the patient in the outpatient or primary care setting may be profoundly constrained by inconstant medication supplies and devastating psychosocial circumstances.

While psychological trauma attracts the media's and donors' attentions, the daily concerns faced by the majority of those with severe mental illness are often unseen. One must also recognize the charge that Western health professionals are guilty of "medical imperialism" when they bring their style of psychiatric diagnosis and treatment to remote corners of the world.

Your host's aspirations

Clearly identifying the host's aspirations is paramount. Although noble, outsiders' intentions to improve mental healthcare may not be well received, in part due to social stigma. If the public does not understand that mental illness is a medical problem, and sufferers are rejected, lawmakers and administrators may assume a general consensus that mental healthcare is regarded as non-essential.

The local mental health liaison

Successful implementation of change in the global health setting hinges on the availability of a local liaison. This individual or organization should have a good understanding of and fluency in the local burden of disease, healthcare system, human and other resources, infrastructure, culture, customs, language, politics, history, and local stigma. We have found that a good local liaison will command respect in their community and be in a position to influence change. Above all, they should be dedicated, empathic, and passionate about mental health. In our experience, this local liaison has been a nurse, a nurse practitioner, a hospital administrator, a physician, and/ or a social worker.

After a disaster

The psychiatric issues of particular concern after a disaster may differ in nature or frequency from those of the everyday.
- "Acute stress reactions" occur days–weeks after and include varied emotional, behavioral, or cognitive reactions:
  - insomnia, low mood, and general anxiety (may be adaptive or pathological, depending on intensity and persistence);
  - unexplained medical complaints (may predominate in non-Western cultures where somatization of distress often prevails over psychologization);
  - dissociative symptoms (not uncommon);
  - substance use.
- Long-term concerns in Western studies include major depressive disorder (MDD), posttraumatic stress disorder (PTSD), and alcohol disorders.

Mental health resources, which may be in especially short supply after the disaster, are further hampered by a poor evidence base guiding the mental health treatment of recently traumatized individuals. However, psychological first aid (PFA) is a clear evidence-informed framework for intervening with recent survivors and can be practiced by non-mental health professionals and non-health professionals. Intuitive, cost-effective, and non-technical, the major tenets of PFA include:
- providing for basic needs;
- protecting from further harm;

- reducing agitation and arousal;
- supporting those in most distress;
- keeping families together and providing social support;
- providing information and fostering communication and education;
- orienting to available services;
- using effective risk-communication techniques.

Common sense and experience suggest the considerable cross-cultural validity of these approaches.

Reading list

Drew N, Funk M, Tang S, et al. Human rights violations of people with mental and psychosocial disabilities: an unresolved global crisis. Lancet 2011;378(9803):1664–75.

Jones L, Asare JB, El Masri M, Mohanraj A, Sherief H, van Ommeren M. Severe mental disorders in complex emergencies. Lancet 2009;374(9690):654–61.

Katz CL. Disaster psychiatry: good intentions seeking science and sustainability. Adolesc Psychiatry 2011;1(3): 187–96.

Patel V. Where There is No Psychiatrist: A Mental Health Care Manual. London: Royal College of Psychiatrists, 2003.

Prince M, Patel V, Saxena S, et al. No health without mental health. Lancet 2007;370(9590):859–77.

Saxena S, Thornicroft G, Knapp M, Whiteford H. Resources for mental health: scarcity, inequity, and inefficiency. Lancet 2007;370(9590):878–89.

Stoddard F, Katz CL, Merlino J (eds). Hidden Impact: What You Need to Know for the Next Disaster – A Practical Mental Health Guide. Boston: Jones and Bartlett, 2010.

Summerfield D. "Global mental health" is an oxymoron and medical imperialism. BMJ 2013;346:f3509.

Thornicroft G. Measuring Mental Health Needs, 2nd edn. London: Gaskell, 2001.

Thornicroft G, Tansella M. Balancing community-based and hospital-based mental health care. World Psychiatry 2002;1(2):84–90.

Thornicroft G, Tansella M. Components of a modern mental health service: a pragmatic balance of community and hospital care. Br J Psychiatry 2004;185:283–90.

van Ommeren M, Barbui C, de Jong K, et al. If you could only choose five psychotropic medicines: updating the Interagency Emergency Health Kit. PLoS Med 2011;8(5):e1001030.

Suggested websites

CDC: Coping with a Disaster or Traumatic Event. http://emergency.cdc.gov/mentalhealth/

WHO Model Lists of Essential Medicines. http://www.who.int/medicines/publications/essential medicines/en/

http://www.who.int/mental_health/policy/essentialpackage1/en/

Additional material for this chapter can be found online at:
www.mountsinaiexpertguides.com/psychiatry

This includes a case study and multiple choice questions.

CHAPTER 45

Symptomatology and Psychopharmacology Across Cultures

Daniella Loh, Olanrewaju Dokun, and Sharon M. Batista
Icahn School of Medicine at Mount Sinai, New York, NY, USA

OVERALL BOTTOM LINE
- Cross-cultural effects occur across psychiatric practice and include differing
  - expressions of emotional distress (which may be through somatic metaphors/symptoms rather than psychologically);
  - help-seeking behaviors;
  - understandings of normal/abnormal;
  - stigmatization;
  - effects on the doctor–patient relationship.
- Culture's role in the expression of personality disorders and substance use patterns is not well understood.
- Biological and environmental factors impact the efficacy and metabolism of psychiatric medications.

Discussion of topic and guidelines
Psychotic illnesses and symptoms
- Although schizophrenia is found worldwide, its manifestations may vary across cultures.
  - Ideas that appear delusional in one culture may be congruent with commonly held beliefs in others.
  - Certain forms of hallucinations may be more prevalent in some cultures than others (e.g., higher rates of visual and tactile hallucinations among African individuals with schizophrenia).
- Cultural differences in non-verbal communication – especially body language and eye contact – should be considered when interpreting affect.
- Patients with foreign backgrounds are frequently misdiagnosed with psychotic disorders when displaying hallucinations, pseudo-hallucinations, or overvalued ideas; however, these may be culturally normative ways of expressing distress.
  - Latino individuals may exhibit higher rates of perceptual disturbances as nonspecific symptoms of distress (and not representing true psychosis).
  - Dissociation could account for psychotic-appearing presentations among immigrants.

Depressive illnesses and symptoms
- Somatic symptoms of insomnia and loss of energy are the most frequently reported symptoms of depression worldwide and often are the most common presenting complaint.

Mount Sinai Expert Guides: Psychiatry, First Edition. Edited by Asher B. Simon, Antonia S. New, and Wayne K. Goodman.
© 2017 John Wiley & Sons, Ltd. Published 2017 by John Wiley & Sons, Ltd.
Companion website: www.mountsinaiexpertguides.com/psychiatry

- In many Asian cultures, emotional symptoms (e.g., depressed mood) are less culturally accepted as signifiers of distress than are somatic symptoms.
- In the US, certain ethnicities carry higher rates of suicide:
  - elderly Asian women, Native Americans, and other indigenous male youths.
- When presented with symptoms that appear to be consistent with a depressive illness, keep in mind that – depending on the context and the meaning that the suffering takes on – this may not represent a medical problem to the patient.
  - For example, although the DSM-IV's bereavement exclusion defined normal bereavement as lasting for 2 months, some ethnic or cultural groups may see an extended period of grief, such as years, as a normal emotional response.

Anxiety disorders

- Panic disorder and attacks occur across cultures, with varying prevalence of defined DSM-5 symptoms, as well as varying culture-specific symptoms (e.g., tinnitus, neck soreness, headache, uncontrollable screaming, or crying).
  - There are higher rates of paresthesias in African Americans and dizziness in certain Asian groups.
  - Cultural syndromes associated with panic disorder include *ataque de nervios* and *khyâl* (see further on).
- Japanese *taijin kyofusho* (see further on) overlaps significantly with diagnostic criteria for social anxiety disorder, but with an important distinction:
  - The patient's primary fear in *taijin kyofusho* is that of upsetting others (with one's gaze or appearance, etc.), as opposed to a central fear of oneself being scrutinized by others, as is found in social anxiety disorder.

Post-traumatic stress disorder (PTSD) and trauma-related sequelae, including trauma-related dissociative disorders and symptoms

- Symptoms of acute stress disorder and PTSD may be differentially expressed.
  - Nightmares may be more commonly reported than other symptoms.
  - Somatic symptoms of anxiety (dizziness, shortness of breath, heat sensations) may predominate.
  - Varying degrees or types of dissociative responses often occur.
- Exposure to trauma is associated with cultural syndromes (see further on) or idioms of distress that may not resemble PTSD (e.g., *ataque de nervios*; *khyâl* attacks).
- Dissociative symptoms are thought to occur ubiquitously across cultures, with the symptom form influenced by cultural and individual background:
  - "Western" dissociative loss of self-cohesion or identity alteration may instead take the form of possession by spirits, deities, demons, animals, or mythical figures.
  - A patient may even be seen as her or his own specific micro-culture, as well (e.g., non-epileptic seizures present in patients with epilepsy).

Culturally accepted, non-pathological forms of possession are common across many cultural traditions and should be distinguished from pathological forms that may be disabling, persistent, and/or uncontrollable.

Somatic symptoms

- Somatic symptoms are a prominent feature of mental distress throughout the world, characterize many of the culture-bound syndromes, and may carry special meanings within a particular cultural context, as idioms of distress (e.g., "burning in the head," "too much heat in the body").

Personality disorders

- Personality styles, forms of "normality," and prevalence of pathologies are influenced by the differential emphases placed on particular values across societies (e.g., sociocentric vs egocentric; child-rearing practices; moral and religious beliefs or traditions; gender roles).

Substance use disorders

- Culture-based behaviors, family structures, and environments have variable effects on risk.
- In some populations, acculturation to the majority culture can mean the adoption of negative health habits and higher mortality, while in others it can be protective.

Cultural concepts of distress

- Formerly known as "Culture-Bound Syndromes" in DSM-IV.
- The term "culture-bound syndrome" has been used to refer to psychiatric syndromes that are closely related to culture and that may or may not fit DSM categories.
- *Amok* (Malaysia): dissociative episode occurring after a perceived slight or insult and marked by an outburst of violent, aggressive, or homicidal behavior directed toward other people and objects.
- *Koro* (southern China): episode of sudden and intense anxiety that the penis will retract into the body and lead to death.
- *Ataque de nervios* (Latino): intense emotional upset, acute anxiety, anger, grief, screaming and shouting uncontrollably, crying, heat in the chest rising into the head, a sense of being out of control, and becoming verbally and physically aggressive. Often occurs following a stressful event, such as news of the death of a close relative.
- *Dhat syndrome* (south Asia): somatic complaints including fatigue, weakness, and anxiety are associated with the loss of semen, as evidenced by discharge or whitish discoloration of the urine. Linked to Hindu ideas that semen is one of seven essential bodily fluids whose balance is necessary to maintain health.
- *Khyâl cap* (*khyâl* attacks) (Cambodia): panic attack-like symptoms including dizziness, palpitations, shortness of breath, cold extremities, anxiety, autonomic arousal, tinnitus, and neck soreness. May occur without warning or be triggered by worrisome thoughts, standing up quickly, specific odors, or going to crowded spaces. Associated with catastrophic cognitions centered on the concern that *khyâl*, a windlike substance, may rise in the body, along with blood and cause a range of detrimental effects (such as pressing on the lungs causing asphyxiation, or entering the cranium causing tinnitus or syncope).
- *Shenjing shuairuo* (China): translated as "weakness of the nervous system" and marked by weakness (e.g., mental fatigue), emotions, excitement (e.g., increased recollections), nervous pain (headache), and insomnia. May often meet criteria for a DSM-5 mood, anxiety, and somatic symptom disorder.
- *Taijin kyofusho* (Japan): translated as "interpersonal fear disorder" and characterized by anxiety about and avoidance of interpersonal situations due to the thought, feeling, or conviction that one's appearance and actions are inadequate or offensive to others. Similar syndromes are found in Korea and other societies that strongly emphasize the self-conscious maintenance of appropriate social behavior in hierarchical interpersonal relationships.
- *Anorexia nervosa* is a condition that has been conceptualized as a culture-bound syndrome of the industrialized world, given its apparent rarity in non-industrialized cultures.

General treatment considerations

- Doctor–patient interactional styles vary between cultures and should always be considered.
  - Recent immigrants may expect a more hierarchical and directed relationship rather than the patient-centered model that is the US norm.

- Consider using linguistically and culturally appropriate diagnostic screening instruments.
- Culturally-adapted forms of cognitive behavioral therapy (CBT) have been developed for different disorders, utilizing imagery or concepts with cultural salience.
  - CBT interventions developed for Cambodian refugees with traumatic stress disorders have integrated relaxation techniques similar to Buddhist mindfulness strategies; culturally appropriate relaxation imagery includes a lotus blossom.
- Due to varying beliefs and customs regarding psychiatric illness, patients commonly seek out spiritual or religious help or alternative treatments prior to or in addition to medical treatment.
- Recognize that stigma may be an issue.

Psychopharmacological principles in specific ethnic groups

Pharmacokinetics

- Pharmacokinetics includes time course of absorption, distribution, protein binding, metabolism, and excretion of drugs. Cross-culturally, metabolism is the most widely studied.
- Cytochrome P450 (CYP) enzymes are responsible for metabolism of 90% of all clinically used drugs. 1A2, 2C19, 2D6, and 3A4 are the most relevant to psychopharmacology. 2D6 metabolizes 80% of antipsychotics and antidepressants, and 2C19 metabolizes a significant number of anti-convulsants and antidepressants.
  - 1A2 and 3A4 activity are the most susceptible to environmental factors.
  - 2C19 and 2D6 activity are related to functionally distinct polymorphisms.
    - High genetic variability (e.g., 70 known functional alleles for 2D6) creates phenotypic differences, with 2D6 activity depending on the number of active versions of the gene. Individuals are characterized as: poor metabolizer (PM), intermediate metabolizer (IM), elevated metabolizer (EM), and ultra-rapid metabolizer (UM).
  - Rates of metabolism influence drug response, likelihood of side effects, and whether its dose form or metabolite is active.
  - Rates of PMs, IMs, EMs, and UMs vary greatly inter- and intra-ethnically.
    - 70% of Caucasians have "normal metabolic activity" compared with 50% of Asians or Africans.
    - The UM phenotype may be more common in Africans (>10–20%) compared with Europeans (<5%).
- Varying in allele frequencies between ethnic groups, polymorphisms within genes encoding for alcohol and aldehyde dehydrogenase isozymes produce different kinetic properties linked to risk.
  - Being a carrier of more than one ADH1B*2 allele has been associated with protection against alcohol dependence in Mexican Americans.

Pharmacodynamics

- Pharmacodynamics refers to the relationship between drug concentration at the site of action and the resulting effects, both desired and undesired.
- Polymorphisms influence the quality/quantity of receptors, second messengers carrying the binding signal within the cell, and/or other regulatory mechanisms influencing the net response to a drug.
  - In Caucasians and to an even greater extent in Asians, homozygosity of the short allele of 5HTTLPR (the serotonin transporter gene) may be linked to poorer response to SSRIs and homozygosity for the long allele with better response.
    - Although the later-occurring STAR*D study did not support this finding, it did not analyze African Americans and Caucasians separately and may therefore be confounded by the potentially poorer response of African Americans to SSRIs on the whole. The STAR*D study did not find any significant difference in response rates due to these alleles in Hispanic populations.

- At present, no other significant finding conclusively links particular polymorphisms to the efficacy of a particular antidepressant/antipsychotic, and none has demonstrated increased frequency of such hypothetical polymorphisms in different ethnicities.
  - This may be due to the existence of multiple genes, each of which has only a partial influence on pharmacodynamics.

Environmental factors in drug effect

- Despite data demonstrating abundant genetic variability *between* ethnicities, *intra-ethnic* genetic (and other) variability may be even more significant.
- "Ethnicity" is a placeholder term meant to account for differences not only in genetics but also in patterns of behavior, shared beliefs, geographic origin, diet, etc.
  - Diet can significantly alter pharmacokinetics:
    - inhibition of CYP1A2 and 3A4 by grapefruit juice;
    - induction of CYP1A2 by cruciferous vegetables (and cigarette smoke);
    - inhibition or induction of CYP1A2 depending on whether diet is predominantly carbohydrate-rich or protein-rich, respectively.
- Alternative and herbal medications may also impact medication metabolism and response.

Reading list

American Psychiatric Association. Section III: Cultural Formulation. In: Diagnostic and Statistical Manual of Mental Disorders, 5th edn. Washington, DC: American Psychiatric Publishing, 2013.

Chaudhry I, Neelam K, Duddu V, Husain N. Ethnicity and psychopharmacology. J Psychopharmacol 2008;22(6):673–80.

Kalra G, Bhugra D, Shah N. Cultural aspects of schizophrenia. Int Rev Psychiatry 2012;24(5):441–9.

Kleinman A. Rethinking Psychiatry: From Cultural Category to Personal Experience. New York: Macmillan/The Free Press, 1988.

Kleinman A. Culture and depression. N Engl J Med 2004;351(10):951–3.

Lim RF. Clinical Manual of Cultural Psychiatry. Washington, DC: American Psychiatric Publishing, 2006.

Sue S, Yan Cheng JK, Saad CS, Chu JP. Asian American mental health: a call to action. Am Psychol 2012;67(7):532–44.

Tseng WS. From peculiar psychiatric disorders through culture-bound syndromes to culture-related specific syndromes. Transcult Psychiatry 2006;43(4):554–76.

Suggested websites

EthnoMed: Mental Health Clinical Topics. http://ethnomed.org/clinical/mental-health

---

Additional material for this chapter can be found online at:
www.mountsinaiexpertguides.com/psychiatry

This includes advice for patients, a case study, and multiple choice questions.

CHAPTER 46

Complementary and Alternative Medicine in Psychiatry

Ellen Vora[1], Amy Aloysi[2], and Rachel Zhuk[2]

[1] Eleven Eleven Wellness Center and One Medical Group, New York, NY, USA
[2] Icahn School of Medicine at Mount Sinai, New York, NY, USA

OVERALL BOTTOM LINE

- Complementary and alternative approaches can offer psychiatric patients low-risk, low-cost treatment options to augment, or to consider in lieu of, conventional treatments.
- Exercise, light therapy, sleep hygiene, stress management, nutrition, St. John's Wort, SAMe (*S*-adenosylmethionine), yoga, meditation, acupuncture, and spiritual practices are supported by varying levels of evidence and may be especially beneficial for patients who have unsatisfactory responses to medications, cannot tolerate certain side effects, or for whom the therapeutic risk/ benefit analysis has additional complexity (e.g., in pregnancy).
- Patients with depression, anxiety, and other mental health disorders often do not reach optimal levels of mental health even if they achieve syndromal remission, and practitioners may employ integrative therapies to help patients build a better foundation for mental wellbeing and resilience.

Discussion of topic and guidelines

The discussion below focuses on the integrative treatment of major depressive disorder (MDD) – a leading cause of disability in the US for those aged 15–44 – in which conventional pharmacotherapy is often limited by inefficacy, side effects, and other concerns. In addition to non-adherence, limited long-term safety data, and the fact that relapse may recur after a medication treatment ends, up to two-thirds of patients with MDD do not achieve remission with conventional medications, and medications may not separate from placebo in mild to moderate depression.

The integrative approach to patients with MDD should include a review of medical history, current physical health, medications, and discussion of a patient's experience with and openness to integrative treatments. Integrative approaches are increasingly evidence-based, but many have not undergone rigorous testing; however, it is the opinion of the authors that when treatments are low-risk and low-cost but have large potential benefit and biologic plausibility, it is reasonable to discuss these options with patients. Practitioners do not need to wait until treatment failure or other challenges occur before considering integrative approaches, but can offer these treatments as options from the outset, if the evidence and clinical indications are supportive.

Mount Sinai Expert Guides: Psychiatry, First Edition. Edited by Asher B. Simon, Antonia S. New, and Wayne K. Goodman.
© 2017 John Wiley & Sons, Ltd. Published 2017 by John Wiley & Sons, Ltd.
Companion website: www.mountsinaiexpertguides.com/psychiatry

Certain integrative treatments should be considered for all patients being treated for MDD, as there is reasonable evidence to support their safety and efficacy: exercise, sleep hygiene, stress management, light therapy, and nutrition. If a patient's depressive symptoms warrant pharmacologic treatment, St. John's Wort (SJW) or SAMe may be considered. Additional modalities for which there is variable evidence include yoga, meditation, acupuncture, and spiritual practices.

Exercise

Several clinical studies have shown aerobic exercise to be as effective as antidepressant medication in the treatment of MDD. A meta-analysis of 11 randomized controlled trials found exercising 2–4 times per week to be a promising treatment for moderate MDD. One study demonstrated that exercising 5 times per week led to remission rates of 47% (i.e., comparable to antidepressant treatment). Aerobic exercise also results in improved learning, hippocampal neurogenesis, alleviation of anxiety, improved sleep, potentially improved global self-esteem, and improved physical health; it may additionally prevent recurrence of mood episodes.

Caveat: the patient must actively participate in this treatment. Exercise studies are inherently difficult to control and blind.

Treatment recommendation: ask patients about their exercise habits, inform patients of the potential impact on mood symptoms, and strongly encourage regular aerobic exercise 2–5 times per week.

Sleep

Several studies have linked lack of sleep with poor mental health. Sufficient deep, restorative sleep on a nightly basis is foundational not only for recovery from MDD and relapse prevention, but also for overall mental health.

Caveat: mood symptoms can be both a cause and effect of sleep disturbances. A chronic sleep disturbance should also prompt the clinician to consider non-psychiatric causes in the differential (e.g., obstructive sleep apnea).

Treatment recommendation: discuss sleep with all depressed patients and encourage patients to adhere to the principles of sleep hygiene, as follows:

- Sleep 7–9 hours nightly.
- Keep a regular sleep schedule, preferably going to sleep around 10–11 pm and rising around 6–7 am.
- Set aside time before bed for winding down *without electronics*.
- Avoid caffeine and stimulants after 12 pm.
- Use the bed for sleep and sex only.
- Minimize TV and computer use in the bedroom (as these associate the bed with stress and activation).
- Avoid exposure to computer, phone, tablet and TV screens before bed, as these have been shown to suppress normal nighttime release of melatonin, leading to delayed sleep onset.
- Sleep in a cool, dark, quiet environment, setting the thermostat to 60–67 degrees Fahrenheit and wearing an eye mask or installing blackout shades.

Stress management

Evidence suggests that chronic stress of various forms directly contributes to MDD. Ways to reduce stress include yoga, meditation, breathing exercises, mindfulness-based stress reduction (MBSR), gentle movement techniques (tai chi, qigong, Feldenkrais), biofeedback, acupuncture, prayer, exercise, engaging in community, spending time in nature, and listening to music. Biofeedback training can specifically enhance self-regulation of the stress response.

Caveat: educating patients about stress reduction can feel like admonishment about something they cannot control, and recommending stress-management techniques can seem like adding one more activity to an already overscheduled lifestyle. It is important to validate this concern and limit recommendations to a few, high-yield activities.

Treatment recommendation: recognize the role of stress in patients' illnesses. Ask patients about stress levels, educate them about the relationship between stress and mood, and review options for stress management. Providers can quickly teach patients 4-7-8 breathing: inhale for a count of 4, hold for 7, exhale for 8.

Light therapy

Originally intended as a treatment for seasonal affective disorder, light therapy may also be used to treat non-seasonal, unipolar depressive disorders, as well as ante- and post-partum depression. (A recent meta-analysis showed bright light treatment of MDD to have effect sizes similar to those found in antidepressant trials.) Light therapy can also be used as an adjuvant therapy along with antidepressants to potentiate an antidepressant response.

Caveat: side effects may include headache, eye strain, nausea, agitation, and risk of inducing mania.

Treatment recommendation: first thing in the morning, patients should sit approximately one foot from a 10,000-lux light box for 20–30 minutes, keeping eyes open but avoiding looking directly into the light source. Most patients should expect to see improvement in mood symptoms within 1–2 weeks, but should continue daily treatment to prevent relapse, especially in the winter months.

Nutrition

Good nutrition, although difficult to define, is essential for physical and mental health. Evidence best supports the efficacy of the Mediterranean diet in the prevention of depression, with growing evidence to suggest that a paleo-template diet can also be therapeutic. It is the opinion of the authors that advising patients to eat real food and avoid processed foods is the most effective way to promote good nutrition. A 5-year longitudinal study of middle-aged subjects found that a processed-food dietary pattern was a risk factor for MDD, while a pattern rich in whole foods was protective. Several individual nutrients are essential to healthy brain function and relevant to psychiatric disease, including thiamine, vitamin B_{12}, folic acid, and vitamin D. Newly emerging research has shown links between the makeup of intestinal bacterial flora and anxiety and depression.

Caveat: any generalized dietary recommendation is inherently oversimplified and potentially controversial, and we make the following recommendations cautiously. The evidence is incomplete and at times contradictory.

Treatment recommendation: encourage all patients to eat a nutrient-dense, whole-foods diet and avoid processed foods. A good rule of thumb: "let half your plate be vegetables"; the other half should be a combination of good-quality protein (wild cold water fatty fish, meat and poultry from pasture-raised animals, properly prepared sprouted legumes, quinoa, tempeh), and starch (sweet potatoes, white potatoes, plantains, rice), as well as nuts, seeds, fruit, fermented foods (sauerkraut, kimchi, miso) and plentiful healthy fats (coconut oil, clarified butter, butter, olive oil). Eliminate processed foods, fried foods, refined carbohydrates and added sugars; reduce consumption of factory-farmed meat, dairy and poultry; and avoid foods prepared with trans fats and industrially processed vegetable oils (corn, soy, safflower, and canola oils). Some patients have dietary intolerances and see improvement in mood symptoms after removing foods such as gluten or dairy. A comprehensive elimination diet is the gold standard for identifying food intolerances. Judicious supplementation of nutrients may also be useful in augmenting the treatment of MDD or other mood disorders:

- Daily probiotic and prebiotic.
- A good quality multivitamin, containing methylated B vitamins.
- Vitamin D_3 (patients should have Vitamin D levels measured and tracked to determine supplementation needs).
- Omega-3 fatty acids (1000–2000 mg daily). Studies have shown that MDD is associated with decreased omega-3 fatty acids and an increased omega-6 to omega-3 ratio. Omega-3 supplementation may be most effective with concomitant decrease in omega-6 consumption.
- Turmeric 400–600 mg three times daily.

St. John's Wort (SJW)

SJW is an herb that has been shown in large, well-designed, randomized, double-blind, placebo-controlled trials to be superior to placebo and comparable to TCAs and SSRIs in the treatment of MDD, with fewer side effects. SJW may be especially useful in patients who have a good response to low-dose SSRI therapy but cannot tolerate side effects such as weight gain or sexual dysfunction.

Caveat: drug–SJW interactions are of some concern, including risk of serotonin syndrome and increased blood levels of medications metabolized by the CYP450 system. SJW should only very cautiously be combined with SSRIs and TCAs, and not used concurrently with MAOIs. Side effects include photosensitivity, and at higher doses resemble those of SSRIs.

Treatment recommendation: SJW is a reasonable choice for monotherapy in the treatment of mild to moderate MDD. Doses range from 500 to 1800 mg/day.

SAMe

SAMe, which occurs naturally in the body, has been shown to outperform placebo and match TCAs in the treatment of MDD. There have been 16 open trials, 13 double-blind placebo-controlled trials, and 19 double-blind controlled trials demonstrating SAMe's efficacy and safety. SAMe is useful as both mono- and adjunctive therapy.

Caveat: SAMe must be taken on an empty stomach. Side effects include nausea and anxiety, and it can precipitate mania in vulnerable individuals. It is expensive at higher daily doses.

Treatment recommendation: doses should be titrated starting at 200 mg/day up to a maximum of 1600 mg/day (higher doses may be necessary in more severe MDD). Folate is involved with SAMe in the methylation pathway leading to the production of biogenic amines, thus supplementation with extra folic acid has been recommended.

Yoga and meditation

By combining the benefits of exercise, meditation, breathing techniques, community, and spirituality into a single activity, yoga targets depressive symptoms from multiple angles, including increasing parasympathetic tone, inducing the relaxation response, and increasing CNS *GABA* activity. Several studies have demonstrated yoga's use in the treatment of MDD. Many studies show that meditation alone has positive effects as an adjunctive treatment for MDD.

Caveat: It can be difficult to find time to build these practices into daily life.

Treatment recommendation: yoga, meditation, and breathing exercises are excellent recommendations for patients suffering from depression and for those wishing to cultivate resilience. If going to a yoga studio is not feasible, recommend yoga DVDs, online yoga classes or guided meditation mp3's at home.

Acupuncture

Acupuncture targets many aspects of well-being, including mood, anxiety, pain, and sleep symptoms. The mechanisms of action are not entirely understood, but may include anti-inflammatory and analgesic effects as well as promoting parasympathetic tone. A 2012 review of acupuncture for MDD found it to be safe, well-tolerated, and effective, both as monotherapy and as augmentation in patients with a partial response to medication.

Caveat: many patients may not be open to acupuncture, may not have access, or may not have sufficient time or money. Acupuncture is inherently difficult to study by randomized, placebo-controlled trials.

Treatment recommendation: we recommend beginning with three sessions and monitoring for improvement. If cost is an issue, patients can seek out community acupuncture.

Spiritual practices

Patients with MDD often feel alienated, isolated, and alone, and spiritual practices can help them regain a sense of connectedness. A cross-sectional study of women with depression history found spirituality may protect against relapse, with up to one-tenth the risk of recurrence of MDD over a 10-year period.

Caveat: these studies show associations but do not prove causality.

Treatment recommendations: explore a patient's openness to developing a spiritual practice or joining a spiritual community.

Summary

Practitioners should consider integrative treatments for patients with MDD. While these approaches are not "one size fits all," it is generally helpful to recommend exercise, light therapy, stress management, sleep hygiene, and to discuss nutrition. St. John's Wort and SAMe could be considered when choosing medications. Practitioners could gauge a patient's openness to acupuncture, yoga, meditation, and the cultivation of a spiritual practice. Ultimately, integrative approaches give patients more tools to help build a foundation of wellbeing and resilience.

Reading list

Brown RP, Gerbarg PL, Muskin PR. How to Use Herbs, Nutrients & Yoga in Mental Health Care. New York: W.W. Norton & Company, 2009.

Hanh TN. Peace Is Every Step: The Path of Mindfulness in Everyday Life. New York: Bantam Books, 1991.

Kabat-Zinn J. Full Catastrophe Living (Revised Edition): Using the Wisdom of Your Body and Mind to Face Stress, Pain, and Illness. New York: Random House, 2013.

Weintraub A. Yoga for Depression: A Compassionate Guide to Relieve Suffering Through Yoga. New York: Broadway Books, 2004.

Suggested websites

National Center for Complementary and Integrative Health:
- Meditation: An Introduction. https://nccih.nih.gov/health/meditation/overview.htm
- Yoga for Health: An Introduction. https://nccih.nih.gov/health/yoga/introduction.htm

---

Additional material for this chapter can be found online at:
www.mountsinaiexpertguides.com/psychiatry

This includes advice for patients, a case study,
and multiple choice questions.

CHAPTER 47

Models for Delivery of Care

Sabina Lim[1] and Joseph M. Cerimele[2]
[1] Icahn School of Medicine at Mount Sinai, New York, NY, USA
[2] University of Washington School of Medicine, Seattle, WA, USA

OVERALL BOTTOM LINE

- Models of mental healthcare delivery have evolved from predominantly inpatient-focused models to ambulatory and community-oriented models.
- New models of healthcare delivery including accountable care organizations (ACOs) and Health Homes have significant implications for mental health services.
- Collaborative/integrated care and integration of mental and physical healthcare are increasingly recognized as key to improving quality of care, outcomes, and healthcare costs.
- Patients treated in collaborative care settings can have significantly improved short- and long- term depression and medical illness outcomes, reduced disability from depression and co-occurring medical illness, improved quality of life, and lower total medical costs compared to patients treated with usual care.

Discussion of topic and guidelines

- Models of mental health services are rapidly evolving in the US.
  - In SAMHSA's 2011 National Survey of Drug Use and Health in the US, 45.6 million adults aged 18 and over (20% of civilian adults) had a diagnosable mental, behavioral, or emotional disorder.
  - Since the movement away from inpatient hospitalization/institutionalization in the 1960s and 70s, and the impact of managed care starting in the 1980s, mental health services have placed greater emphasis on ambulatory and community-based services.
  - Although long-term psychiatric hospitals are still present, current models include a broad continuum of outpatient-based services, including: (1) partial or intensive hospital programs; (2) clinics providing psychopharmacological treatment, individual and group psychotherapies, and case management; (3) community-based services, such as assertive community treatment, mobile crisis and outreach services, and peer support services.
- Such models of care typically serve individuals with severe acute and/or chronic and persistent mental illness.
  - Individuals with less severe illnesses are more often treated by private psychiatric practitioners or in primary care settings.
  - Upwards of 80% of psychotropic medications are prescribed by non-psychiatric practitioners.

Mount Sinai Expert Guides: Psychiatry, First Edition. Edited by Asher B. Simon, Antonia S. New, and Wayne K. Goodman.
© 2017 John Wiley & Sons, Ltd. Published 2017 by John Wiley & Sons, Ltd.
Companion website: www.mountsinaiexpertguides.com/psychiatry

- There is also increasing evidence of the relationship between mental health and physical health, with a significant percentage of patients seen in primary care settings with concurrent mental illnesses.
  - Despite the growth of ambulatory psychiatric services over the past decades, issues of access and quality of care still persist, with an over-reliance on acute psychiatric services (namely, emergency and inpatient-based care).
  - Physical health and mental healthcare service delivery remain separate and distinct, despite the increasing evidence of the strong interplay between mental and physical health problems.
  - Services are delivered in physically separate locations, and reimbursement mechanisms differ for physical and mental healthcare. In many states, behavioral health services are "carved out" from physical health insurance plans as a separate set of benefits and often managed via a separate contracted vendor.

Current models

- The primary care physician of a patient with depression would typically refer out to a psychiatric clinic.
- The patient is usually given the information of the provider to whom she or he is being referred, and it is up to the patient to ensure follow-up appointments.
- A similar pathway exists for patients seen first in a psychiatric setting who require assessment and/or treatment for physical illnesses. The patient would be referred to a medical clinic, group practice, or private practitioner, depending on the patient's insurance plan.
- The patient may or may not receive assistance from staff to set up the appointments.
- Communication, formal or informal, between providers may or may not occur.
- There is little incentive for collaboration and coordination of care between specialties, and care pathways are provider-centric rather than patient-centric. Referral no-show rates for either setting are generally reported as more than 50%.

The Affordable Care Act (ACA)

- Since the passage of the ACA a variety of new models of healthcare delivery and reimbursement have arisen, many incorporating conceptually and operationally different models of mental health services.
  - ACOs and Health Homes are two of the most widely discussed models of care delivery in the ACA.
  - ACOs are groups of providers (hospitals, physician groups, etc.) who agree to collaborate with each other to be responsible for the management and coordination of the entire healthcare needs in a defined population of individuals.
- The ACO model is based on the expectation that when a group of providers work together to coordinate and manage the whole health of a population, healthcare costs will go down, while the quality of care and patient experience will improve. ACOs must have enough primary care professionals to care for at least 5000 Medicare beneficiaries, care management services, and the ability to manage financial risk.

Health Homes

- A Health Home is a model of care organization where a provider, usually the primary care physician, coordinates the entire healthcare needs of the individual.
- Health Homes must have health promotion services, care management and coordination, and a robust information technology system to coordinate care between all providers.

- Health Home enrollees must have: (1) two serious chronic medical conditions; (2) one serious chronic medical condition and risk for developing a second; or (3) one serious and persistent mental health condition.
- ACOs and Health Homes are focused on the whole health of populations/individuals, and embody a framework of service delivery that incentivizes and promotes jointly managed care of illnesses.
- The prominence of ACOs and Health Homes exemplifies the increased interest in integrated care of both physical and behavioral health needs.
  - The case study (on the companion website) for this chapter involves a patient with two of the most common chronic illnesses encountered in primary care populations – depression and diabetes.
  - These two conditions co-occur in approximately 10% of primary care patients.
  - Depression increases the risk of complications from diabetes, increases medical symptom burden, and contributes to other clinical outcomes such as doubling the risk of dementia.
  - Diabetes negatively influences the course of depression by shortening time until depression recurrence and increasing disability.
- All-cause mortality is elevated in patients with depression and diabetes compared to patients with diabetes alone.

Integrated physical health and behavioral health programs

- These have gained prominence as a successful treatment intervention that can be used by Health Homes and ACOs to integrate care for patients with concurrent physical and mental health problems.
- There are several models of integrated care, ranging from "co-location" to "collaborative care" to "full integration".
- At its most mature form, the "fully integrated" care system represents a completely merged and integrated practice between providers of different disciplines, all in the same physical space and functioning together as one large care team. Most programs that employ this intervention, however, are not yet at this advanced stage.
- Five principles of collaborative care have been described:
  - patient-centered team care;
  - population-based care;
  - measurement based treatment to target;
  - evidence-based care; and
  - accountable care; (see http://aims.uw.edu/collaborative-care/principles-collaborative-care).
- In general, successful models of collaborative care emphasize case identification using techniques such as screening with standardized tools, and subsequent systematic tracking of patients diagnosed with chronic illnesses such as depression and diabetes.
- A care manager interacts often with the patient and addresses patient education, self-management support, and close follow-up to ensure that patients do not fall out of treatment. A consulting or in-team psychiatrist reviews the registry of patients and hears additional information about patients from the care manager.
- The psychiatrist can then make treatment recommendations to the care manager who then tells the primary care physicians the recommendations.
- The psychiatrist can then follow up on patients, implement stepped-care approaches, and see the patients who do not improve over 12–16 weeks.
- In this model, compared to usual care, a greater number of primary care patients are exposed to the psychiatrist's specialty knowledge and treatment recommendations.

- When the patient's care is managed in a highly coordinated manner by the primary care physician and the care team, the possibilities for gaps or delays in services are decreased, long-term costs of care are expected to decrease due to earlier and more effective management of chronic illnesses, and the patient is likely to have a more satisfying care experience.

Reading list

American Hospital Association. 2010 Committee on Research. AHA Research Synthesis Report: Accountable Care Organization. Chicago: American Hospital Association, 2010.

Cummings NA, O'Donohue WT, Cummings JL. The financial dimension of integrated behavioral/primary care. J Clin Psychol Med Settings 2009;16(1):31–9.

Kaiser Commission on Medicaid and the Uninsured. Mental Health Financing in the United States. California: The Henry J. Kaiser Family Foundation, 2011.

Katon W. Epidemiology and treatment of depression in patients with chronic medical illness. Dialogues Clin Neurosci 2011;13:7–23.

Katon W, Lin EHB, Von Korff M, et al. Collaborative care for patients with depression and chronic illnesses. N Engl J Med 2010;363:2611–20.

Katon W, Russo J, Lin EH, et al. Cost-effectiveness of a multicondition collaborative care intervention: a randomized controlled trial. Arch Gen Psychiatry 2012;69:506–14.

The National Council for Community Behavioral Healthcare. Partnering with Health Homes and Accountable Care Organizations: Considerations for Mental Health and Substance Abuse Providers. Washington, DC: National Council for Community Behavioral Healthcare, January 2011.

National Survey on Drug Use and Health. Results from the 2011 Summary Report. Available at http://www.samhsa.gov/data/NSDUH/2k11MH_FindingsandDetTables/2K11MHFR/NSDUHmhfr2011.htm#2.5

Thota AB, Sipe TA, Byard, GJ, et al. Collaborative care to improve the management of depressive disorders: a community guide systematic review and meta-analysis. Am J Prev Med 2012;42:525–38.

Suggested websites

Aims Center. http://aims.uw.edu

Mental Health Integration Program. http://integratedcare-nw.org/

SAMHSA-HRSA Center for Integrated Health Solutions. http://www.integration.samhsa.gov/integrated-care-models

https://www.amazon.com/Integrated-Care-Working-Interface-Behavioral/dp/1585624802

https://www.amazon.com/dp/1118900022/ref=pd_lpo_sbs_dp_ss_3?pf_rd_p=1944687542&pf_rd_s=lpo-top-stripe-1&pf_rd_t=201&pf_rd_i=1585624802&pf_rd_m=ATVPDKIKX0DER&pf_rd_r=SACXJG846YNNNWG2KXR8

The new APA Toolkit. https://www.psychiatry.org/psychiatrists/practice/professional-interests/integrated-care/integrated-care-track

---

Additional material for this chapter can be found online at:
www.mountsinaiexpertguides.com/psychiatry

This includes a case study and multiple choice questions.

Index

Page numbers in *italic* refer to figures. Those in **bold** refer to tables.

Mount Sinai Expert Guides: Psychiatry, First Edition. Edited by Asher B. Simon, Antonia S. New, and Wayne K. Goodman.
© 2017 John Wiley & Sons, Ltd. Published 2017 by John Wiley & Sons, Ltd.
Companion website: www.mountsinaiexpertguides.com/psychiatry